AYURVEDA

Asian Secrets of Wellness, Beauty and Balance

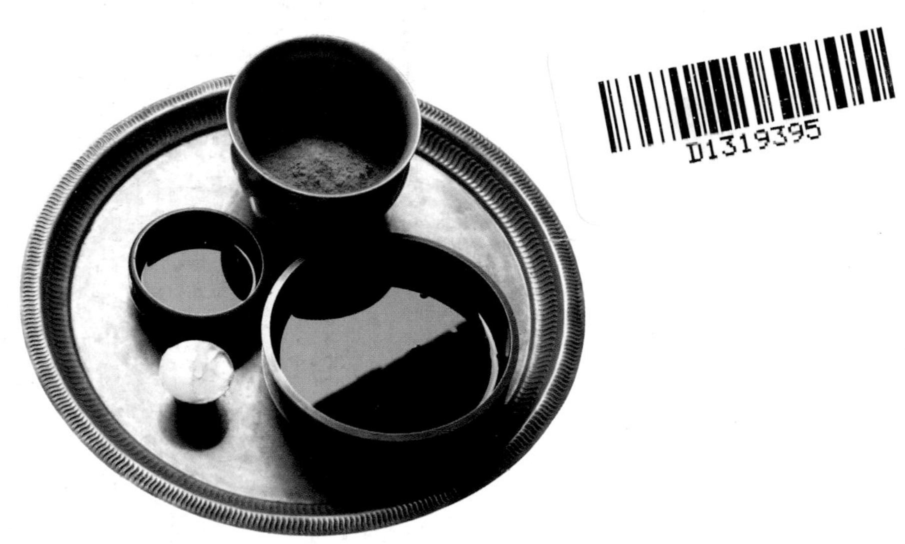

AUTHOR KIM INGLIS
PHOTOGRAPHER LUCA INVERNIZZI TETTONI

TUTTLE PUBLISHING
Tokyo • Rutland, Vermont • Singapore

Published by Tuttle Publishing, an imprint of Periplus Editions (HK) Ltd., with editorial offices at 364 Innovation Drive, North Clarendon, Vermont 05759, USA and 61 Tai Seng Avenue, #02-12, Singapore 534167

ISBN: 978-0-8048-4087-3

Distributed by

North America, Latin America & Europe
Tuttle Publishing
364 Innovation Drive
North Clarendon, VT 05759-9436, USA
Tel: 1 (802) 773-8930
Fax: 1 (802) 773-6993
info@tuttlepublishing.com
www.tuttlepublishing.com

Japan
Tuttle Publishing
Yaekari Building, 3rd Floor
5-4-12 Osaki
Shinagawa-ku
Tokyo 141 0032
Tel: (81) 03 5437-0171
Fax: (81) 03 5437-0755
tuttle-sales@gol.com

Asia Pacific
Berkeley Books Pte. Ltd.
61 Tai Seng Avenue, #02-12
Singapore 534167
Tel: (65) 6280-1330
Fax: (65) 6280-6290
inquiries@periplus.com.sg
www.periplus.com

12 11 10 09
6 5 4 3 2 1

Printed in Singapore

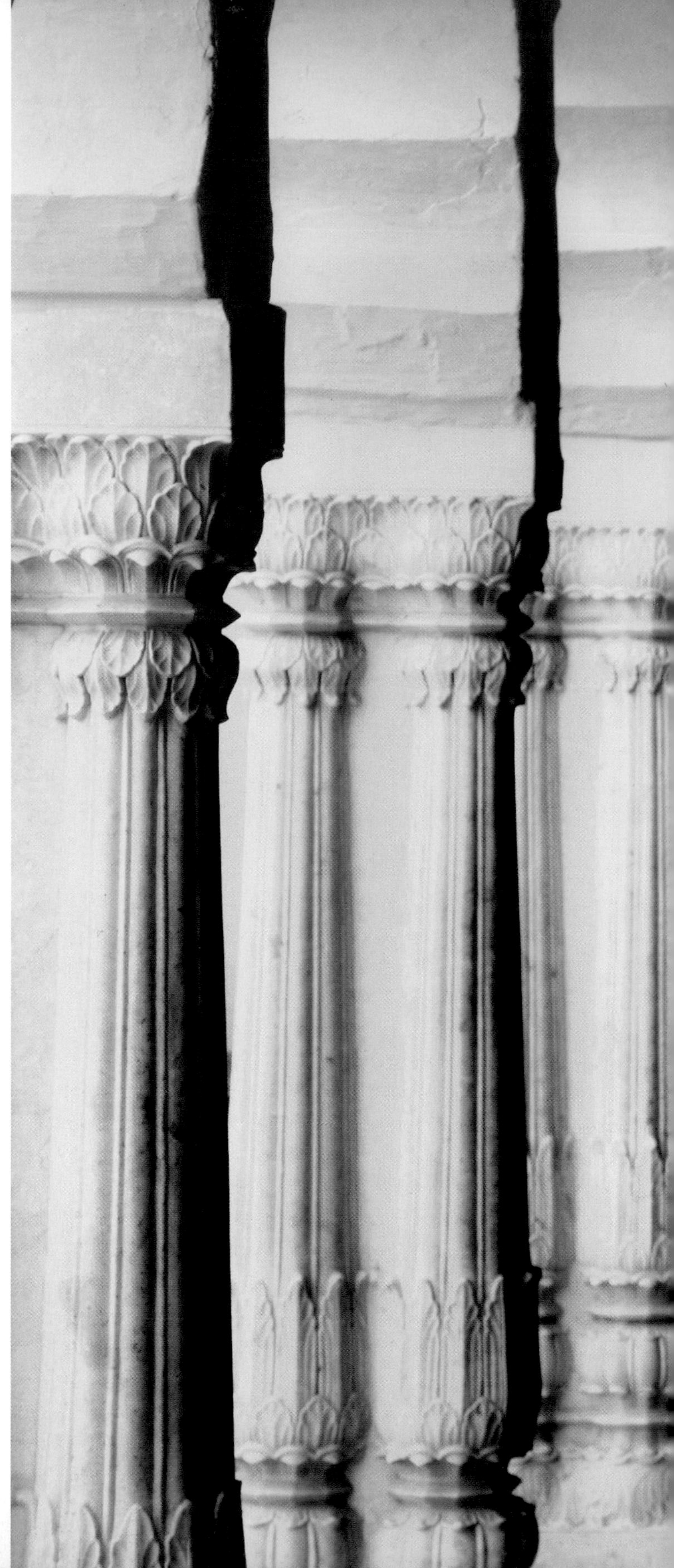

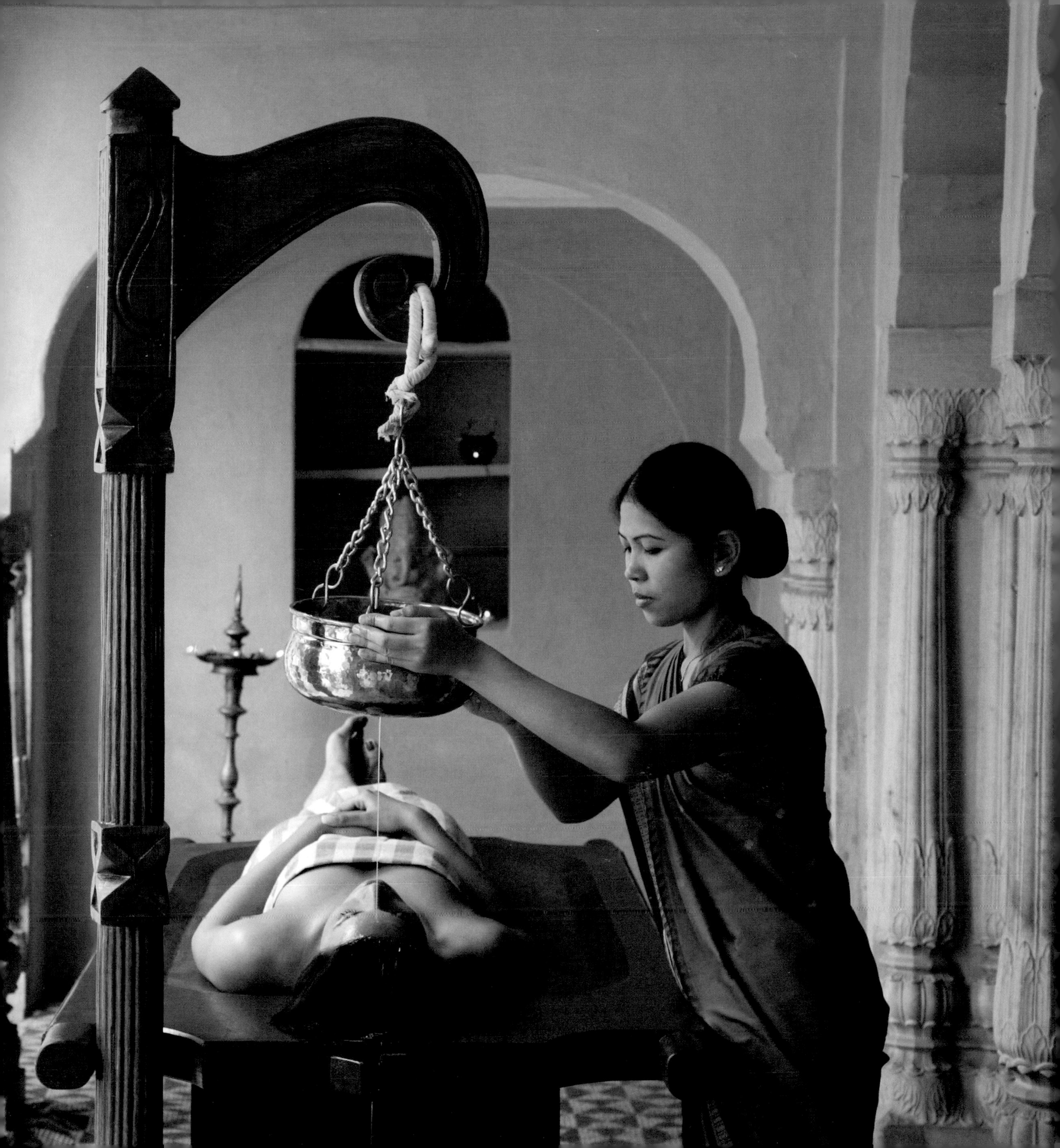

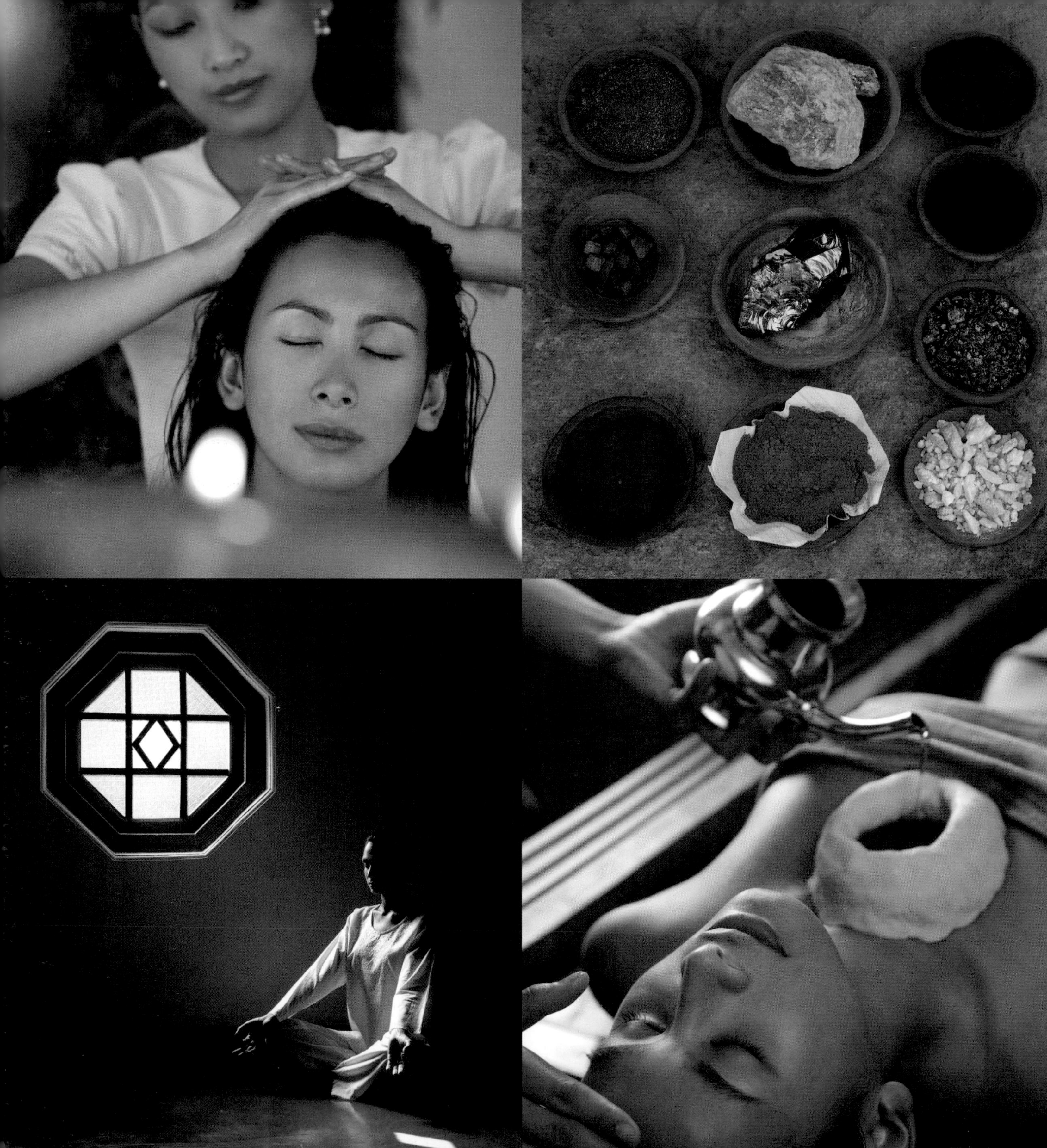

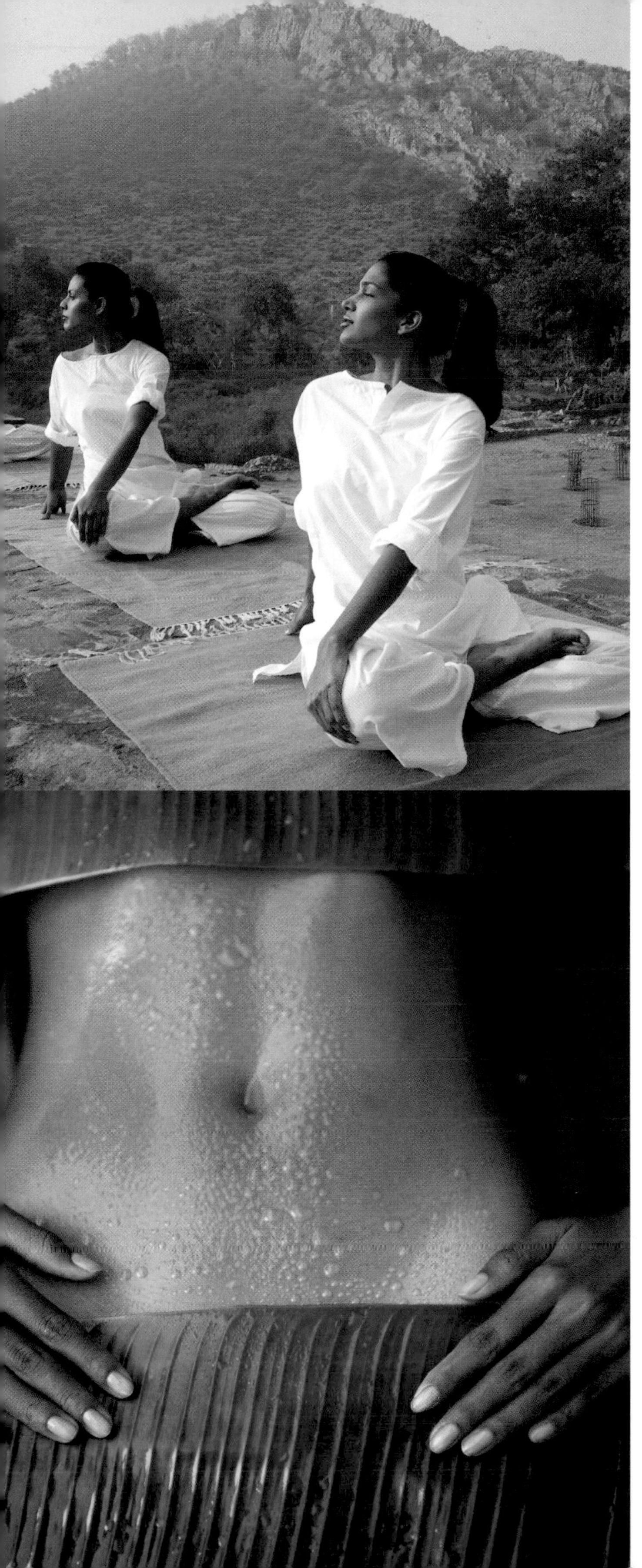

CONTENTS

Utilizing the purifying properties of mud is an ancient practice that continues in India to this day. Taking the earth element from the *panchamahabhut* or "five great elements", it cleanses skin and boosts metabolism.

ancient wisdoms, today's practices

At no time in the history of the planet have India's stress-busting, all-encompassing therapies had more importance. While we strive to improve material gains, we often neglect the spiritual, the physical and the mental. However, with stressful lifestyles taking their toll, taking time out to concentrate on ourselves is no longer a treat — it's a necessity. This is where India's age-old traditional practices come in.

Whether you travel to India to visit a spa, to try to "find yourself", to experience some medical care, or to spend some relaxing time with friends or family, you are almost certain to come across some of these ancient practices. Even though the country is modernizing at a rapid rate, everyone — on some level or another — is tied to its deep-rooted traditions.

Ancient Healing

Many of these age-old traditions are explored in this book. We get to the core of the country's medical systems — Ayurveda, Unani and Siddha — and explore its history of herbal healing and ancient beauty procedures. The mind, body, spirit practices of yoga, meditation and *pranayama* are showcased in depth, while related cultural phenomena such as temple and household habits and gemology are also considered. Some of these ideas will be familiar to readers, others will be totally new. We'll take you through the myriad of wonders that has emerged from this extraordinary, exotic subcontinent, all the while explaining how past wisdom has relevance in today's world.

Ayurveda and yoga are probably the most well known of the ancient modalities outside India — and both seek to encompass much more than physical wellbeing. They are covered in depth in the ancient texts or Vedas and there are countless written instructions for both. Even though they weren't traditionally practiced together, today they are finding synergy. "What's interesting about India's systems," explains one Ayurvedic physician, "is that they often incorporate more than one regime. Methods of healing like Ayurveda include a lifestyle regimen, yoga, aroma, meditation, gems, amulets, herbs, diet, *jyotishi* (astrology), color and more." It is this holistic approach that is so exciting.

History of Ayurveda

Translated from Sanskrit as the "Science of Life", Ayurveda was first mentioned in the verses of the *Rig Veda*, the first of the Vedas or Hindu sacred texts. Here there is reference to *panchamahabhut* (the five basic elements of the entire creation), and the three *doshas* or primary forces of *prana* or *vata* (air), *agni* or *pitta* (fire)

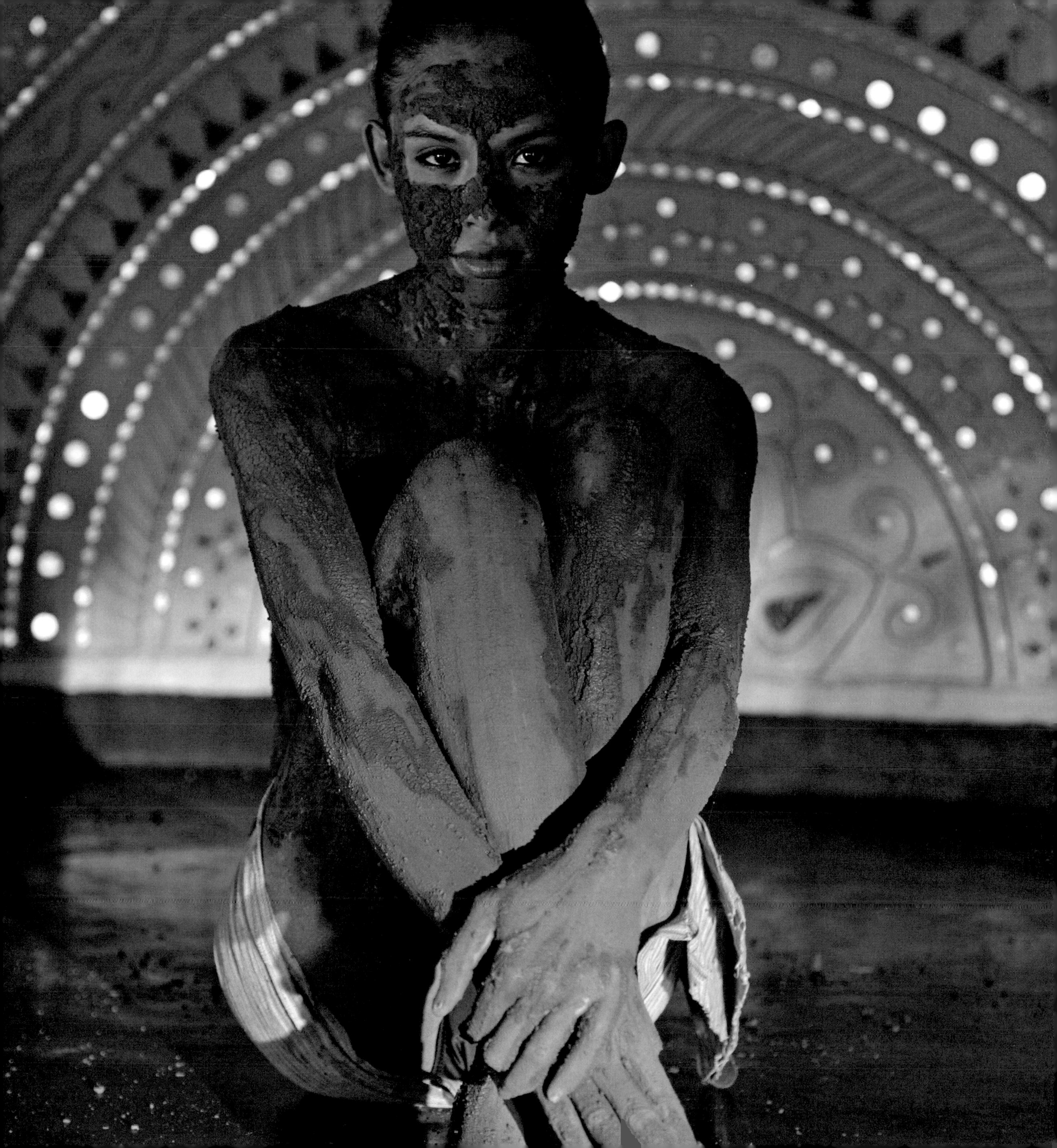

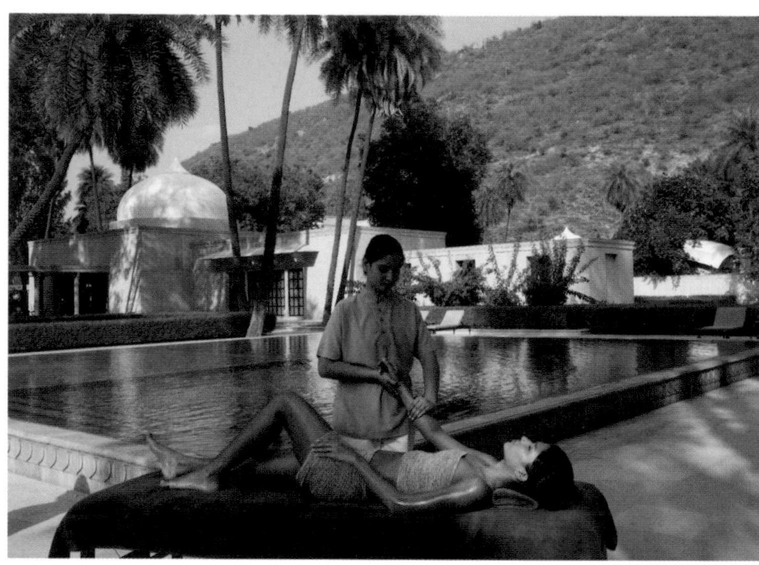

Wellness treatment being administered at the luxury spa at Amanbagh.

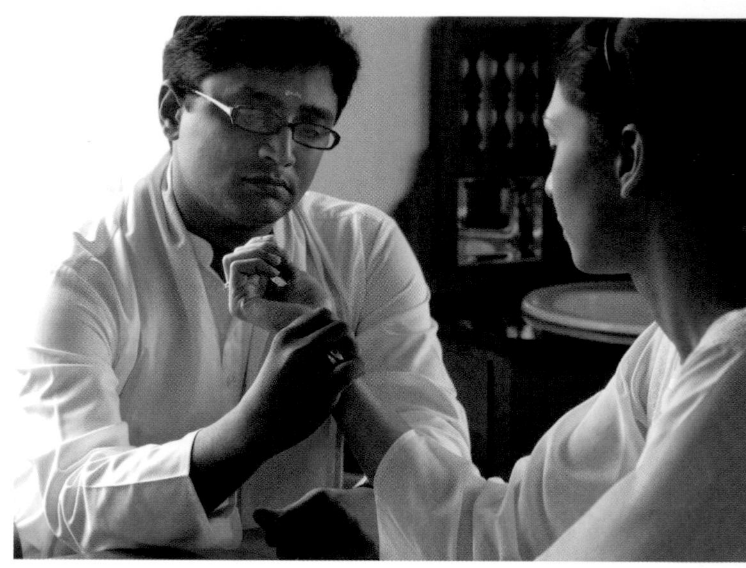

Taking the pulse is one of the first indicators in Ayurvedic diagnosis (see below also).

and *soma* or *kapha* (water and earth) as comprising the basic principles of Ayurveda. However, there is much more detail in an *upaveda* (subsection) of the *Atharva*, the fourth Veda, written some time during 3,000 to 2,000 BC. Here, Ayurveda is documented more specifically: it is described as knowledge of self-healing or holistic healing, with the idea that everything is interrelated, yet still unique. The texts stated that if Ayurveda was applied on an individual basis in people's everyday lives using diet, massage, oils, herbs and exercise, practitioners could be healthy and disease-free.

Around the turn of the first millennium BC the treatise known as the *Charaka Samhita*, the most referred Ayurvedic text on internal medicine, appeared. Believed to have been written by the great sage-physician Charaka, it explained the logic and philosophy of Ayurvedic medicine. Written in the form of a symposium wherein groups of Ayurvedic scholars take up a series of topics for discussion, it is written in verse in keeping with the Vedic oral tradition of conserving knowledge. It therefore seems likely that Ayurveda had been in existence for many hundreds, if not thousands, of years beforehand.

A spiritual ascetic or *sadhu* attends to a supplicant.

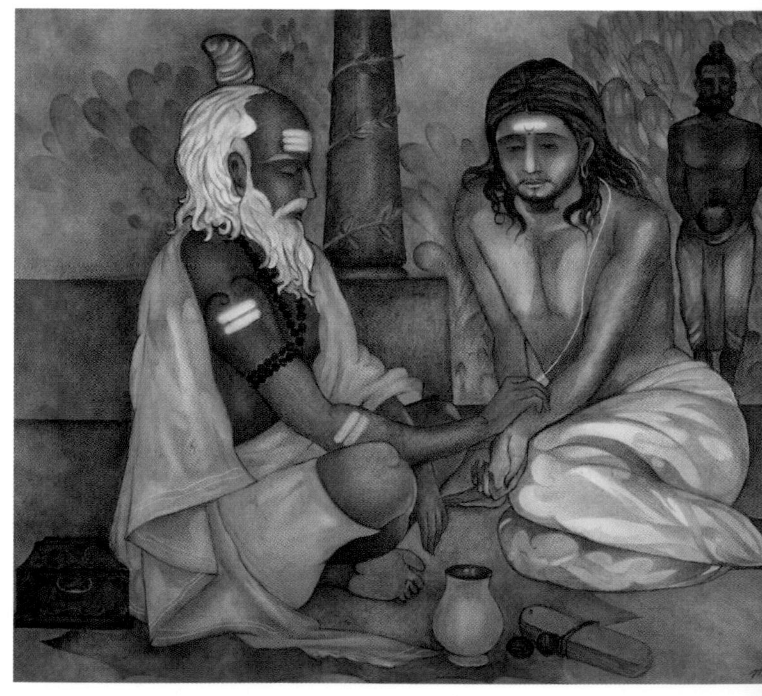

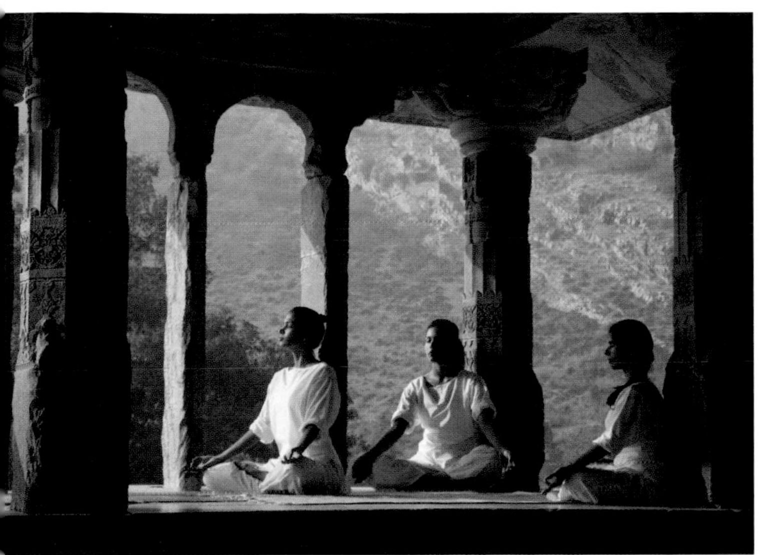

Yoga is recommended along with Ayurveda for total wellbeing.

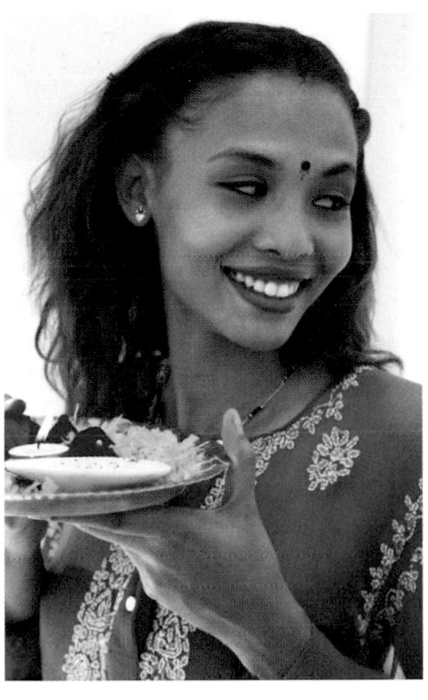

A traditional Indian welcome.

Around the same time, the *Sushruta Samhita* appeared. It comprised knowledge about prosthetic surgery to replace limbs, cosmetic surgery, caesarian operations and even brain surgery. Sushruta is famous for his innovation of cosmetic surgery on the nose known as rhinoplasty, an interesting fact as he lived two centuries before Hippocrates, the Greek father of Western medicine. Around 500 AD, Vagbhata compiled the third major treatise on Ayurveda, *Astanga Hridaya*. It contained knowledge from both previous books, but also new information on diseases and cures. It is the text of choice for many practicing Ayurvedic physicians because it is a precise condensation of the two earlier texts.

There were, of course, many other useful reference texts, and it is documented that Ayurveda became entrenched in Indian life between 1,000 BC and 800 AD. Both Hindus and Buddhists maintained the academic progress of Ayurveda, and also ensured that the science was made as publicly available as possible. Medicinal herbs were planted, hospitals were formed, and the art of nursing (as described by Charaka) was widely systematized. But it wasn't until the Buddhist period (323 BC to 642 AD) that Ayurveda began to be exported outside India's shores. During this time Buddhist missionaries and monks took knowledge of Ayurveda, along with other aspects of Indian culture, to Europe (Rome and Greece), the Middle East (Baghdad) and China. Closer to home, the neighboring countries of Sri Lanka, Tibet, Thailand, Burma and Indonesia all accepted its teachings. In fact, its influence can still be seen in many of their healing systems: Acupressure, for example, is a direct descendent of *marma* massage.

In India, Ayurveda's heyday was probably from the 6th century to the 10th century AD: During this time, many universities and teaching hospitals were founded to cater to students from all over the world, and there are numerous references to the efficacy of the Indian system of medicine. But by the 12th century, Ayurveda's influence began to wane. Waves of Muslim invaders in northern India from the 10th to the 12th centuries burned books, destroyed hospitals and libraries, and slaughtered Hindu sages and Buddhist monks as infidels. They brought with them their own *hakims* or Unani doctors (a form of medicine formulated by Arabian physicians, see pages 36–37) — so the system fell into decline.

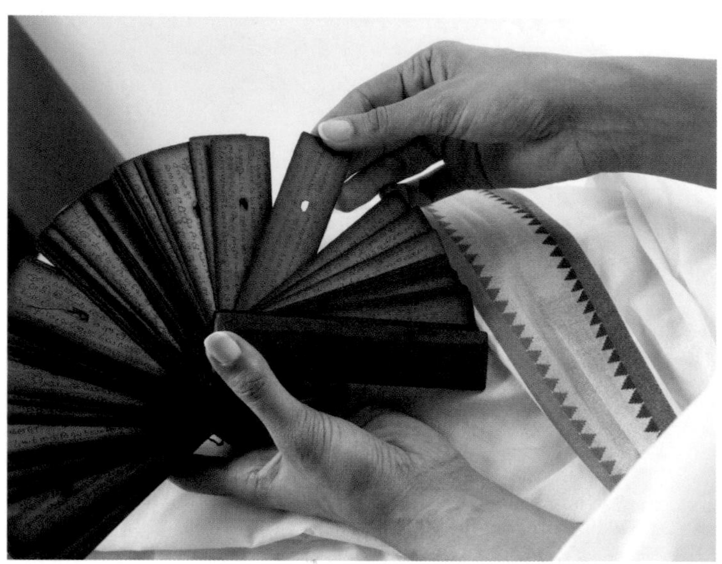

Early Ayurvedic texts were engraved on palm leaf manuscripts.

Opposite *Shirodhara* or the pouring of medicated oil on to the forehead or "third eye" is one of Ayurveda's best known therapies outside India.

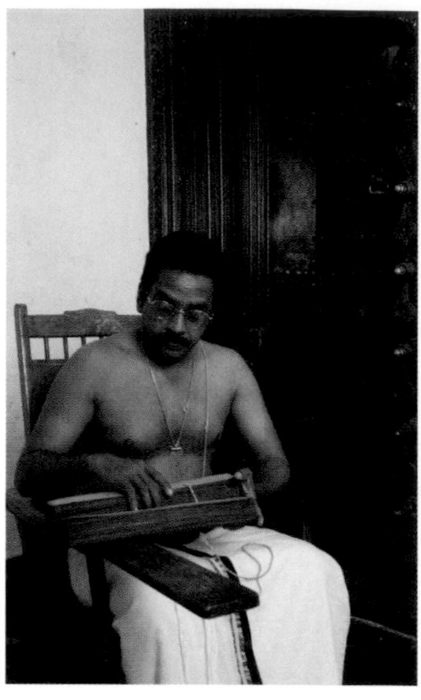

Ayurvedic physician in Kerala.

This was further exacerbated by the arrival of the British. The East India Company denied state patronage to Ayurveda, closed down existing schools and government medical colleges, and substituted it with Western medicine. Of course, at a local level, Ayurveda continued to be practiced, but it wasn't until Indian Independence that official initiatives were taken to revitalize indigenous medical forms — and Ayurveda once again began to rise.

What is Ayurveda?

Ayurveda advocates that each person is born with a basic constitution or genetic make-up called *prakruti* in Sanskrit. If there is a changing nature or situation in the body during one's life (*vikruti*), imbalance occurs. This may pass over time or may become a disease. The aims of Ayurveda are *ayus* ("long life") and *arogya* ("diseaselessness") with ultimate spiritual goals. Health is achieved by balancing what are known as the bodily humors or *doshas* at all levels, according to an individual's constitution, lifestyle and nature. There are many similar holistic medical systems in other communities, including the Chinese, American Indians, Africans and South Americans.

Diagnosis

Before any Ayurvedic treatment is prescribed, patients first of all undertake a consultation with an Ayurvedic physician to ascertain their body type and present health status. "Body type is the variation in percentage of *vatha, pitta* and *kapha* (air, fire and water) in our body," explains Ayurvedic physician Dr Yogesh. "Based on the present *dosha* state or *vikruti*, suitable therapies, oils, medications, advice or more may be prescribed."

Most Ayurvedic physicians point out that Ayurvedic treatments vary from place to place, doctor to doctor and according to the nature of the client/doctor relationship. This makes it confusing to many, and difficult to analyze, research and compare with other medical systems. "However, the purpose is always the same," explains Dr Renja Raphel, "Each body has its own defined constitution from birth to death that is affected by many different things. We doctors try to bring the body back to equilibrium: we find out what is lacking and modify it, we add things and we request changes in diets, climates, stress levels, lifestyle habits and more." He goes on to add that the body has the power to help itself; Ayurveda simply helps it with the healing process.

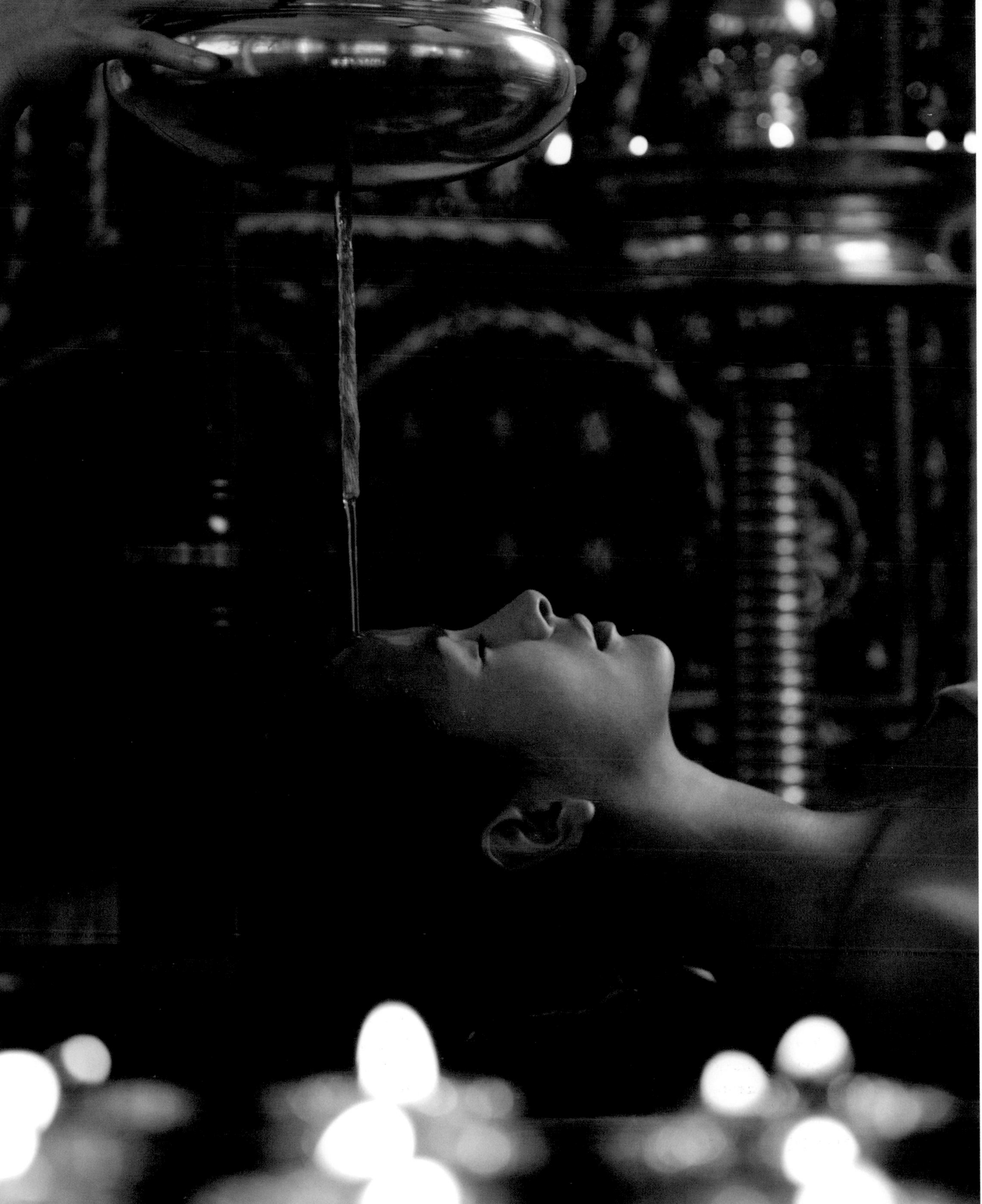

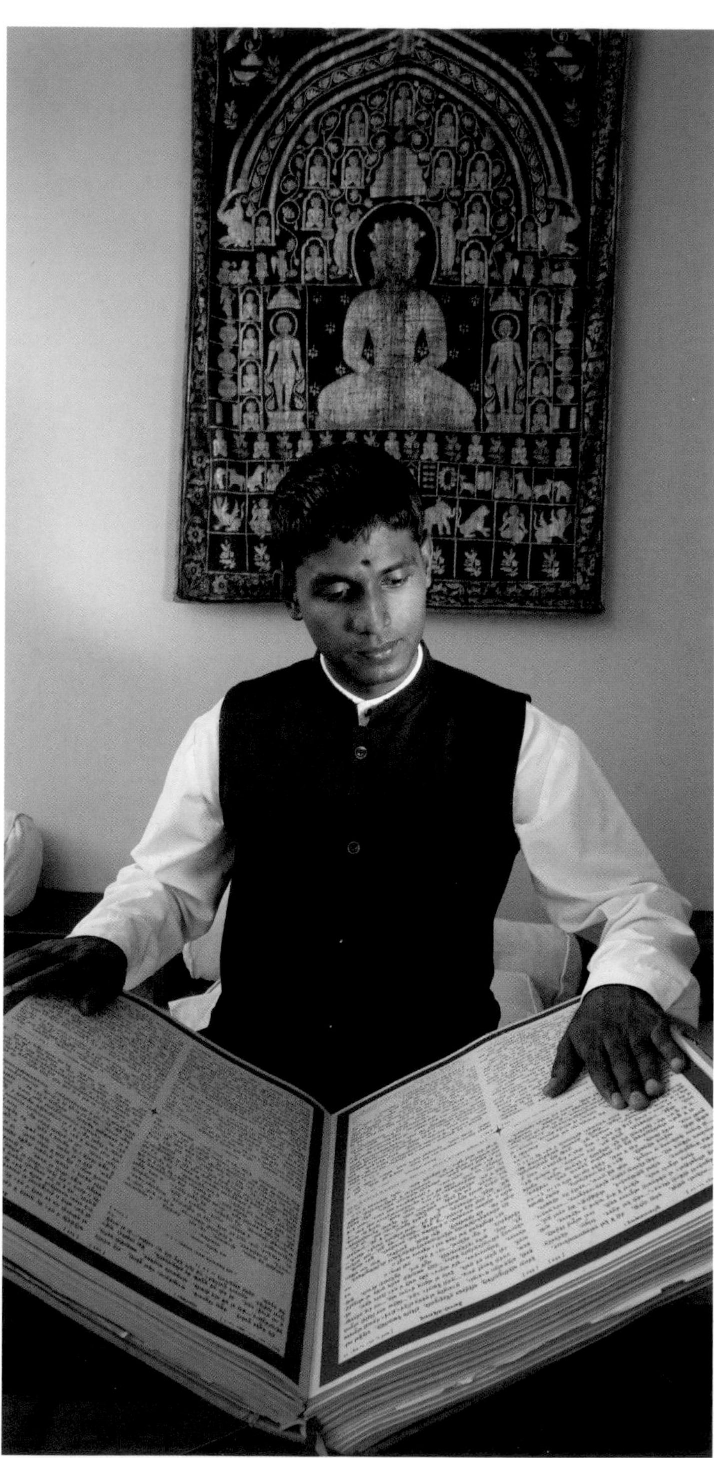

Left A student of the Vedas seeks understanding through a copy of one of the treatises in Sanskrit.

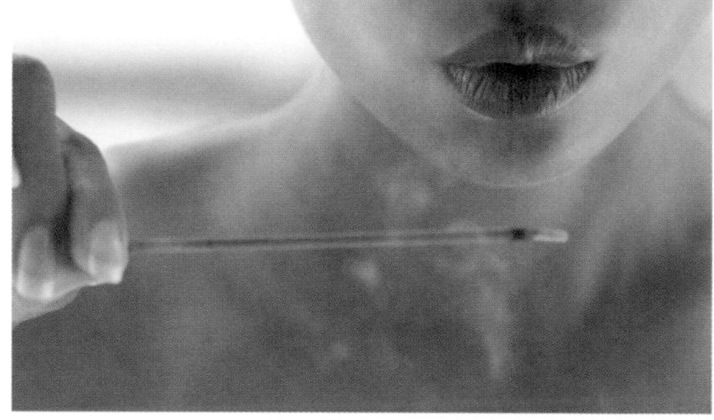

The use of *agarabathi* or incense sticks to promote clean air is an age-old practice.

Diagnosis is an extremely important part of Ayurveda. In a clinic or hospital, it is undertaken first thing in the morning before the patient has consumed anything. The doctor inspects the tissues and the skin; examines the "nine doors" (two eyes, two ears, two nostrils, mouth and throat, anus and penis or vulva) and their secretions; takes faeces and urine samples to assess the *analam* or digestive fire; takes the patient's pulse and assesses body temperature; interrogates the patient on their sleep patterns, health, lifestyle habits, climate preferences and more; and generally takes a great deal of time to consider the patient as a whole. Nothing can be prescribed without this extremely thorough consultation.

Many visitors to India aren't seeking medical treatment, but are intrigued by this ancient wellness system and want to try a treatment. This is perfectly possible in a spa whre the consultation is shorter, but still important. "At a spa, we look at *darshana* or appearance, *sparshana* or touch ie pulse and body temperature, and undertake *prasnai* or discussion," explains Dr Yogesh, "this gives us enough information to decide on a patient's basic imbalances and which medicated oils we should use in a treatment."

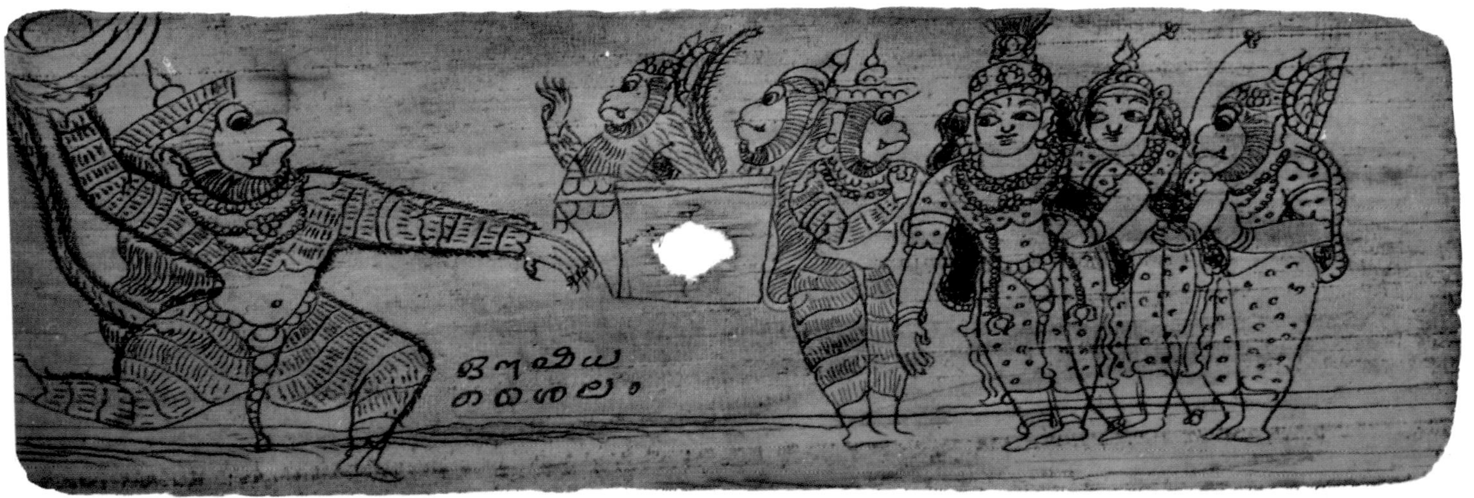

A leaf from the *Ramayana* in Mahalayam called "Medicine Mountain": it depicts the monkey god Hanuman using a mountain of medicinal herbs to help his fellow monkeys. Even in the Epics, much is made of India's healing heritage.

Ayurvedic equipment from Kerala: medicine box, oil containers, mortar and pestle.

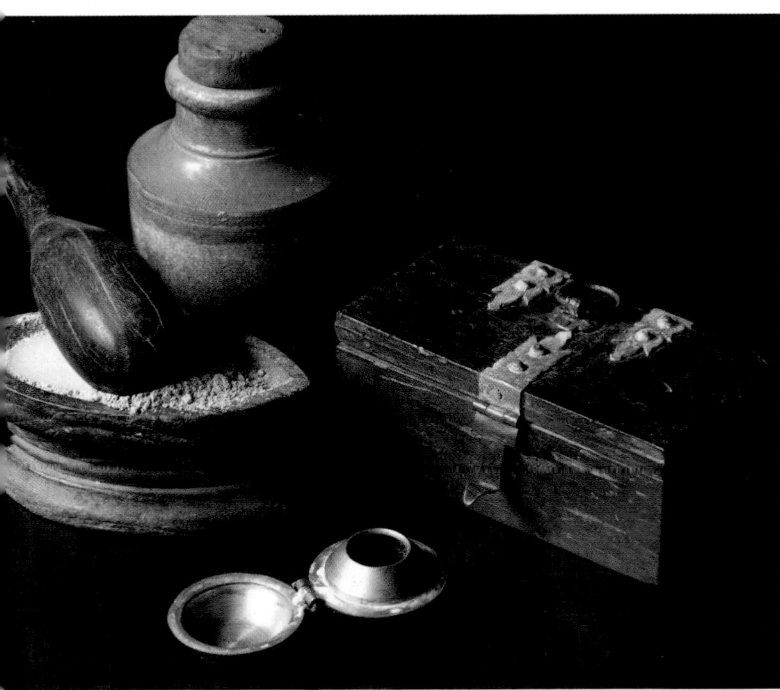

Prognosis and Treatment

After the diagnosis, the doctor decides whether the disease falls into one of four categories: Curable with ease, curable with difficulty, ameliorable, or incurable. At this point an astrologer may be consulted to find the best time and place for treatments to take place. Sri Krishnakumar, the managing director of one of the most famous Ayurvedic hospitals in India, the Arya Vaidya Chikitsalayam in Coimbatore, says that every avenue must be pursued for the benefit of the patient. "Everything is inter-related," he explains, "the mind and the body, the person and the universe, the disease and the lifestyle. A consultation with an astrologer may bring up something that the doctor has not noticed."

This is one example of how Ayurveda may be difficult for non-Indians to grasp. Skepticism of such practices runs high in the West, even though looking holistically at patients and problems is increasingly gaining credence. Another difficulty may be had with some of the treatments.

These are literally multi-faceted and depend on a huge number of factors including disease, client personality and habits, work practices, *dosha* imbalance, climate, and many more. The basic

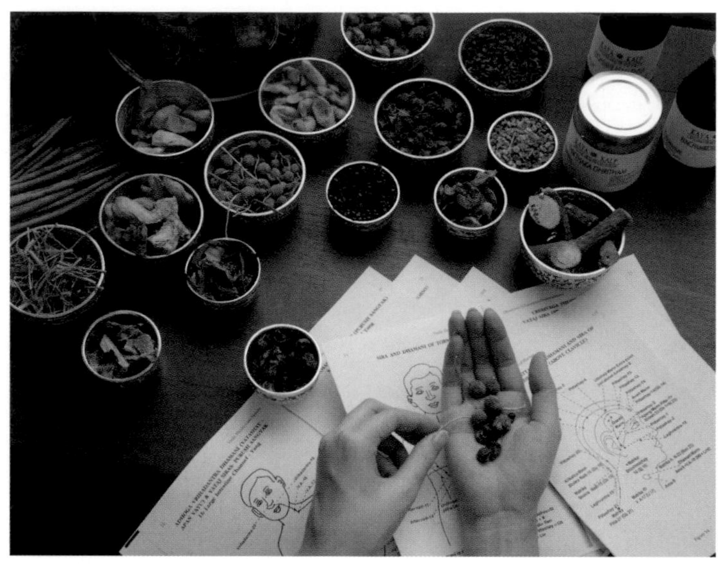

India is home to a vast cornucopaeia of healing plants; many of Ayurveda's ancient recipes are now supported by modern scientific research.

Opposite An old map of India transposed with the body of Shiva, the god of yoga. His head, symbolizing intellect, is found in the Himalayas (his spiritual home), whilst his feet, used for grounding, are found at the tip of the subcontinent.

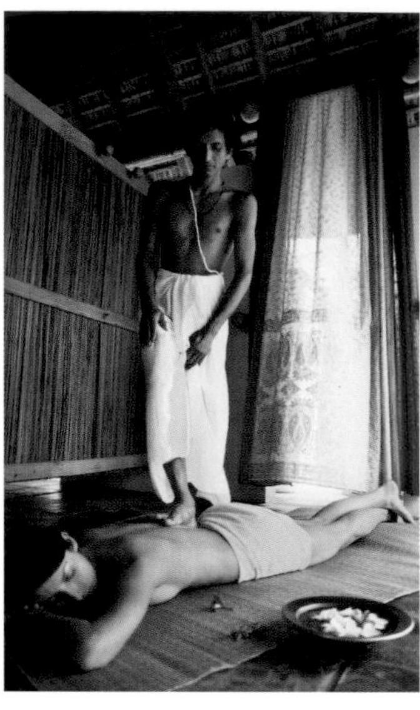

Ancient form of pressure point massage.

premise is to cleanse and detoxify the body and balance the *doshas*, restoring them to their original state of equilibrium. But how this is achieved varies hugely. There are hundreds of levels of practice, from official to folk, and thousands of prescriptions — and no treatment is a panacea. One thing is for sure though: a course of treatments is rarely shorter than three weeks, and after the course is completed, follow-up is very important.

In the following pages, information on some common therapies is given, but if you visit an Ayurvedic doctor, you may expect to be prescribed any — or many — of the following: purification therapies, medication, special diet, herbs and minerals, massage and other body work, exercise, yoga, meditation, aromatherapy, flower and gem essences, advise on lifestyle, work and climate change, and acupressure.

All the medicines, oils and powders used in treatments are 100 percent natural and rely on India's huge pharmacopoeia. "Ayurvedic texts contain the details of a staggering number of plant ingredients, minerals, metals and other natural substances, along with their properties, their methods of collection and extraction, as well as specific combinations of complementary herbs," says Shahnaz Husain, herbal ambassador and producer, "The specific processing methods and well-known combinations enhance the efficacy of the treatments. Many of the formulations are still used with great success today."

Ayurveda in Spas

Even though some treatments are less common nowadays, many are still to be found both at grassroots level and in the country's 2,100 Ayurvedic hospitals. They are also increasingly finding their way into spas and retreats. Husain notes: "Ayurvedic treatments are ideal for spa treatments, because they counteract degenerative processes, environmental pollution, toxic build-up and mental stress, all of which have become undesirable features of modern life." She notes that many people visit a spa particularly to address such modern-day afflictions, and with Ayurveda taking total wellbeing into consideration, its treatments are in line with the aims of most spas.

Some diehard Ayurvedic doctors, with their emphasis on authenticity and historical accuracy, frown on this relatively new spa phenomenon. They believe that Ayurveda should remain in the realm of medicine. Others, however, feel it is a trend to be encouraged — as it advertizes the benefits of this ancient healing

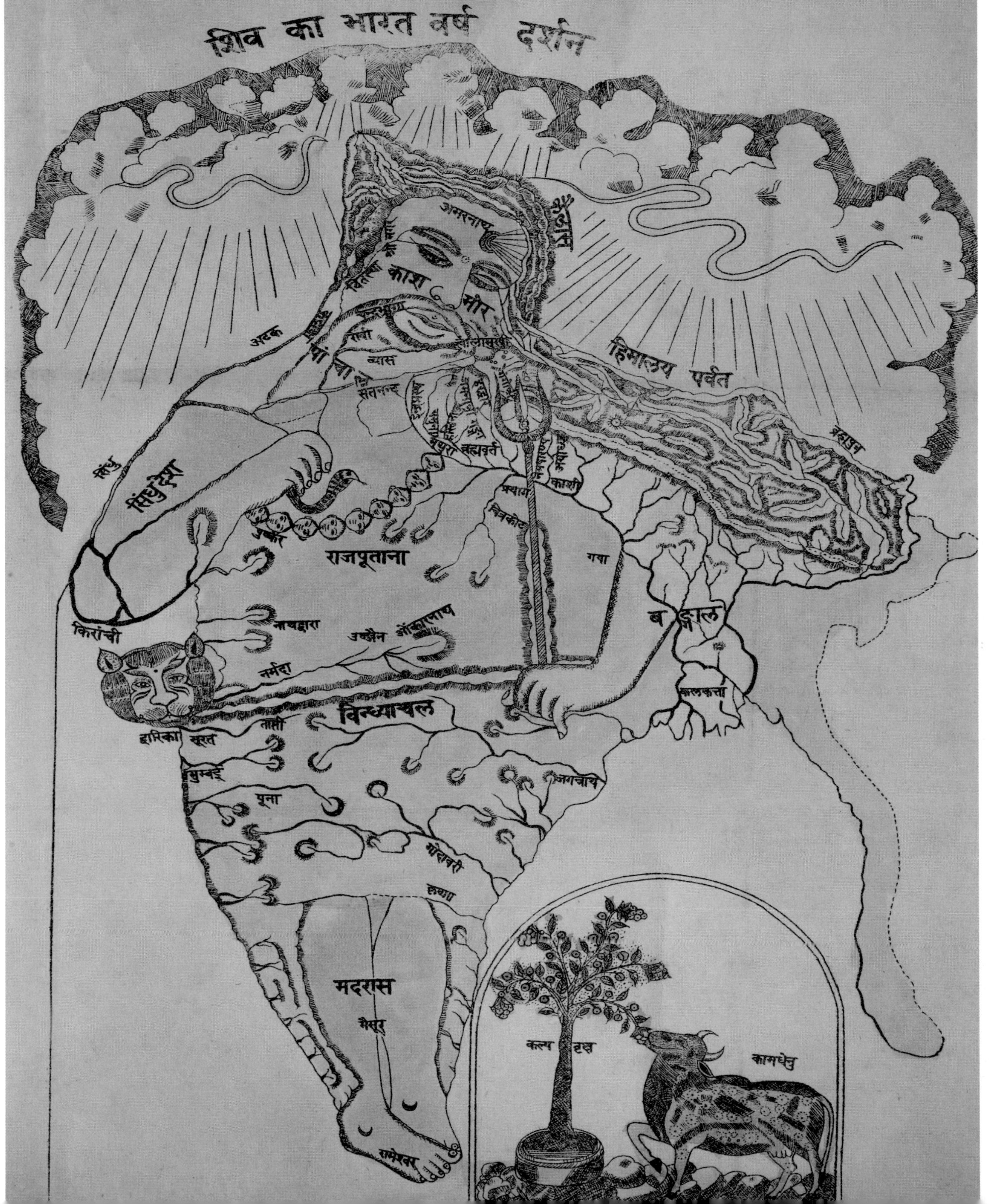
शिव का भारत वर्ष दर्शन
अमरनाथ
कैलाश
काश
मीर
अटक
व्यास
हिमालय पर्वत
सिंधु
सिंधुदेश
राजपूताना
प्रयाग
काशी
गया
ब ङ्गाल
नाथद्वारा
उज्जैन
किरांची
नर्मदा
कलकत्ता
विन्ध्याचल
द्वारिका
सूरत
ताप्ती
बम्बई
पूना
जगन्नाथ
गोदावरी
कृष्णा
मदरास
मैसूर
रामेश्वर
कल्प वृक्ष
कामधेनु

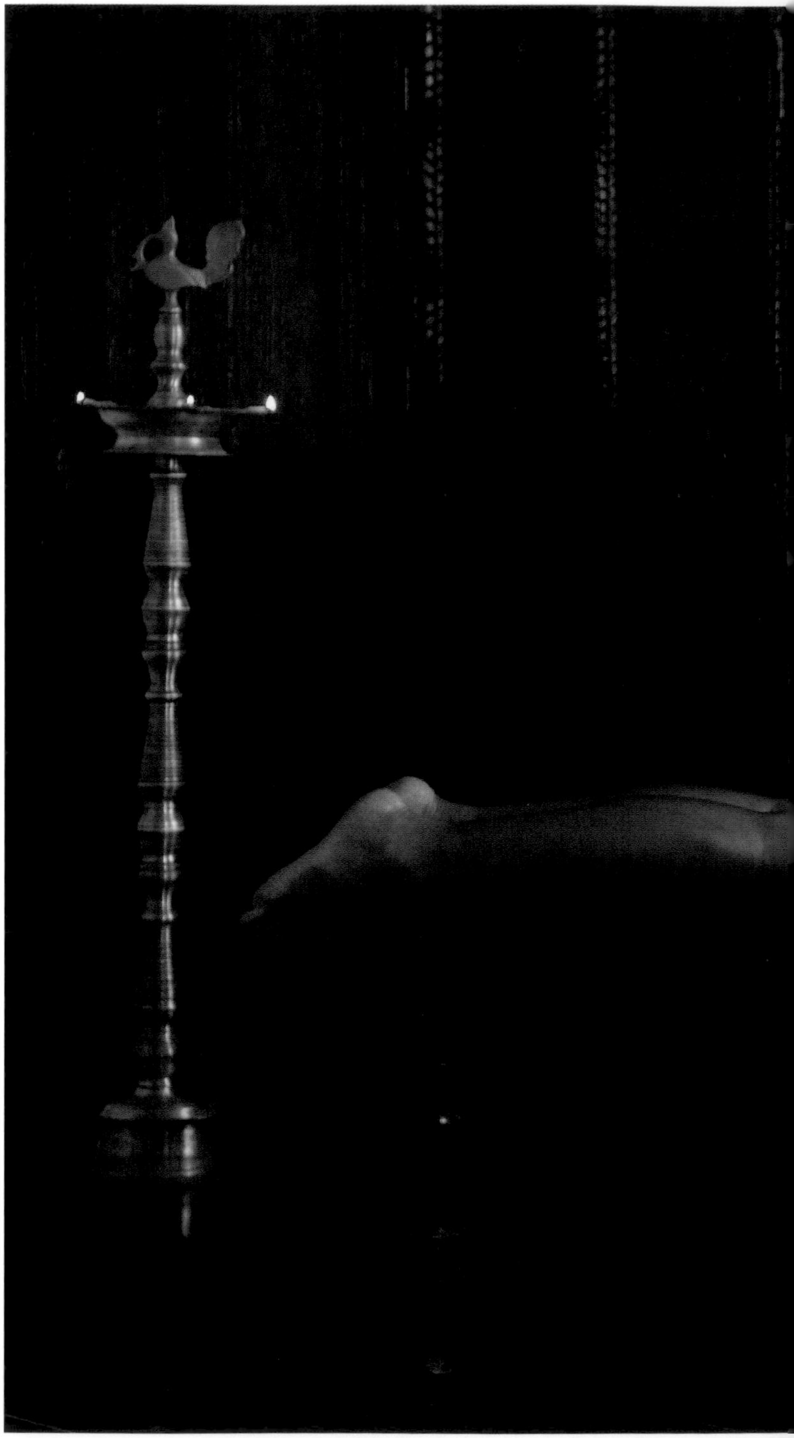

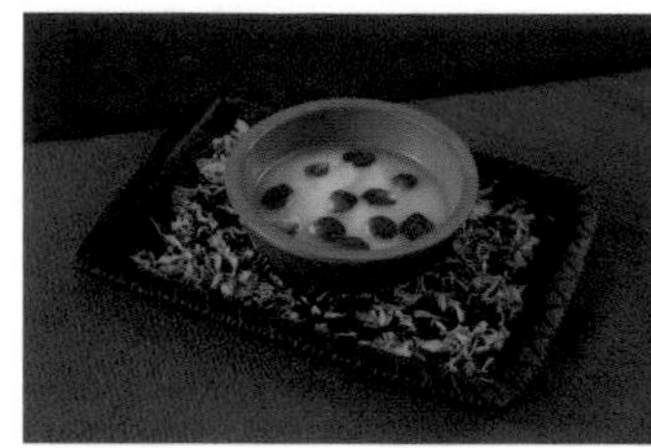

Scented body lotion with rose petals.

Right *Abhyangam* or Ayurvedic massage given by a Keralan therapist at the spa at Neemrana Fort Palace.

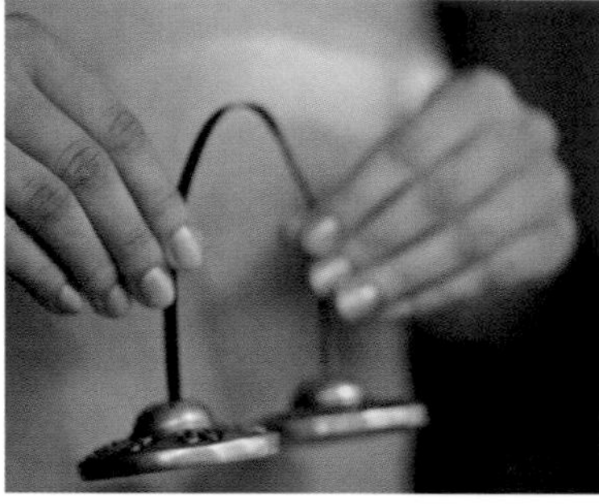

Tibetan chimes rung before a treatment starts.

system. "As long as the doctors who run such spas differentiate between the clinic and the spa, it is fine," one doctor told me. He also admitted that the country's Ayurvedic experiences ricochet wildly from by-the-book, clinical treatments to unhygienic, back-room practices and others that are driven purely by monetary gain.

Unfortunately, there is a problem with standardization, but the government and the medical community are working on ways to rectify this. This book only recommends reputable spas, retreats, clinics and hospitals, and differentiates clearly between the medical and the recreational. With the right environment, proper and safe medicinal care, high standards of cleanliness and pure medication, Ayurveda is a force to be reckoned with.

Rejuvenating the body, soothing the mind, nurturing the spirit — India's therapies open up possibilities we never realized we had. Many aim to help a person reach their maximum potential, while others utilize the country's pharmacopoeia for relaxation, beauty care and rejuvenation. It's the aim of this book to delve into all of the above; to explain, illustrate and, hopefully, inspire. It isn't a medical or scientific treatise, more an overview of ancient wellness practices that — finally — are beginning to be appreciated on the global stage.

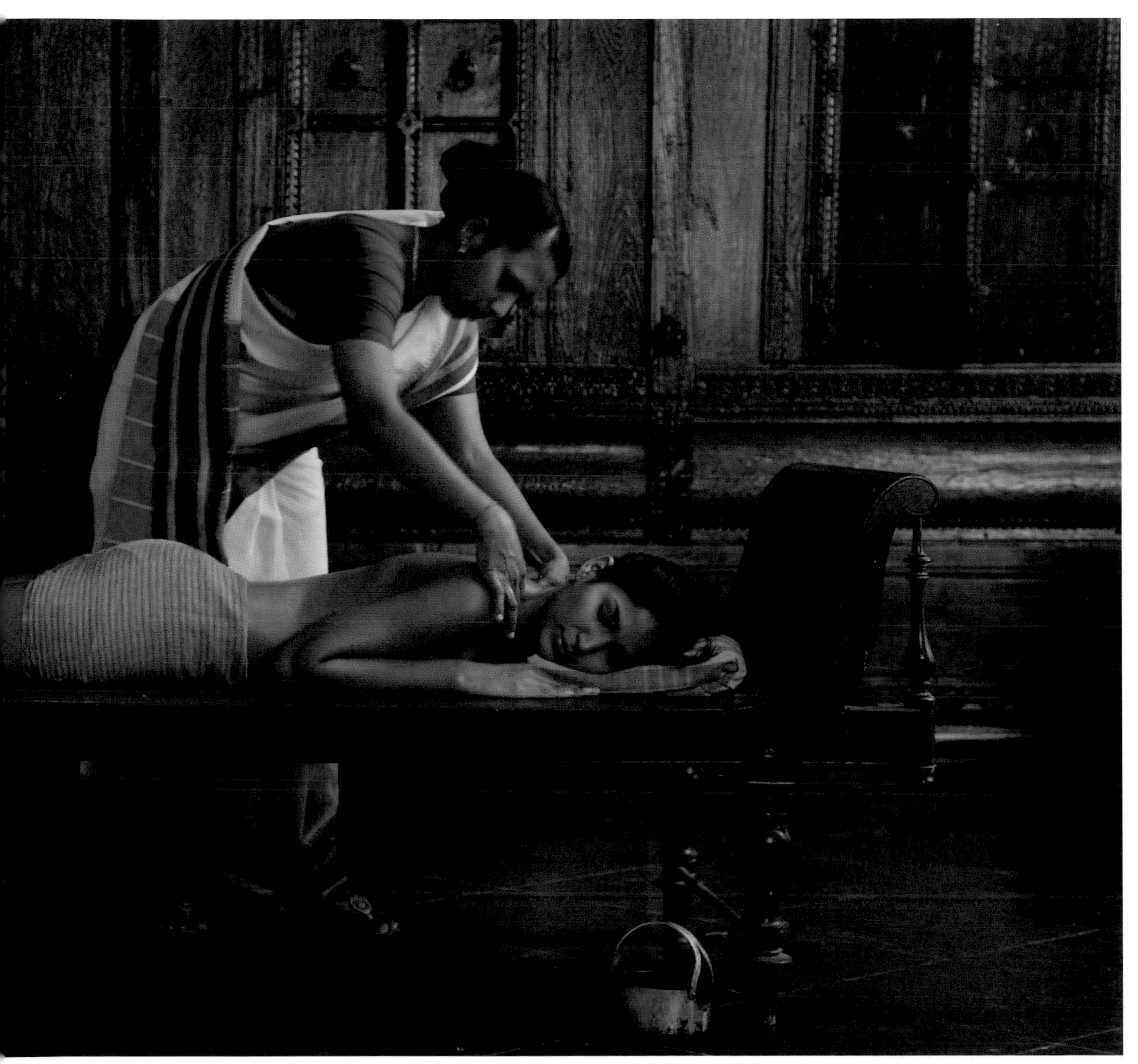

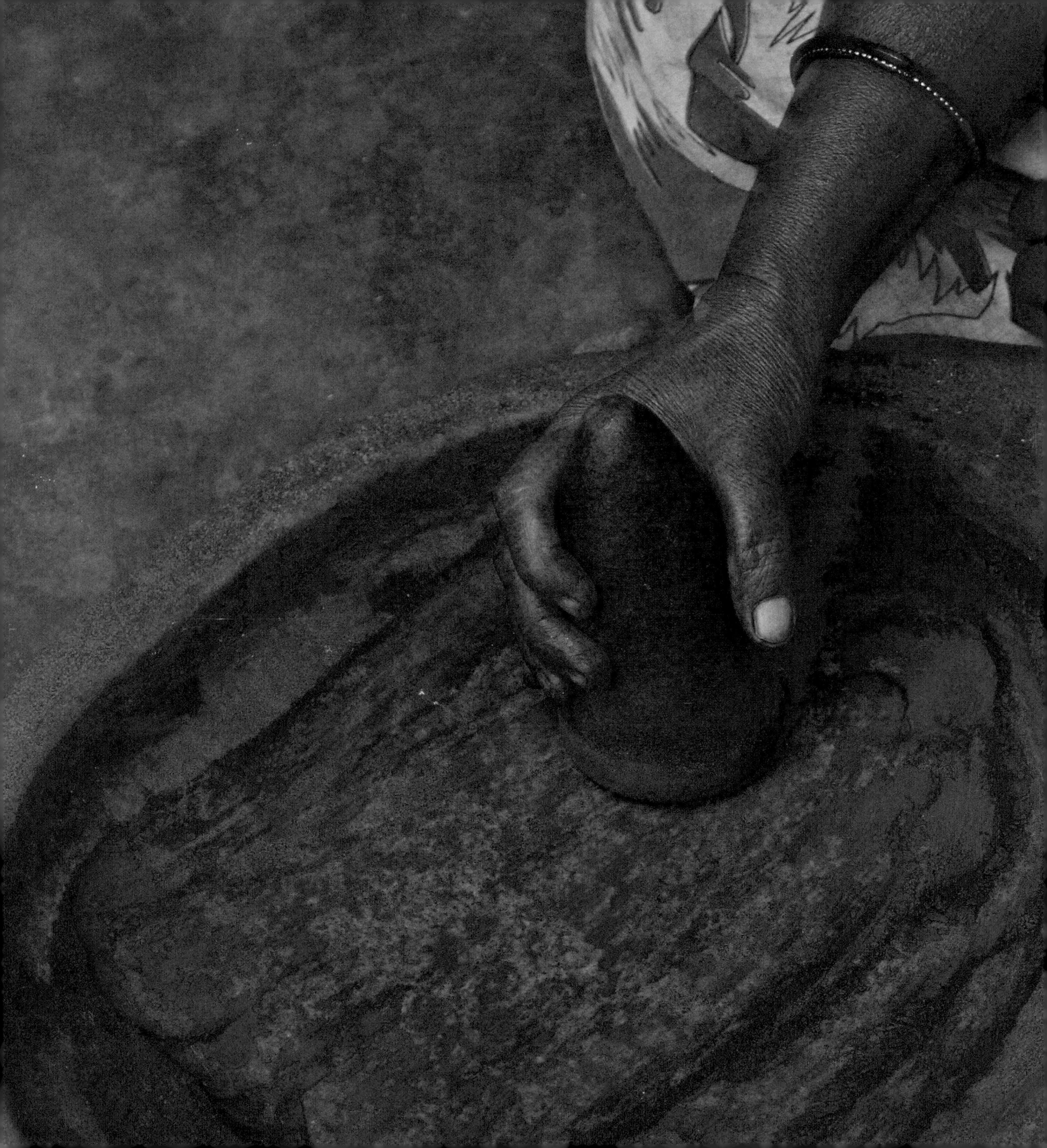

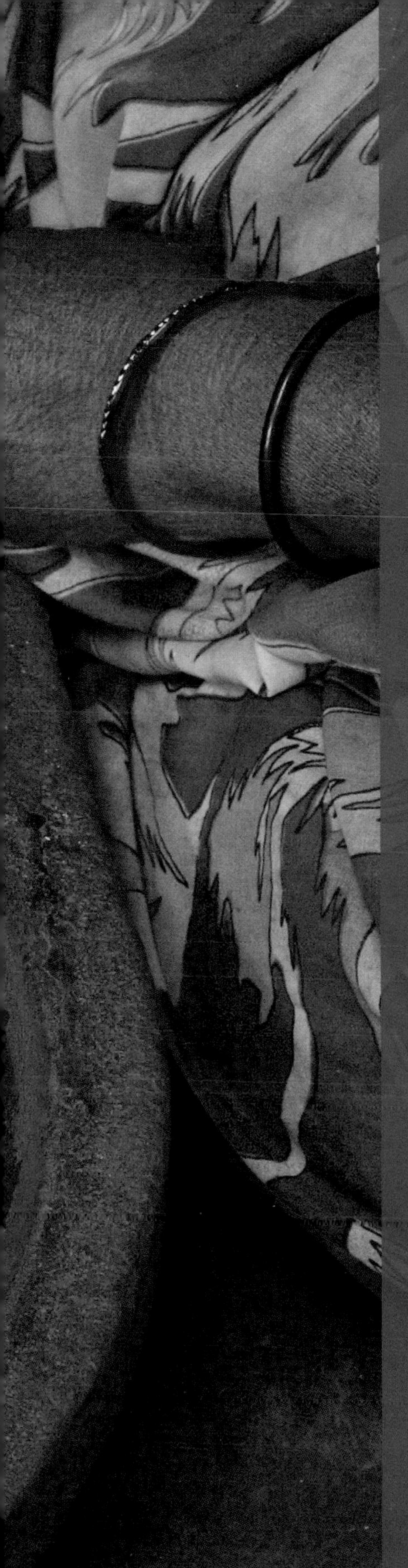

wellness

Ayurveda is the principal health system in India, but other forms such as Unani, Siddha and Tibetan medicine are also practiced. This chapter considers all these, along with many specific therapies from each. A variety of therapeutic massages is covered, as well as heat and steam therapies, and more obscure treatments for eye or skin health. All are geared towards detoxification, both internal and external, with the ultimate aim being good health, longevity and spiritual enrichment.

abhyangam

Traditional Ayurvedic Massage

The *Charaka Samhita*, one of the foremost Ayurvedic texts, advises that every person should have an Ayurvedic massage or *abhyangam* on a daily basis, preferably in the morning. "It is nourishing, pacifies the *doshas*, relieves fatigue, provides stamina, pleasure and perfect sleep, enhances the complexion and the luster of the skin, promotes longevity and nourishes all parts of the body," it says. A therapeutic massage, not a relaxation tool, *abhyangam*'s primary aim is to encourage the movement of toxins from the deeper tissues into the gastrointestinal tract where they can be efficiently eliminated. It is also given to stimulate circulation of the blood and lymph.

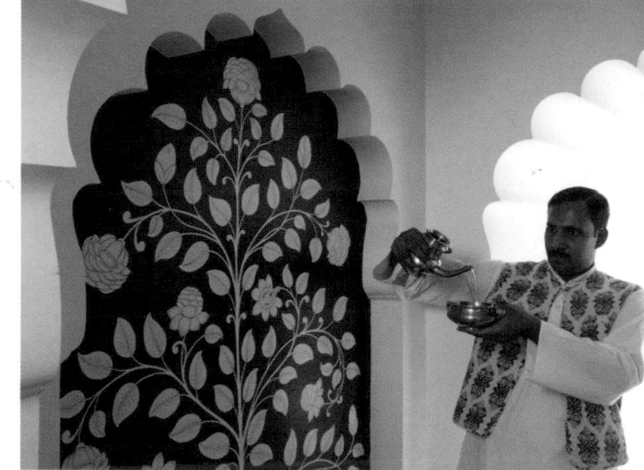

Abhyangam is traditionally performed with lashings of medicated herbal oil chosen according to one's *dosha*, and is meant to be performed by one, two, four, or more therapists simultaneously. It employs long strokes, mainly with full palm involved, and all the pressure movements are in the direction of blood circulation, from the trunk to the extremities and up to down. The reverse hand movements are passive (without pressure).

The classic texts outline five different positions that the client should adopt during *abhyangam*, with the first two postures being repeated at the end, thus making a total of seven. These are: 1) Seated with both legs extended. 2) Lying on the back. 3) Lying on the left side. 4) Lying on the stomach. 5) Lying on the right side. 6) Seated with both legs extended (a repeat of 1). 7) Lying on the back (a repeat of 2).

Therapists generally spend an equal amount of time on each posture, but if there are particular areas that need more attention, they will take precedence.

If you have *abhyangam* at one of the Oberoi Spas, the therapist soon gets a feel for your body, and concentrates on repeated strain injured areas (RSIs) to increase benefits. The idea is that the physical therapy has a direct connection to the mental and the spiritual: by the end, you should be physically and mentally relaxed — yet alert and rejuvenated also. Benefits of good *abhyanga* massage include increased circulation, improvement in muscle tone, calming of the nerves, increased mental alertness, soft, smooth skin and, of course, the elimination of impurities and toxins from the body.

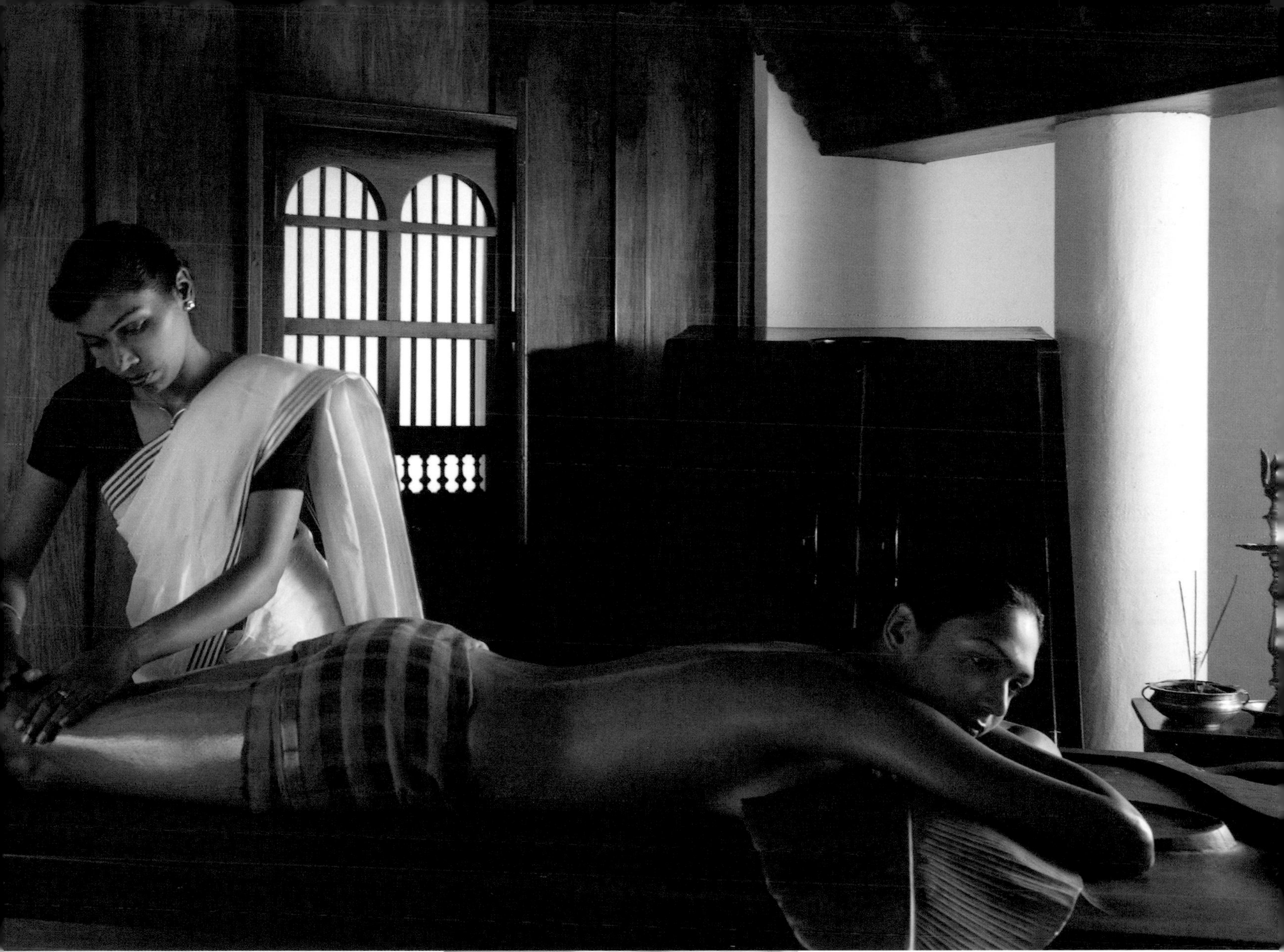

Opposite Dr Renja Raphel, the Keralan-trained Ayurvedic doctor at the spa at Rajvilas in Rajasthan, prepares an oil mix with medicated herbs for a client.
Right Ayurveda tends to advocate the use of brass vessels for oils, although clay containers are also used. As metal was considered extremely pure as well as hard-wearing, it is a sensible choice.

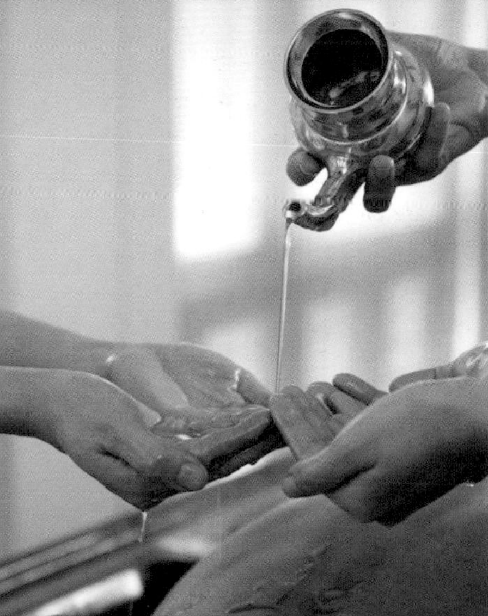

Above The Ayurvedic center called Ayurmana at Kumarakom Lake Resort in Kerala was believed to have been bestowed with the grace of the both Kodungalloor goddesses and Narasimhamoorthy — so is as close to a sacred structure (barring a temple) as you are likely to get. Therapy rooms including this prayer room glow with polished wood and the sanctity that comes with total peace and seclusion.

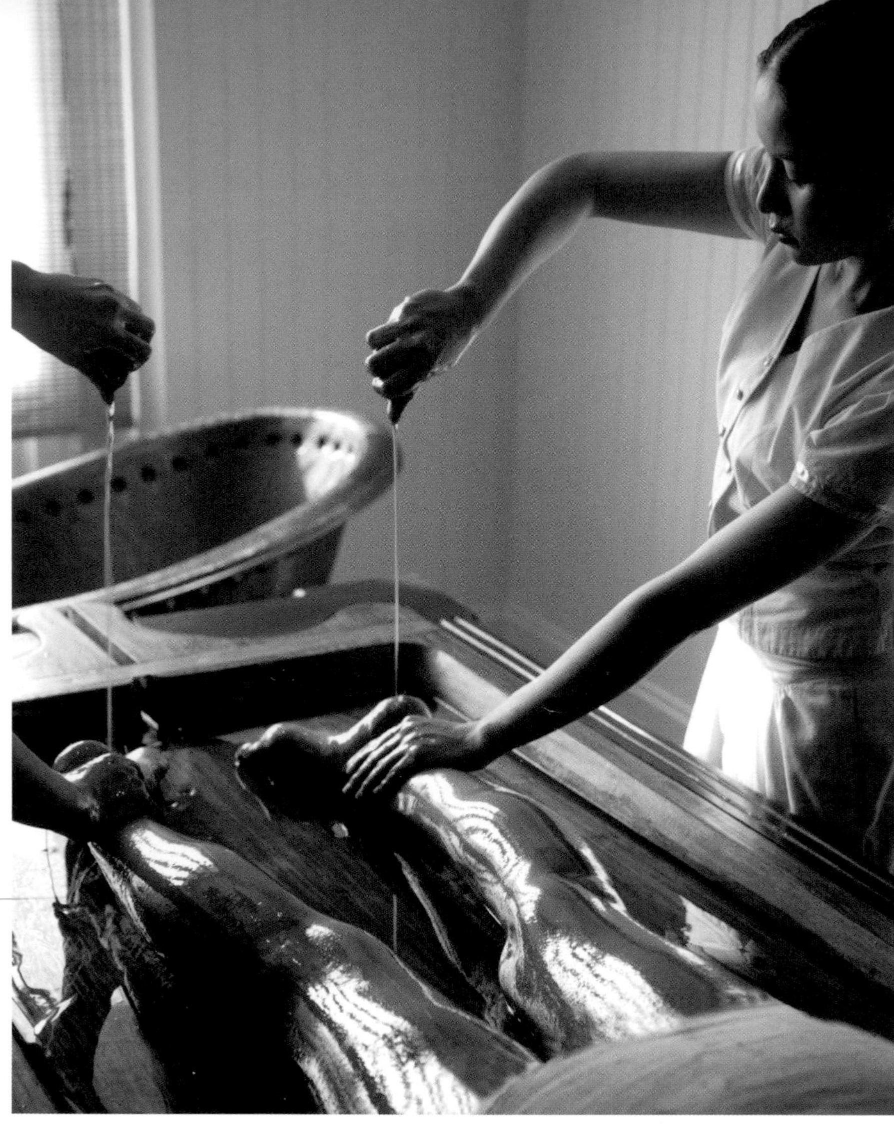

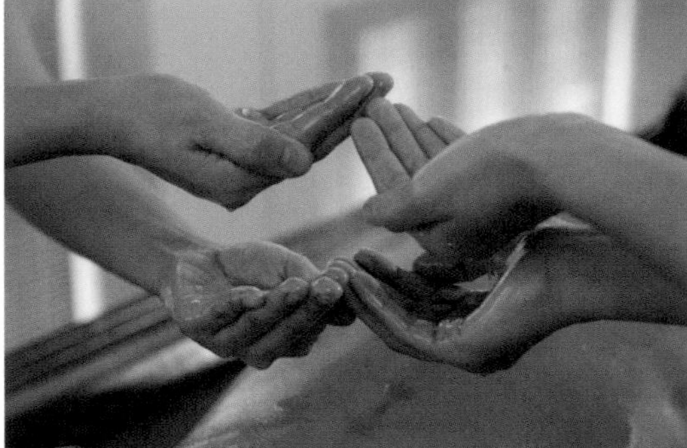

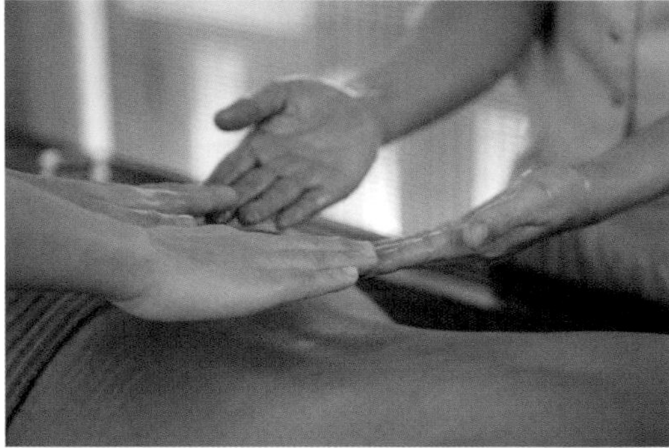

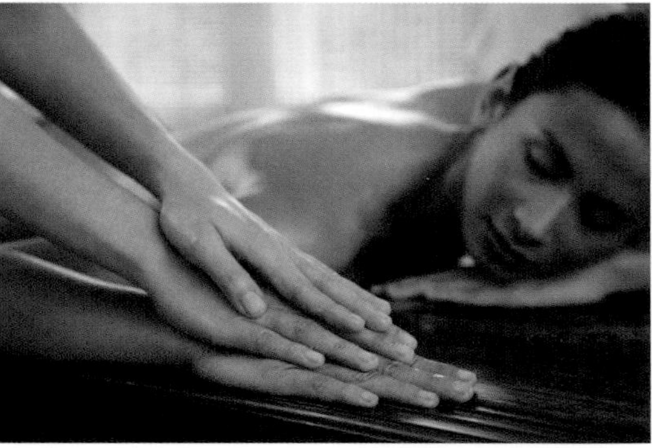

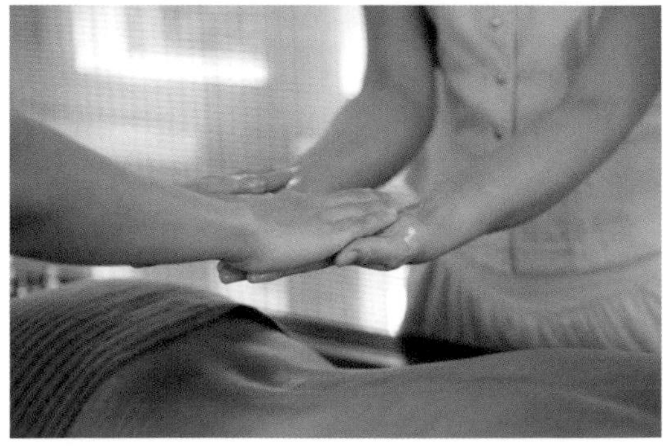

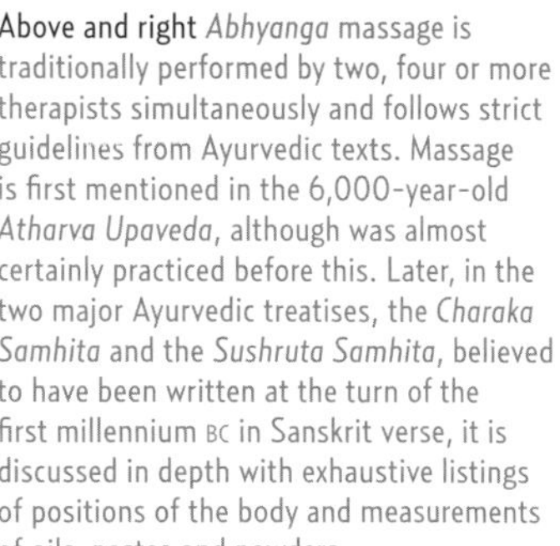

Above and right *Abhyanga* massage is traditionally performed by two, four or more therapists simultaneously and follows strict guidelines from Ayurvedic texts. Massage is first mentioned in the 6,000-year-old *Atharva Upaveda*, although was almost certainly practiced before this. Later, in the two major Ayurvedic treatises, the *Charaka Samhita* and the *Sushruta Samhita*, believed to have been written at the turn of the first millennium BC in Sanskrit verse, it is discussed in depth with exhaustive listings of positions of the body and measurements of oils, pastes and powders.

In the *Charaka Samhita*, discussion of massage as a purification means to alter the chemical processes in cells is detailed and comprehensive. This comes in the chapter on *panchakarma* (see pages 46–49), whereby methods for the evacuation of toxins and the restoration of *prana* or cosmic energy to the body via lymphatic drainage are outlined. The *Sushruta Samhita*, on the other hand, is a treatise on surgery; it is here that methods of acupressure on the Meridian points, magnetism on the *chakras* and the positive spiritual and mental effects of massage are covered.

chavitti thirumal

Pressure Point Massage with Feet

Ayurvedic texts indicate that exercise, be it cardiovascular, involving stretching and breathing, or therapy, must be practiced on a daily basis for total wellbeing. Exercise is necessary to raise the metabolism, increase oxygenation, improve the function of the heart and circulatory system, and expel toxins.

For martial art and dance pupils, exercise and body conditioning are particularly important. In the past, pupils were taught (often individually) by gurus in what is known as the guru-*shishya* tradition; their education didn't just include the one particular activity, but involved a thorough grounding in the classical texts, as well as such disciplines as yoga and *pranayama*. Nowadays, this tradition continues, but there are both residential and non-residential dance, drama and martial arts' schools as well.

Kalari payattu gurrukal (master or teacher) Tomy Joseph stresses the importance of conditioning the body to stay in shape. "*Gurrukal* need to master both preventative and curative techniques too," he notes. He says that *chavitti thirumal*, a very particular massage technique done with bare feet with the masseuse hanging from ropes tied to the ceiling, are mandatory for a *gurrukal*. Teachers routinely massage their pupils in this way to prepare the body for the stresses of the martial art, to maintain suppleness and to treat pain and swelling caused by combat.

The treatment is also given to those with neuro-muscular and skeletal disorders as well as to help clients reach beyond their psycho-physical limitations. Based on a precise knowledge of the body's energetic channels *(nadis)* and vital spots *(marmas)*, the therapist suspends his weight from ropes overhead and applies pressure with long strokes of the soles of his feet, after the client's body has been prepared with specially medicated oil. There is usually some manipulation of the joints and limbs also.

What distinguishes *chavitti thirumal* from other massage treatments is the application. The foot of the masseur is able to give a deeper, more thorough pressure and is able to cover the whole length of the body from the tips of the fingers to the tips of the toes, with long continuous graceful strokes. Therapists need to undergo many years of training: learning the *chavitti* art requires a certain type of calling and certainly a deep dedication to the wellbeing of clients and their physical, emotional, mental and spiritual upkeep.

After placing a foot in some medicated oil, the *chavitti* therapist balances his or her weight via ropes hanging from the ceiling, and presses deep into *marma* points along the client's back and legs.

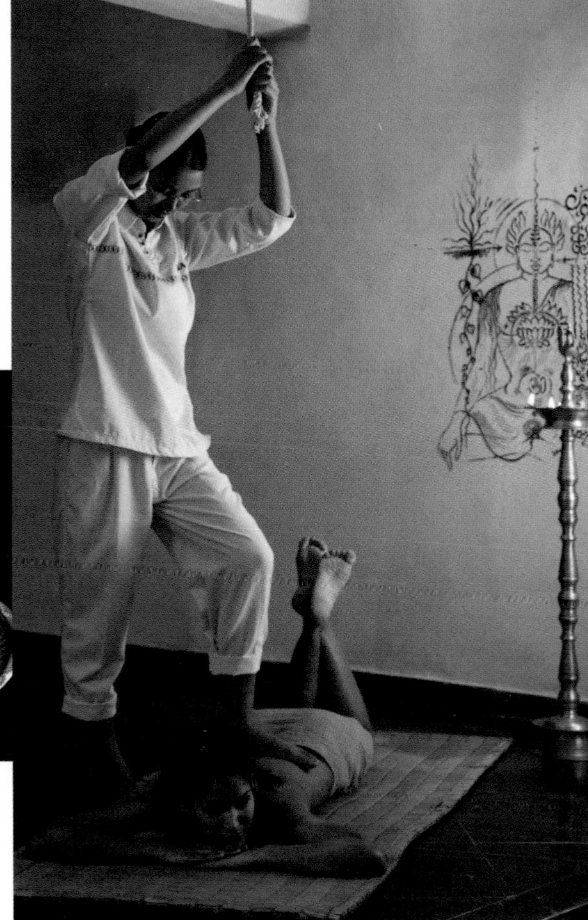

hot stone abhyangam

This deeply penetrating, all-over body blast is an example of how Ayurveda may be integrated with other healing traditions from elsewhere in the world. Developed by therapists at the world-famous Soukya International Holistic Health Center near Bangalore, it employs the healing medicated herbal oils and massage movements of Ayurveda with the warmth and nurturing qualities of hot stones developed by both Native American Indians and Tibetans (separately of course!). It is one and a half hours of pure bliss.

There is both a therapeutic element and a feel-good factor to this treatment, so you can relax cocooned in the warmth emanating from the hot stones knowing that what is taking place is good for you. The long, firm strokes of the masseuse encourage the elimination of toxins from the deeper tissues and also stimulate peripheral circulation of both blood and lymph. This, along with the heat from the stones, enables the medicated oils to be absorbed to do their work. Naturally, as with all Ayurvedic treatments, oils are chosen according to the client's constitution and/or ailment.

One therapist is in charge of heating and re-heating the stones, while the other alternates between oil massage, stone massage with oil, and placing stones at key points on the body. As the treatment progresses, a rhythm is established. One part of the body is being massaged, while a strategically placed stone sends heat deep into another part of the body; as the stone cools, it is replaced or taken away and another stone is placed elsewhere. After the back, legs and arms have been seen to, the client turns over, and is then invited to lie down on eight stones that run up either side of the spine. The heat is then twofold: coming up through the back, and down from stones on the front.

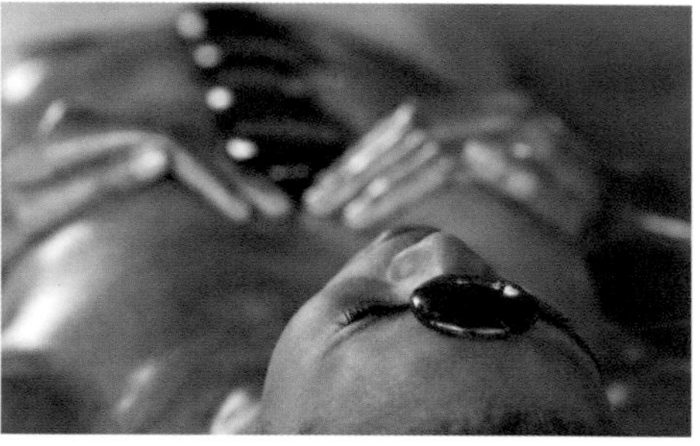

Stones are often basalt, a black volcanic rock with a high iron content, that absorbs and retains heat well. Such stones are believed to improve energy flows in the body.

With soothing music, firm massage strokes and the wonderfully nurturing warmth from the smooth stones, this is an experience to savor. The mind wanders and returns, the body sighs in acceptance, the spirit is soothed. Unfortunately, it seems all too soon when the treatment comes to an end. Nonetheless, the benefits linger and if this therapy is prescribed as a daily treat during a long-term stay, the effects are magnified considerably.

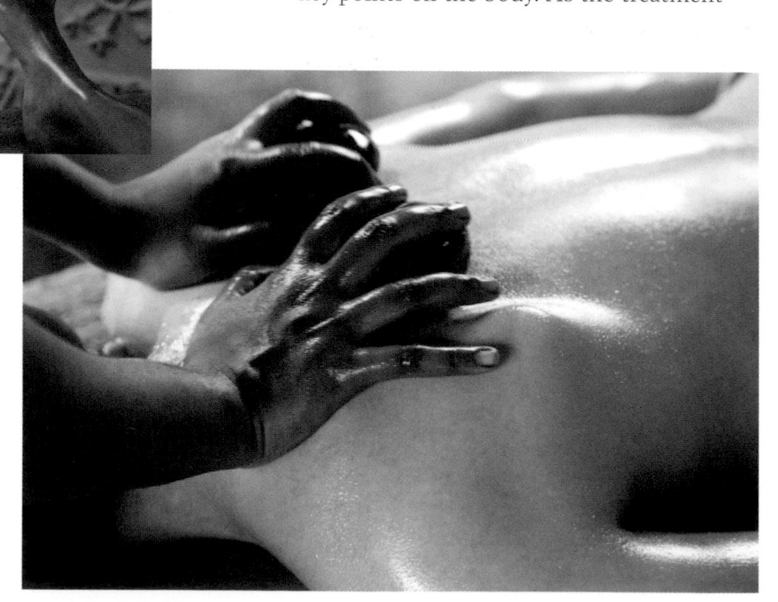

Small stones placed between the toes are delightfully indulgent, while larger ones are used for the massage itself. Feelings of warmth and security emanate from them; all the while the medicated oil does its detoxifying work.

marma massage Pressure Point Massage

Indian pressure points are known as *marmas* and are similar to Chinese acupressure points. Translating from the Sanskrit as "secret" or "hidden", they are found at junctures of the body where two or more tissues, muscles, veins, ligaments, bones or joints meet.

In Traditional Chinese Medicine (TCM), there are thousands of such points, but only 107 exist in the Ayurvedic system. Consisting of major points that correspond to the seven *chakras* and minor points that radiate out along the torso and limbs, they are measured by finger units *(anguli)* to detect their correct locations. There are 22 points on the lower extremities, 22 on the arms, 12 on the chest and stomach, 14 on the back and 37 on the head and neck. The mind is considered the 108th *marma* point. In the *Sushruta Samhita* each point has a Sanskrit name.

Ayurveda states that every *marma* point is placed at a junction of different channels of *prana* movements in the body. *Prana,* similar to *chi* in TCM, is considered the subtle vital energy that pervades every part of the body, nurturing the cell systems. If *marma* points become blocked or ruptured, *prana* flow is interrupted and organs may become diseased. If they are clear, *prana* is free to travel the meridians or *nidas* unchecked — and the body is healthy.

The idea of massaging the *marma* points began in Kerala at around 1500 BC when masters of *kalari payattu* first used the *marma* points as points for injury. It was only a matter of time before Ayurvedic physicians realized that these points could also be used for healing — and began to experiment with massaging the points to trigger a healing flow of energy. Today, *marma* massage is practiced at clinics and spas for a number of different reasons, be it therapeutic, relaxing or revitalizing.

Marma massage generally combines soft, flowing movements (*abhyangam*) with pressure point therapy. For the latter, the therapist uses one or more fingers depending on the size of the *marma* point, and either presses directly or in circular motions on that particular point. It is believed that clockwise movements stimulate and energize a *marma* point, while counterclockwise motions break up blocked energy and toxins held within a point. The practice is quite similar to Chinese acupressure or Japanese *shiatsu*, the origins of which lie in Ayurvedic practice. Benefits of regular *marma* massage are a general balancing — emotional, spiritual and physical — resulting in clarity, calmness and confidence.

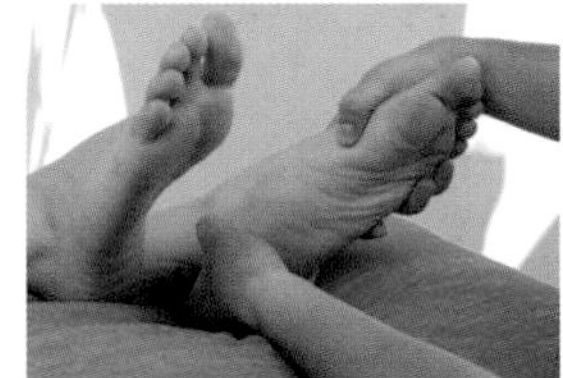

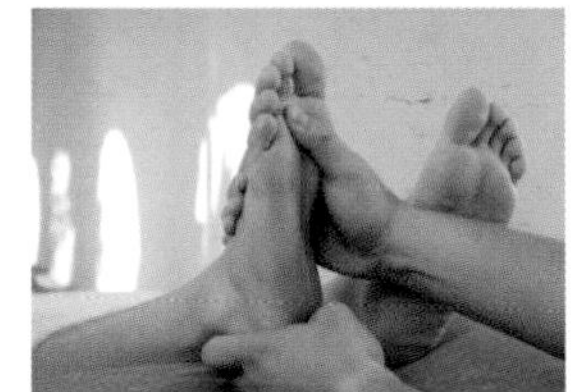

Showing both *chakra* points and meridians, this educational drawing (**left below**) shows how *prana* or the vital force needs to flow around the body. Specific points (**left and below**) are pressed to release blocked *prana*.

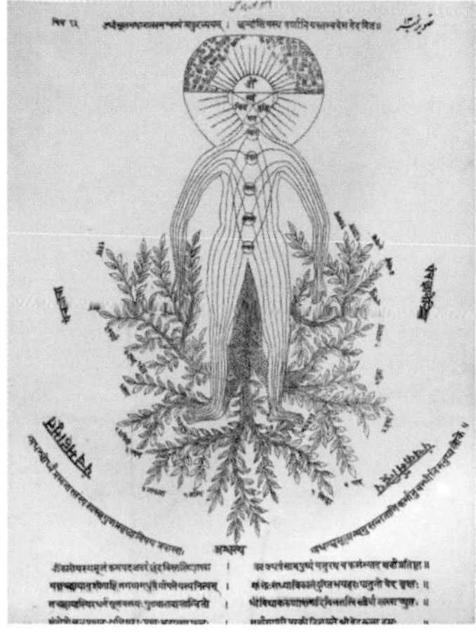

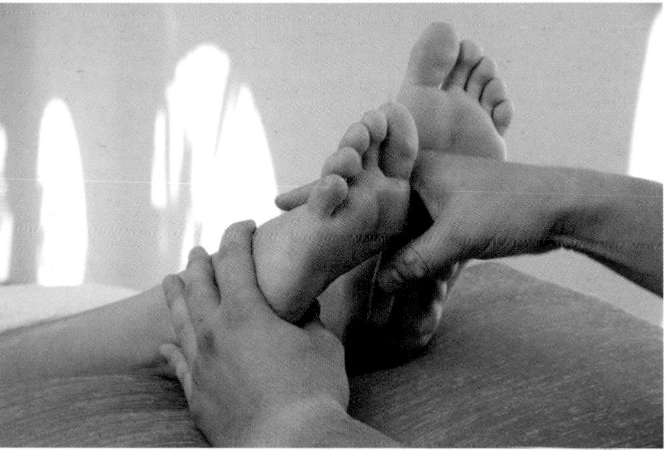

champi Indian Head Massage

In spite of its name, Indian head massage involves work not only on the head but on the upper back, shoulders, neck, scalp and face too. In much the same way that Traditional Chinese Medicine dictates that certain points on the feet are directly aligned to internal organs, Ayurvedic texts relate certain parts of the head to other body parts and/or symptoms or diseases. Therefore, a *champi* or head massage does not only affect the immediate areas massaged: it can be a healing, rejuvenating and thoroughly stimulating experience as well.

The moment a baby is born, the fontanel on the top of its head is covered immediately with cloth soaked in oil with a *bala* root decoction to strengthen the head, sight and intelligence. Mothers massage their babies' heads to facilitate strong skull and brain development, and later, give their daughters head massages to stimulate the scalp and infuse conditioning oils into the hair. Men are used to receiving a sharp rubdown at the barber's shop and another place you are likely to receive an Indian head massage is in a salon or spa.

The massage normally takes 30 to 60 minutes and is given seated in a chair. It may be dry or oils may be used to both condition hair and calm the nervous system, as hair roots are connected to nerve fibers. Techniques vary, but the therapist usually start by gently kneading upper back, shoulder and neck muscles, then works up to the head. Here, the scalp is squeezed, rubbed and tapped and hair may be combed or pulled. The therapist locates the *marma* points along the head and spends time tugging and pressing earlobes, before moving on to the face. Facial massage is usually a mixture of acupressure and gentle manipulation, ending with soft stroking.

People who suffer from vertigo, head-aches, migraines, insomnia, tinnitus and depression are all reported to find *champi* helpful. As the therapist works on the three higher *chakras*, the *vissuddha* (the base of the throat), *ajna* (the forehead) and *sahasrara* (the crown), mental and emotional stress is immediately released. In addition, the localized massage improves the supply of glucose and blood to the brain, improves the circulation of cerebrospinal fluid, dissipates accumulated toxins and opens pranic channels. Results include improved memory, clarity of mind, better eyesight and concentration, and clearing of the sinuses.

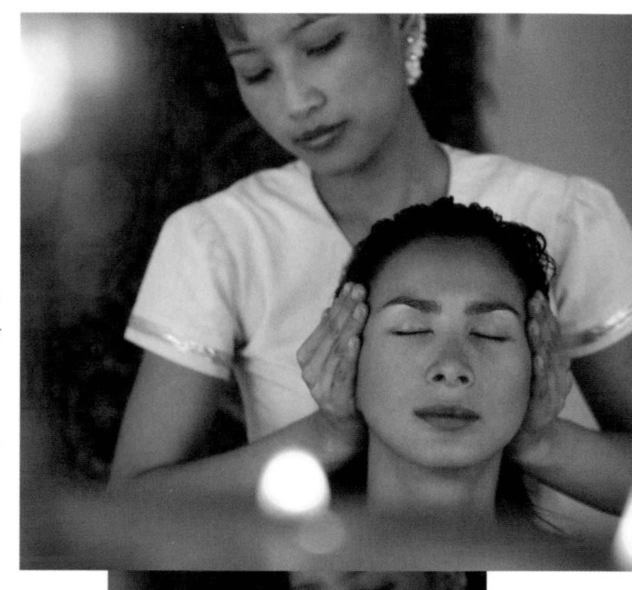

Above and left The therapist at the Ayurvedic Penthouse at Mandarin Oriental in Bangkok, first prepares for a 60-minute Indian head massage session by creating an atmosphere of calm with candlelight and aromatic oil burners. Then, she starts the therapy with pressure point massage to stimulate the vital energy points in the skull, thereby increasing the flow of subtle energies in the body. The result is a client comforted, nurtured and relaxed.

udwarthanam Dry Massage with Herbal Powder

A stimulating massage that uses dry powders not oil, *udwarthanam* is vigorous, energizing and not for the faint hearted. Dry herbal powders, chosen according to one's *dosha*, are rubbed into the skin in the opposite direction to hair growth with strong repeated movements. The friction of the powder during the massage creates body heat that increases circulation, breaks down cellulite, firms muscle tone and reduces fat by improving the metabolism of the muscles. It is recommended for those who want to lose weight, as it reduces cholesterol levels and adipose tissue and promotes better digestion and. It also removes toxins and exfoliates the skin, leaving skin tingling, soothed and soft.

Most Ayurvedic massages tend to use long, flowing strokes that go away from the heart and from bottom to top, but *udwarthanam* employs short, sharp superficial rubs that go in the opposite direction, away from the heart towards the extremities and from the top of the body downwards. This is the opposite of the *dosha* flow. According to Ayurvedic physician, Dr Ajitha of Soukya, the powder helps to open up the micro-channels in the body, so reduces fat accumulation, tautens up muscles, reduces bad body odor and exfoliates dead surface skin cells. In a clinical setting, *udwarthanam* is usually prescribed for 10 to 14 days for those with *ama twan* or slowness of flow in the channels, and as a means to reduce fat. However, the massage type is increasingly finding its way into spas and retreats, where its invigorating style is gaining popularity.

At the spa at Udaivilas, a beautiful resort on the shore of Lake Pichola in Udaipur, one of three Ayurvedic powders or *choornam* are used: the popular *triphala choornam* or three fruit powder, a powder composed from *Terminalia chebula* or *Terminalia bellaruca*, or *kola kula thadhi choornam*, made from a variety of pulses and herbs. The massage is quite rough and the powder enters the superficial bloodstream, but also enters nasally as it flies about in the air. This cleanses the internal system too. Afterwards, the client is encouraged to spend 10 minutes in the steam room and further massage any residual powder into the skin. As sweating occurs, toxins are released through the skin's pores, and the skin is left feeling soft, extremely smooth and rejuvenated.

Another place that offers *udwarthanam* is Soukya International Holistic Health Center. Here it is prescribed for guests who are obese and the powders are prepared on site. They differ from patient to patient, but may contain *vacha* (*Acorus calamus*) to alleviate swelling, the Ayurvedic all-round wonder fruit *amalaki* or Indian Gooseberry (*Emblica officinalis*), green gram powder and/or basil. All the herbs are washed, cut into small pieces, dried and pulverized on site to make either a fine or coarse powder, which is then strewn on to the body and massaged in by two therapists simultaneously.

Below Some of the powders used at Udaivilas; they contain what doctors call *madagna* properties that reduce fat and help clear blockages.
Bottom Two therapists at Soukya massage a client with powder made on site. *Udwarthanam* is also useful as a depilatory because the short, sharp rubs tend to pluck hairs from the roots.

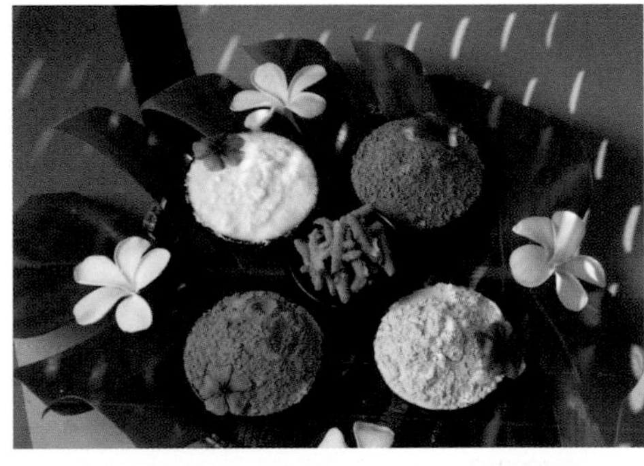

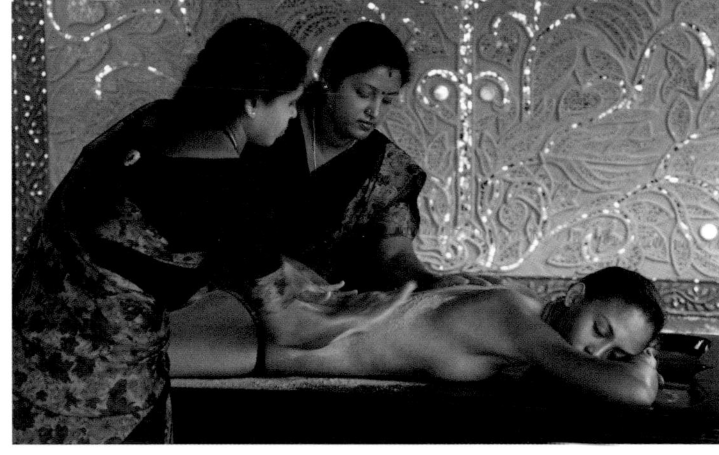

sirodhara Oiling the Third Eye

Surprisingly, *sirodhara* is the most widespread Ayurvedic therapy offered at spas outside India. Why this is the case is unclear, as it is not prescribed for many ailments in a clinical environment. It invariably comes top of the Ayurvedic menu, and even spas without an Ayurvedic department offer bastardized versions. Many people have tried it, and even if they haven't, they will almost certainly have heard of it.

Coming from *siro* ("head") and *dhara* ("pouring of herbal liquids on specific body parts"), *sirodhara* denotes the continuous pouring of herbal oils, milk, buttermilk or ghee over the head and scalp. The patient lies on his or her back on a wooden treatment table, cocooned in warm towels, while a therapist trains a steady rhythmic stream of warm liquid from a perforated vessel made of clay, wood or metal on to the forehead. The table is made from one of seven therapeutic woods and is designed to catch the oil for recycling on the same client.

Oil stroking the "third eye" has a balancing effect on the deepest recesses of the brain and is profoundly relaxing. In Ayurveda, it is seen as a stimulating procedure for the nervous system and is prescribed for bringing down aggravated *vata* conditions such as insomnia, headache, insecurity, fear and nervous strain. Irritable *pitta* predominant people with overactive minds can experience a cooling, calming benefit from a session or two and *kaphas* often fall asleep. Used in conjunction with other therapies, *sirodhara* has been practiced for thousands of years to treat many and varied conditions such as ear, nose and throat disturbances, glandular problems, psychiatric disorders, hypertension, skin diseases, facial paralysis and more. During a session, the nervous system unwinds, busy brains become clear, and tired bodies are refreshed.

In a clinical environment, the choice of liquid and duration of treatment varies according to the individual. *Vata* patients are generally prescribed medicated herbal oil, *pitta* types receive herbal milk, ghee or coconut oil, and buttermilk is often recommended for *kapha* patients. Ancient texts denote 53 minutes for *vatas*, 43 minutes for *pitas* and 31 minutes for *kaphas*! It is suggested the best time to receive *sirodhara* is early in the morning for a period of 21 consecutive days, depending on the client. A variation of *sirodhara* is *deha-dhara*, where two to four therapists pour a continuous flow of oil over the entire body.

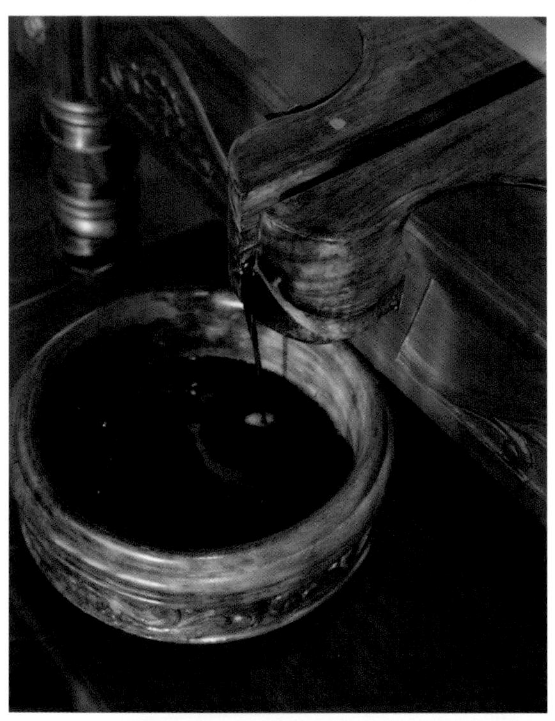

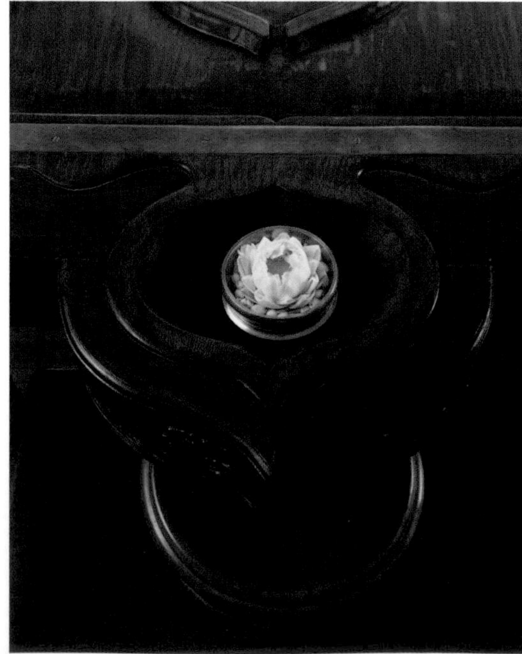

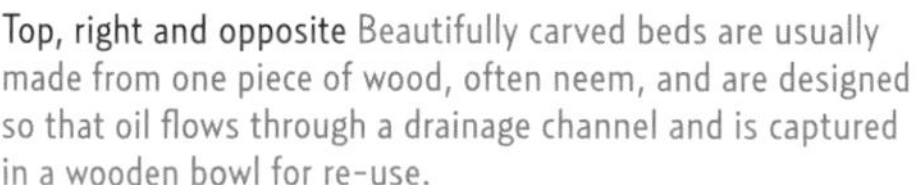

Top, right and opposite Beautifully carved beds are usually made from one piece of wood, often neem, and are designed so that oil flows through a drainage channel and is captured in a wooden bowl for re-use.

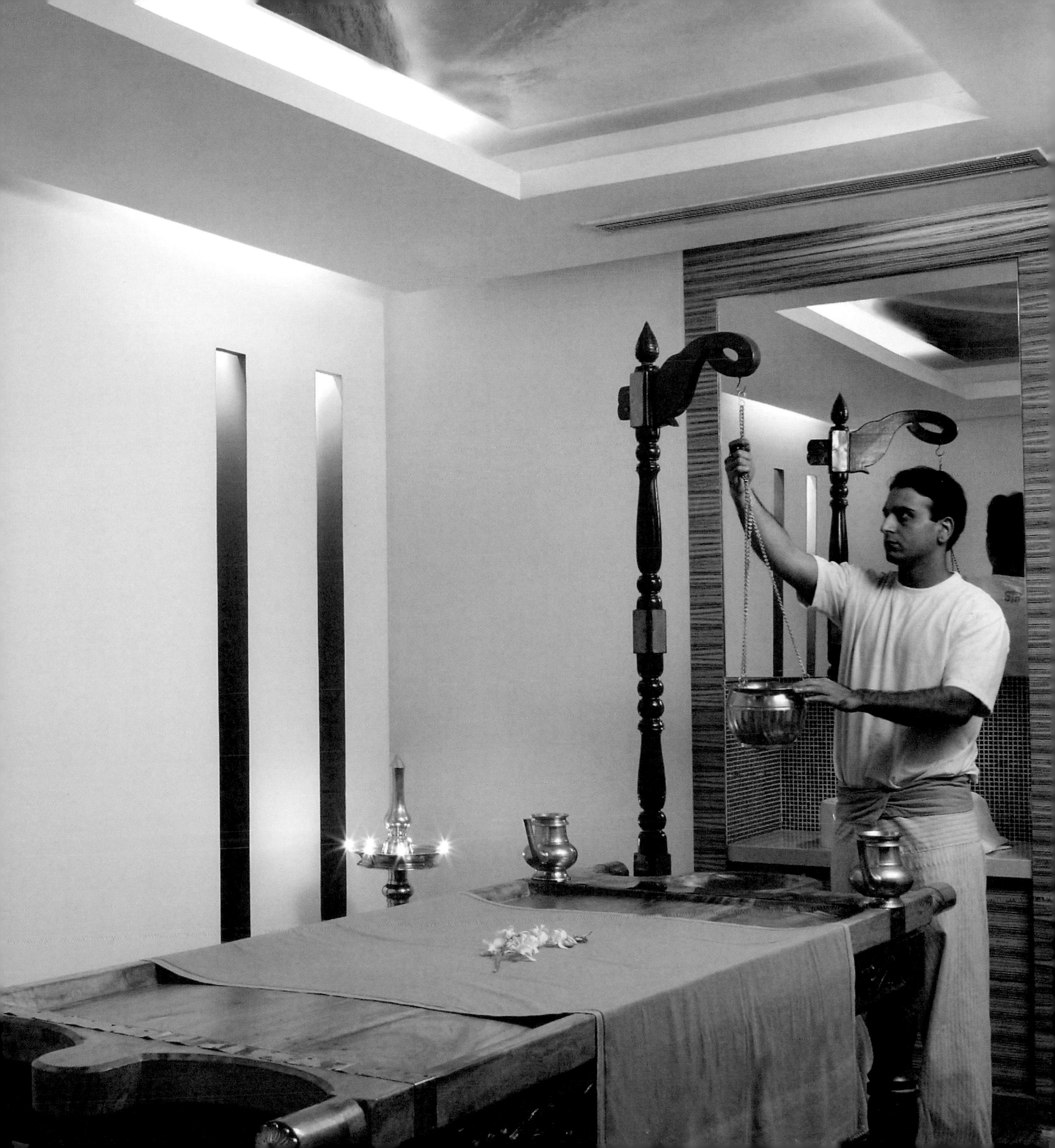

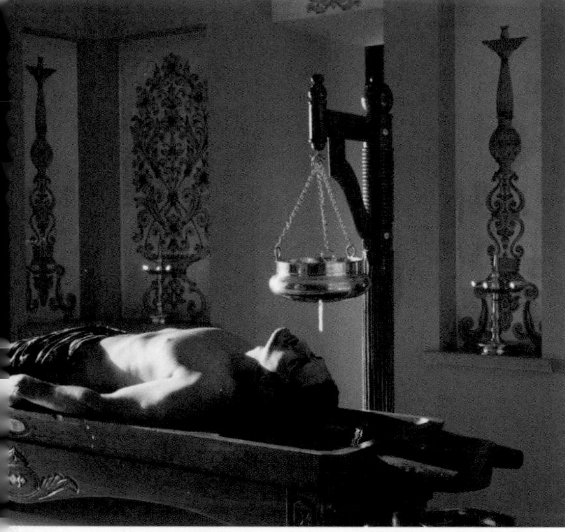

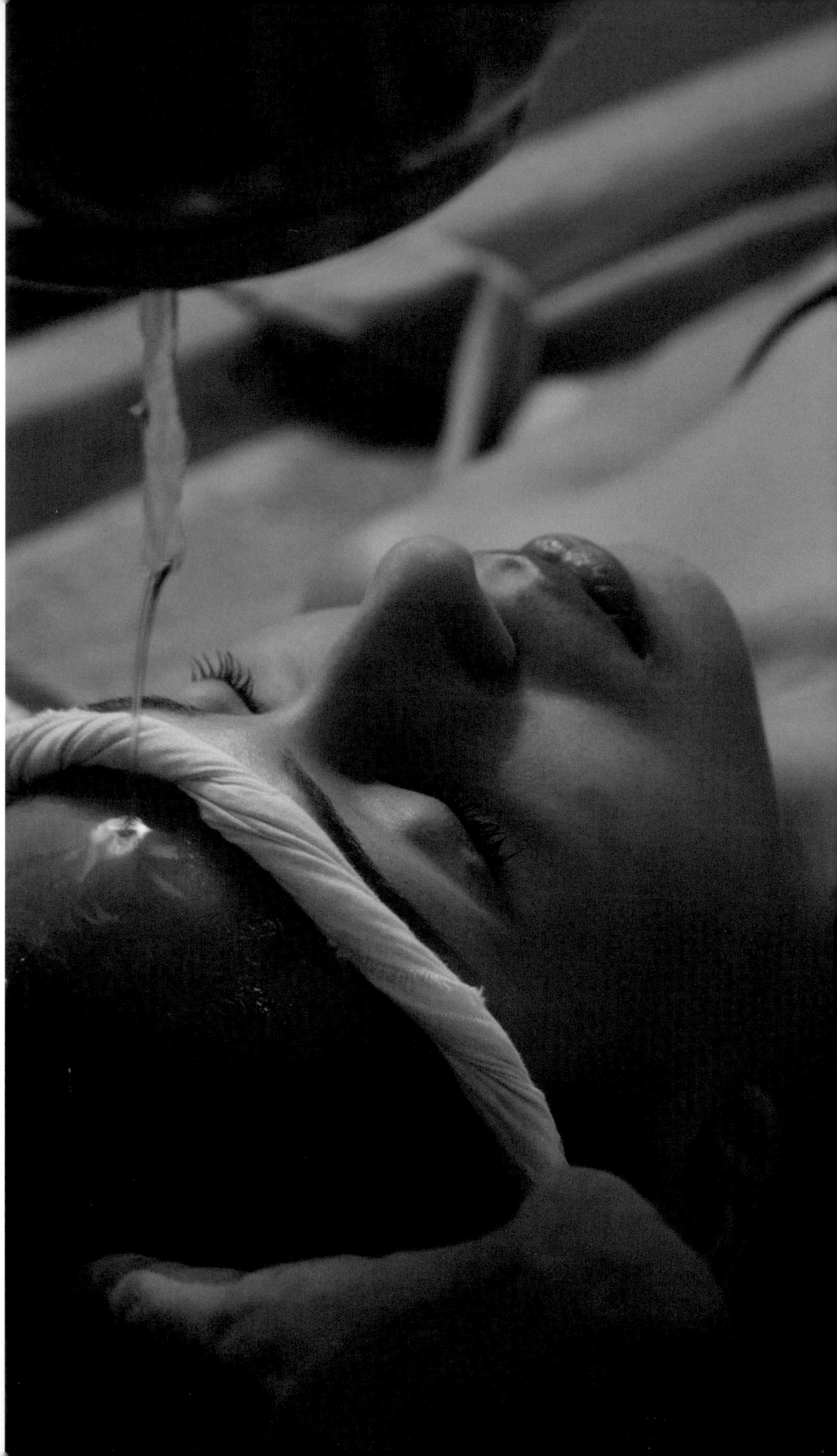

Opposite, top and below The *Charaka Samhita* specifies seven types of wood for an Ayurvedic bed or *patti* with the emphasis being on the wood having no joins. Because of the quality of the wood, beds are often works of art in themselves; often inlaid with copper or tin inserts, the more elaborate ones have evocative carvings as well.

Left At Quan spa in the JW Marriott Mumbai, oil at a *sirodhara* session is forced to flow back over the forehead down to the bed with the fastening of a piece of cloth just below the "third eye".

Right The palatial surrounds of Neemrana Fort Palace's courts and halls are highly conducive to healing. Here, a therapist trains the flow of oil on to the forehead of a client.

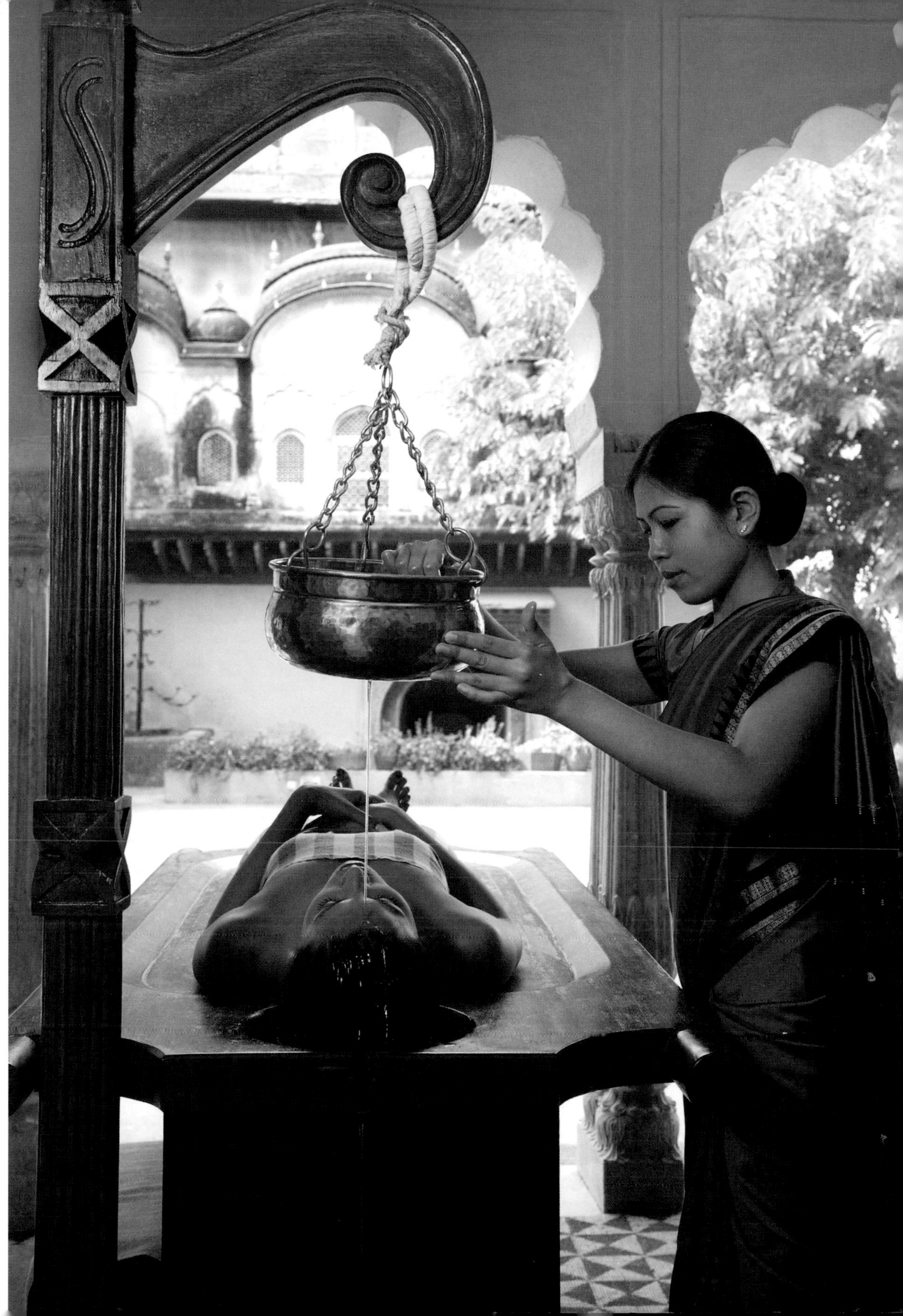

vasthi The Medicated Enema

To most Westerners the subject of enemas is one to be avoided, at best; subjected to, at worst. This probably stems from an innate squeamishness, but, be that as it may, the insertion into the anus, urinary organs and genitals of various kinds of enemas such as water, medicated and non-medicated oils and milks, and herbal decoctions is an integral part of Ayurvedic practice. This is because Ayurveda states that the status of the alimentary canal and other internal organs is of vital importance to one's overall health.

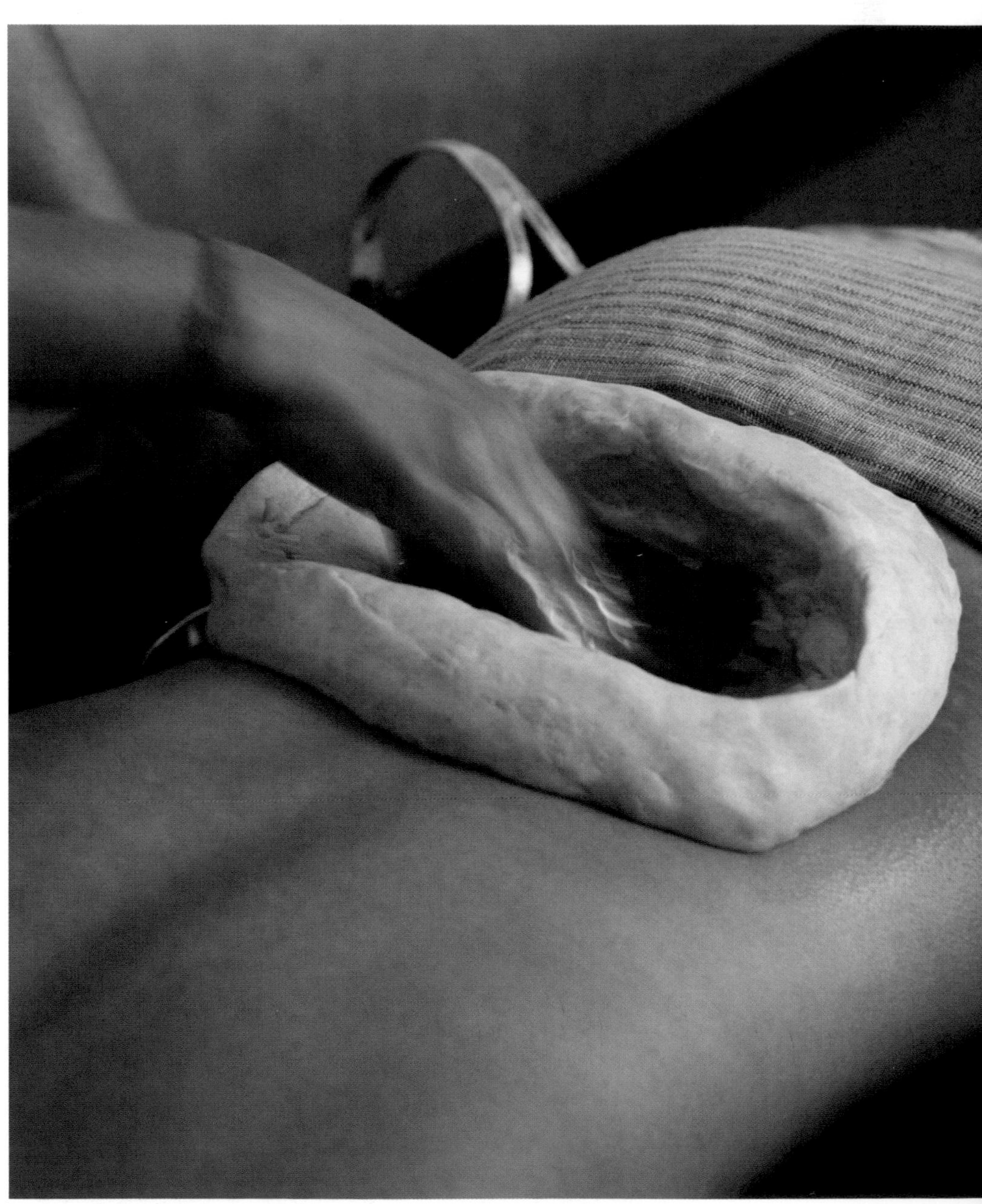

Vasthi (*basti*) is the word for a medicated enema, and in Ayurveda *vasthi* involves the introduction of herbal and medicinal concoctions in a liquid medium into and also *on to* the body. Sites where *vasthi* may be administered therefore also include external areas such as the eyes, lower back, head and the chest region. It is believed that these medicinal *vasthi* remove wastes and toxins from the body (either internally or externally), balance the functions of the *doshas*, provide nourishment and raise the body's mmunity.

Vasthi is most effective in the treatment of *vata* disorders, although many enemas over a prescribed period of time are usually required. There are different types of *vasthi* given for many vastly differing ailments, including constipation, chronic fever, cold, sexual disorders, kidney stones, heart pain,

Left After a doughnut-style mix of gram flour and water is placed on the lower back and deemed watertight, warmed medicated oil is poured into the "container". It is left to seep into the client's sacro-lumbar region or "foment" as Ayurvedic physicians call it.

Right The nurturing Ayurvedic Penthouse at the Oriental Spa in Bangkok offers a number of *vasthi* treatments including *hrid* or *uro vasthi*, an effective therapy for complaints of the heart and respiratory organs. Warm medicated oil, chosen according to the client's complaint and doshic imbalance, foments on the chest area for 40 minutes or so.

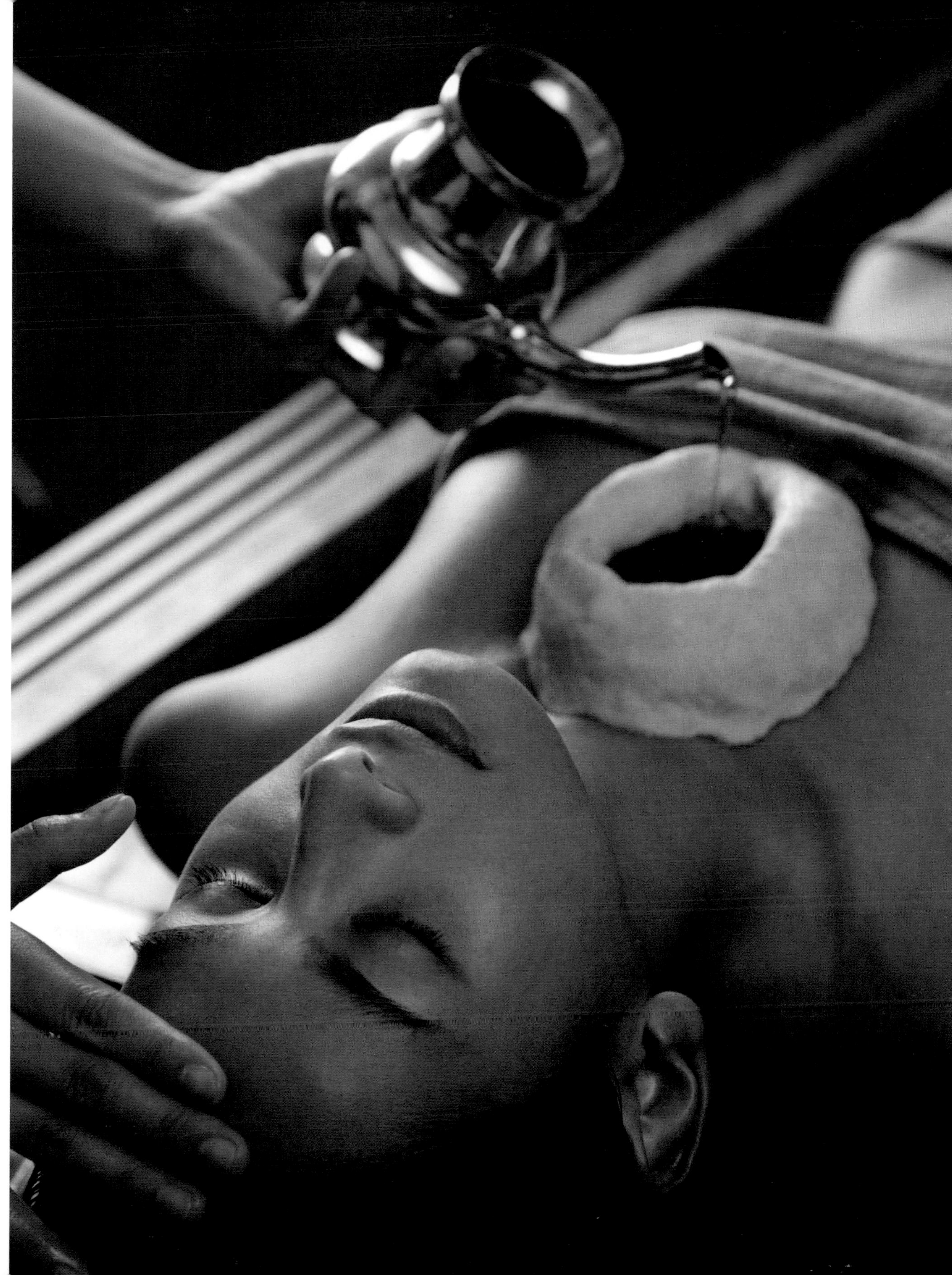

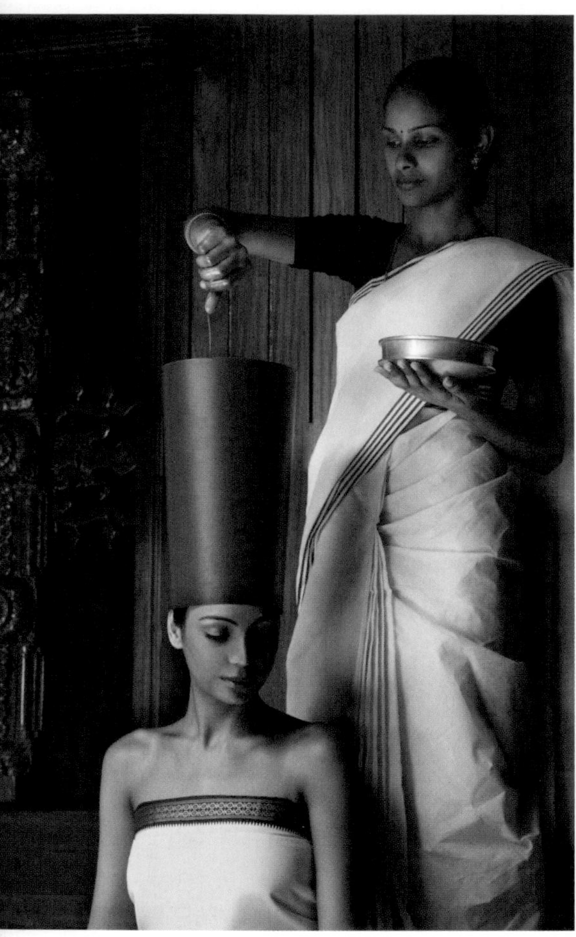

backache, sciatica and other pains in the joints. Many other *vata* disorders such as arthritis, rheumatism, gout, muscle spasms and headaches may also be treated with the varying *vasthi*.

Vasthi is one of the five main procedures of the famous (or infamous) *panchakarma* therapy (see page 46), but it may also be used in localized areas for neck complaints *(greva vasthi)*, knee joint conditions *(janu vasthi)* and heart disease or asthma and respiratory diseases (*hrid* or *uro vasthi*). In Indian spas, a couple of *vasthi* therapies are offered for one-off "try-outs":

Siro Vasthi

Usually offered for conditions such as facial paralysis, depression, insomnia, dryness of nostrils, mouth and throat illnesses and severe headaches, *siro vasthi* is on some Indian spa menus as a relaxing, stress-relieving and hair-conditioning therapy. *Siro vasthi* (*siro* means "head") involves the application of lukewarm herbal oils poured into a cap fitted on the head for any time between 15 to 60 minutes. The oils are left to stagnate on the scalp for the time required; according to one's *dosha*, current imbalances and/or medical conditions, medicated herbs will have been added to the oil. An antioxidant medicated oil called *dhan wantharam* that contains 28 herbs and an earthy fragrance is often used as it has rich pain-relieving properties.

Kathi Vasthi

A *vasthi* treatment that concentrates on the sacro-lumbar region of the back (*kathi)*, this is a curative treatment useful for lower back problems. It is also used for complaints that affect the abdomen, such as irritable bowel syndrome, endometriosis, menstrual and urinary tract disorders. It involves the pouring of warm medicated oil into an enclosed area of the lower back, created with a reservoir of dough (see right).

In some spas, *kathi vasthi* is used as a rejuvenative therapy to de-stress, relieve exhaustion or help with localized lower back pain. Providing the *kathi vasthi* is administered by a qualified Ayurvedic physician who has chosen the correct medicinal oil, a 20- to 60-minute session should not do any harm — and the gentle administering of warm, soothing oil on the back can be extremely pleasant.

Left A Keralan therapist at the atmospheric Ayurmana facility at Kumarakom Lake Resort pours warm medicated oil on to the skull of a client. Prior to this therapy, which is thought to relieve stress and regulate brain function, it is recommended the head be shaved.
Below and right A therapist prepares a dough mixture, then places it on the back for a *kathi vasthi* session in the soothing surrounds of the Deva spa at Mandarin Oriental Dhara Devi in Chiang Mai, Thailand.

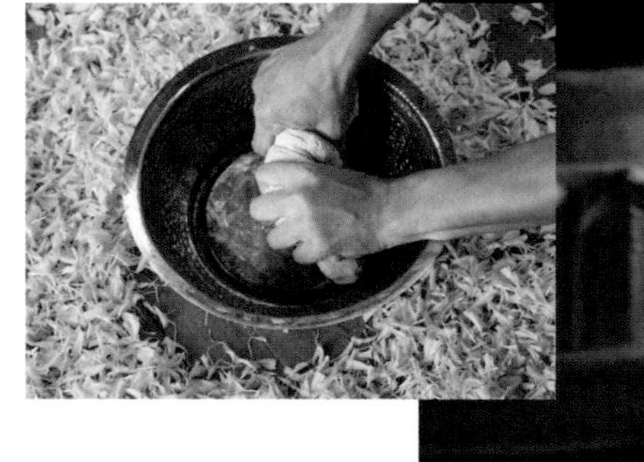

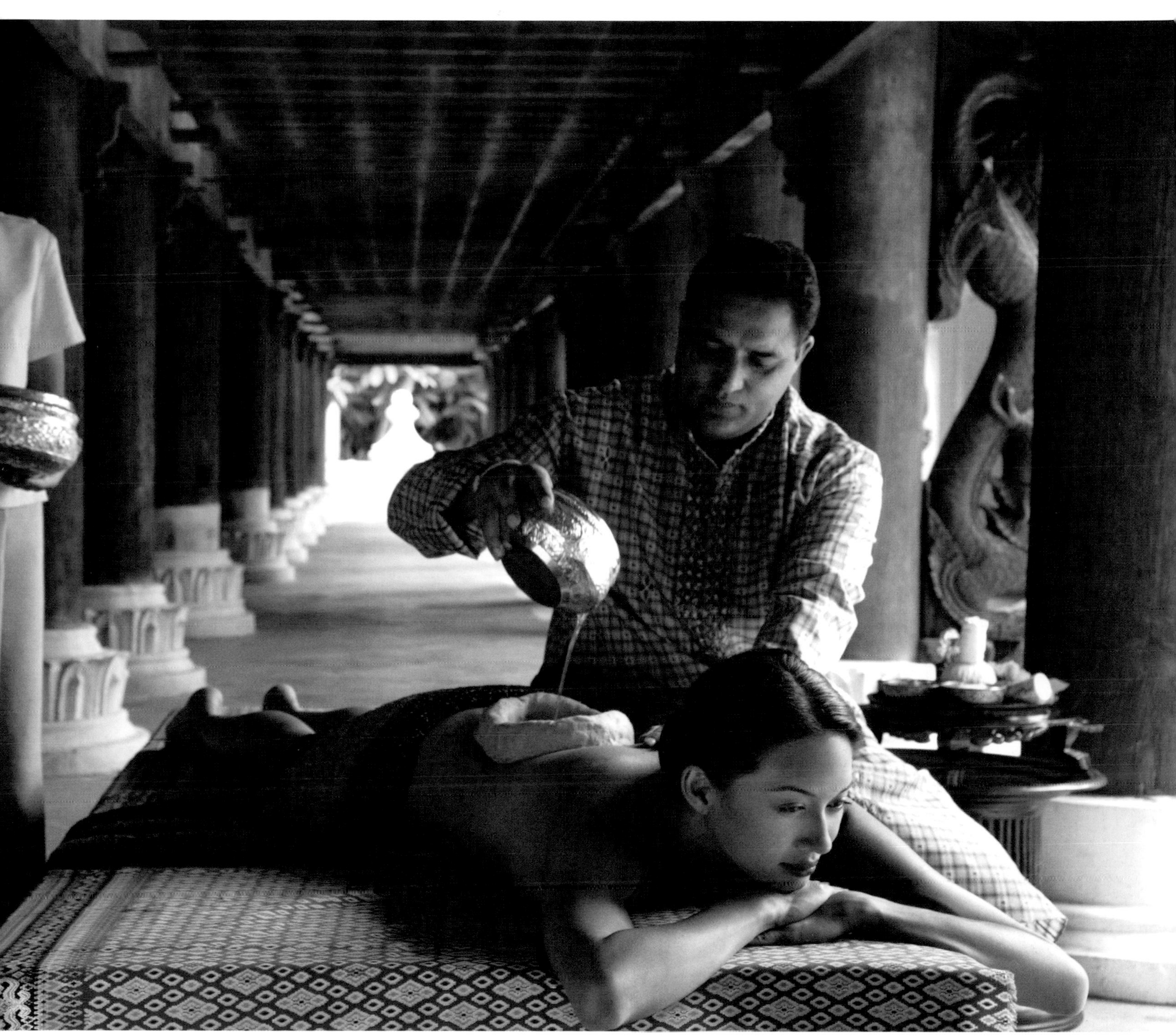

vasthi

unani An Holistic Graeco-Arab Medical System

Although most spa-goers in the West will have heard of Ayurveda, they may not be so familiar with another branch of medicine known as Unani that is practiced extensively in India. Unani originated in Greece with the philosopher-physician Hippocrates (460–377 BC) and was formulated over time by various Islamic scholar physicians in what is now the Middle East. Noted Arab physicians such as Rhazes (850–925) and Avicenna (aka Ibn Sina 980–1037) further developed Unani and, by the European Middle Ages, it had became the authoritative basis for the study of medicine. It was instrumental in introducing professional standards of practice to medicine all over Europe.

Unani was introduced to India during the medieval period, and over time, mass acceptance and continuous use led to many Unani hospitals, research centers and clinics being built. Its heyday in India lasted from the 13th to the 17th centuries, as the Delhi Sultans, the Khiljis, the Tughlaqs and the Mughal emperors provided patronage to Unani scholars, often employing them as court physicians.

During this period, many drugs and herbs native to India were added to the existing apothecary of Unani remedies. Clinical trials and experimentation resulted in expansion, and even though Unani suffered setbacks during the colonial period, it had become entrenched in Indian life. Today, India has the largest number of educational, research and health care institutions of Unani medicine in the world with over 20,000 registered Unani practitioners (*hakims*) and countless non-registered ones who practice on a hereditary basis.

Unani is recognized by the World Health Organization (WHO) as a holistic traditional medical system. In 1977 when the WHO established its traditional medicine program, it declared: "There is no doubt that this branch of medicine is making and will continue to make a very significant contribution to our efforts to achieve health for all."

Unani's goal is the preservation of health, the encouragement of self-healing and the restoration of the body's equilibrium. In its infancy it was a rigorous system that eliminated superstition and harmful folk practices, and as developments and discoveries were made, it added to its repertoire of remedies and practices. Nowadays, Unani practitioners combine herbal medical remedies with dietary advice, regimental therapy, psychological practices, surgery and spiritual discipline.

As with other holistic practices, a Unani *hakim* tends to look at the patient as a whole — mentally, physically, emotionally and spiritually — before prescribing a course of treatment. Dr Mathai of the integrative medicinal retreat called Soukya explains: "Unani aims to promote positive health and prevent diseases and is based around six essentials: good air and water,

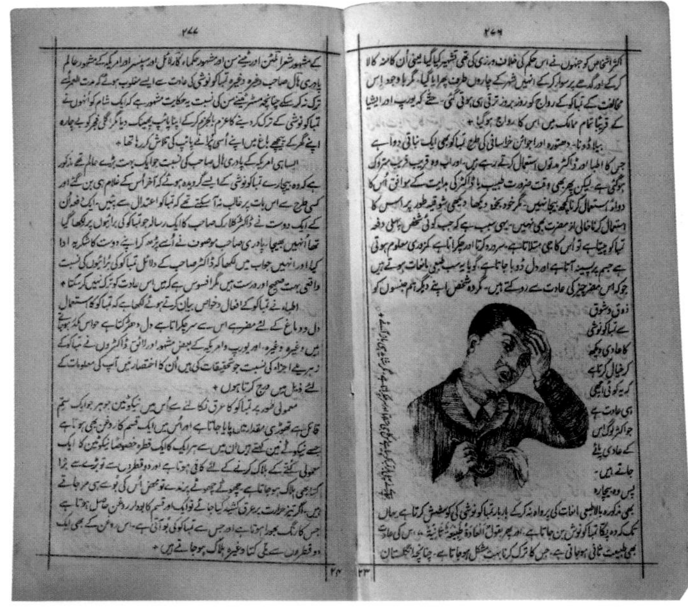

A copy ofthe *Makhzan-i-Hikmat* or *The Family Doctor and Hakeem: An Encyclopaedia of Domestic Medicine and Surgery* by Dr H Ghulam Jilani in Urdu. It is open on a page that deals with medication for migraine.

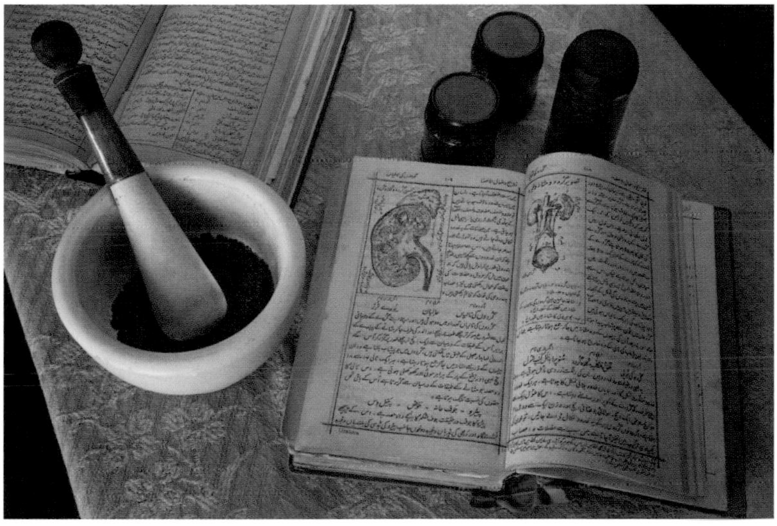

Above All Unani medicines are made from 100 percent natural ingredients including plants, herbs and minerals. This *mufaras* or medicine made by Hakim Sayed Riazuddin in Mysore contains musk, amber, silver, gold and *zafaran* leaf. It is reputed to be helpful for excessive palpitation of the heart.

Right A Unani application used on the skin to help with white pigmentation marks. Made at Soukya mainly from *bakuchi* or *Psoralea corylifolia* seeds, it is anti-fungal and anti-protozoal. Repeated applications over a period of time result in a gradual fading of the discoloration.

a balanced diet, exercise and rest, psychic movement and rest, sleep and wakefulness, and evacuation and retention. Remedies are usually herbal, although ingredients of animal, marine and mineral origin are used. Humoral theory (the presence and balance of blood, phlegm, yellow bile and black bile) is at its heart, and the temperament of a person is accordingly expressed by Sanguine, Phlegmatic, Choleric and Melancholic. According to Unani theories, any change in these humors brings about changes in the status of health of a human body."

Many herbal preparations in India are as likely to be Unani in origin as they are Ayurvedic, as historically the two overlap significantly. Unani herbology is well documented and spa treatments such as body polishes and wraps often use ingredients from the Unani pharmacopoeia. There are a number of pastes, formulated from fresh herbs, seeds and roots, suitable for ailments such as vitiligo, eczema, psoriasis, bronchial asthma and arthritis. This is good news for sufferers, as many such ailments do not have a cure in Western medicine.

A case in point is a thick herbal paste used at Soukya to reduce skin pigmentation or leucoderma. *Psoralea corylifolia* seeds are boiled in milk, then dried (not in direct sunlight), with the process being repeated seven times in total. Afterwards, the mix is ground into a powder, some other ingredients are added and a little bit of water makes it into a paste. Over a period of a month, the paste is applied on to the specific areas of the skin daily for 20 to 45 minutes and the area held in direct sunlight. Afterwards, it is washed off. Patients report a diminishing of the bright white spots with time. However, as with Ayurvedic remedies, there is no quick fix!

siddha Tamil Herbal Healing

Perhaps not so well known outside India as Ayurveda, Siddha is an ancient form of natural medicine that has been practiced in Tamil Nadu for centuries. Taking its name from 18 Tamil *siddhars* (devotees of Shiva who attained *siddhi* or perfection), it shares with Ayurveda the theory of five elements and three *doshas*, which are referred to as *muppini* in Tamil. However, unlike Ayurveda, Siddha divides the body according to the five elements. So, earth corresponds to the legs, water to the abdomen, fire to the chest, air to the neck and space to the head. It also relates the five elements to bodily fluids.

The fundamental principles of Siddha medicine are encapsulated in several Tamil texts. Like all Hindu philosophers, the *siddhars* believed, that all life should seek oneness with God, so a productive long life was to be encouraged. Their basic premise was that the universe consists of two essential entities — matter and energy — that are found in five primordial elements: *munn* (solids), *neer* (fluids), *thee* (radiance), *vayu* (gas) and *aakasam* (ether). If these elements are maintained in equilibrium, the result is health; if there is disruption, the result is disease.

Alchemical ideas dominate Siddha medicine, with its *materia medica* consisting of herbs, roots, salts, metals and mineral compounds. The 18 *siddhars* classified 4,448 diseases and prescribed medicines accordingly. Nevertheless, *bhasmas* (fine powders made from incinerated and purified metals and minerals) are at the forefront of their prescriptions. However, as with Ayurveda, other common preparations include *choornam* (powders), *kashayam* (decoctions), *lehyam* (confections), *gritham* (ghee preparations) and *tailam* (oils). Siddha specialities are *chunna* (metallic preparations that become alkaline after purification), *mezhugu* (waxy preparations) and *kattu* (preparations that are impervious to water and fire). The medicines are generally taken internally, although there are some external applications also.

The Siddha system includes not only medicine and alchemy but also yoga and philosophy. Diet is an important part of Siddha, as doctors identify and associate different food types with different *doshas*, and the pursuit of longevity without illness and a useful, spiritual life is its ultimate aim. The spiritual aspect of healing, wellness and being at one with the Divine cannot be under-emphasized: it lies at the heart of all Siddha discipline.

It is not often that visitors to India come across Siddha practices outside Tamil Nadu, but sometimes you will be lucky. Aura spas at the forward-looking Park Hotels offer a type of *marma* massage prescribed mainly for rheumatics that dates from pre-Vedic times in Siddha culture. Using medicated herbal oils it targets the *marma* points to release stored emotions in order to restore mental, emotional and spiritual equilibrium. Each point is related to a particular concept: for example, shoulder points store emotions of responsibility and sternum points relate to the heart, so the masseur concentrates on different areas for different effects. It is an extremely powerful treatment that sometimes results in intense emotional outpouring and tension release.

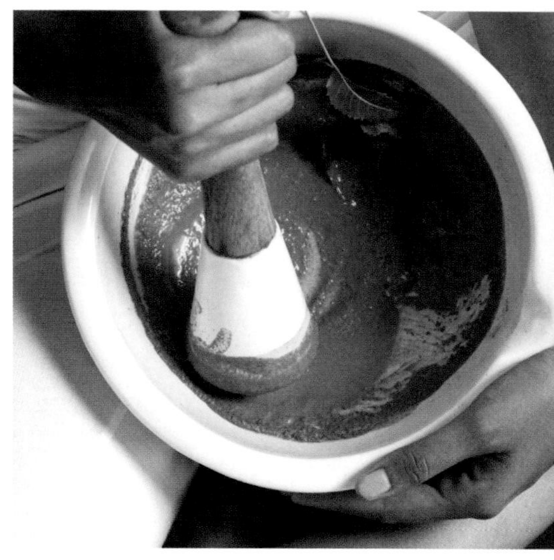

Above A Siddha preparation made at Soukya from neem leaves and turmeric used as an external paste in the treatment of psoriasis. **Right** A selection of minerals in raw, incinerated, semi-cooked and purified form, all used in Siddha formulations. They include iron, mercury, arsenic and sulphur.

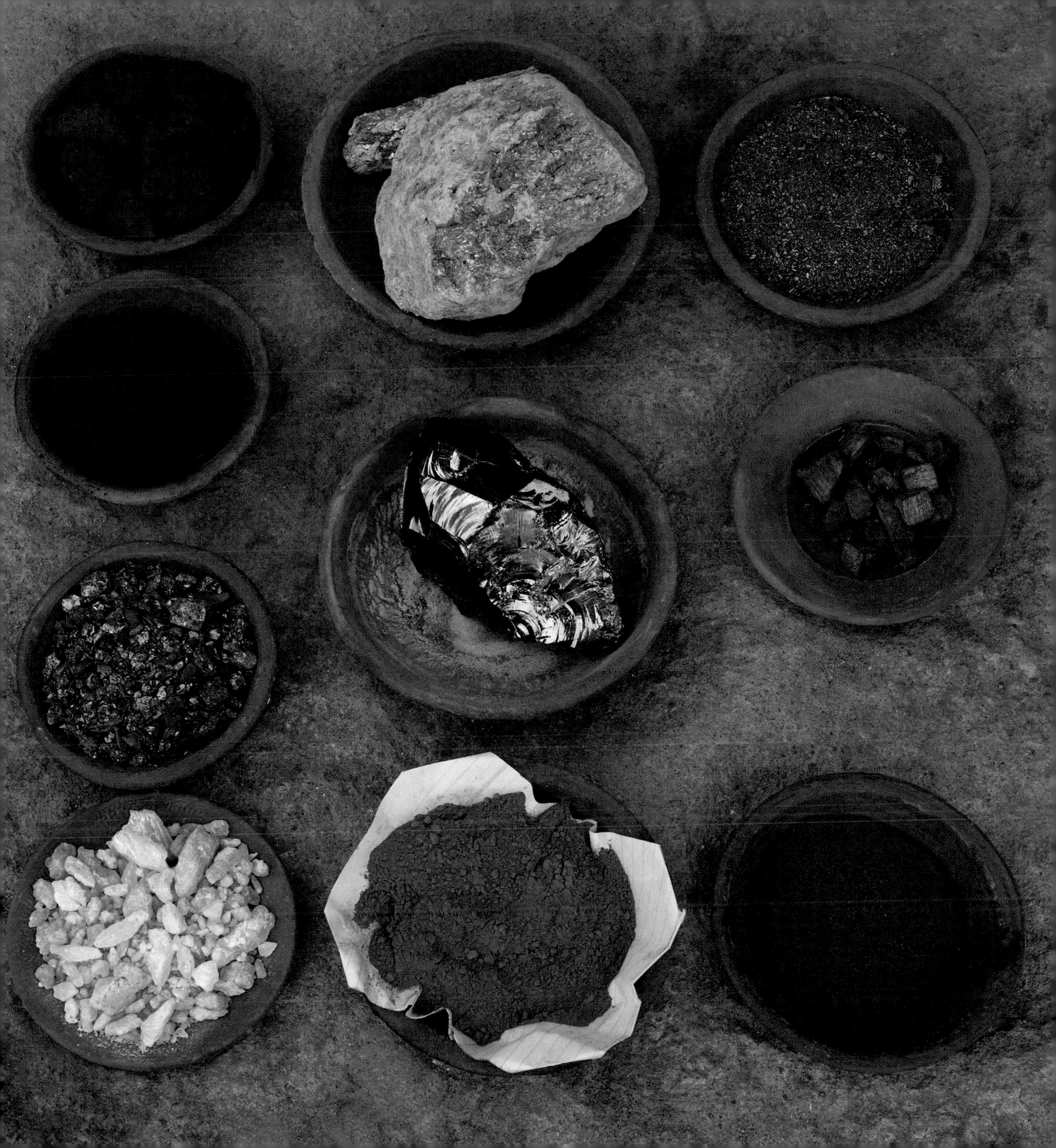

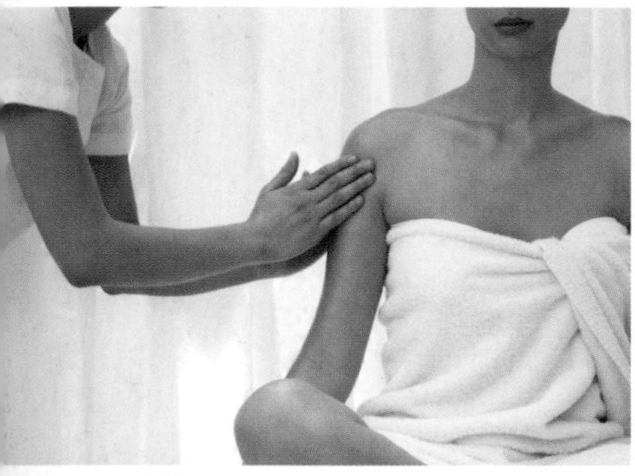

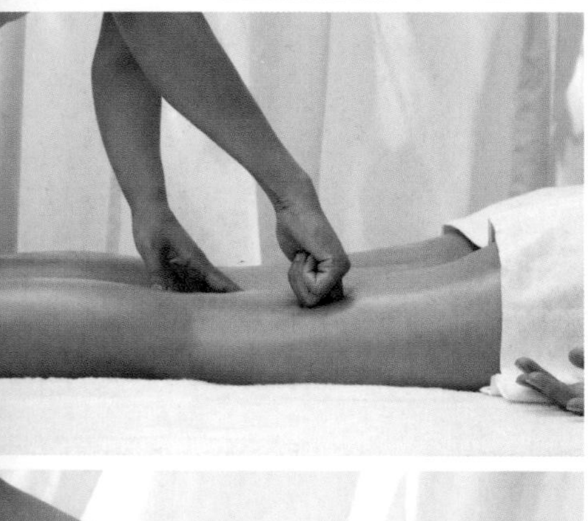

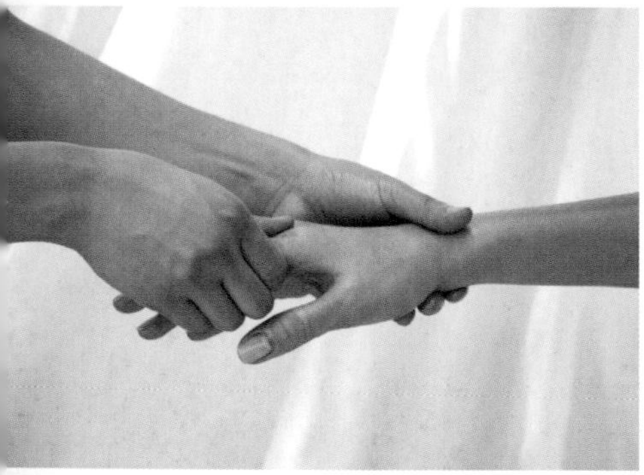

The photos on these two pages show various pressure positions given in a type of *marma* massage that dates back to pre-Vedic times in Siddha culture. Using medicated herbal oils, it was prescribed mainly for rheumatics. Here, it has been resurrected at Aura spas in the forward-thinking Park Hotels. "The 107 *marma* points are targeted to release stored emotions in order to restore mental, emotional and spiritual equilibrium," explains spa director Megha Dinesh. "Each point is related to a particular concept: ie the knee is related to death, that's why so many older people get arthritis in the knee. Shoulder points store the emotions of responsibility and the sternum points are related to the heart, so people with hunched shoulders may be loveless." She goes on to add that the treatment is very powerful and can have long-lasting effects especially if particular areas are targeted for very specific results.

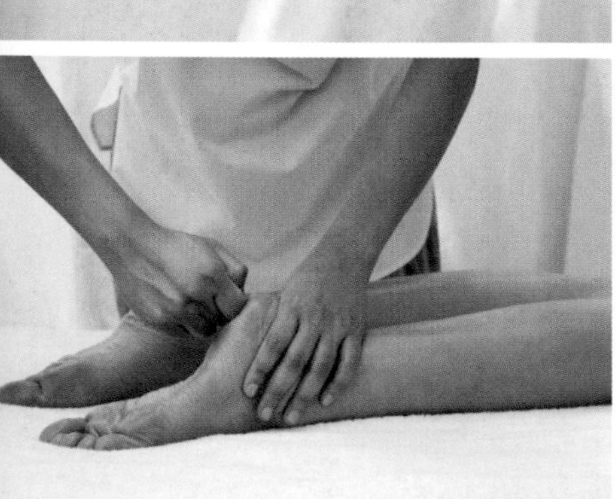

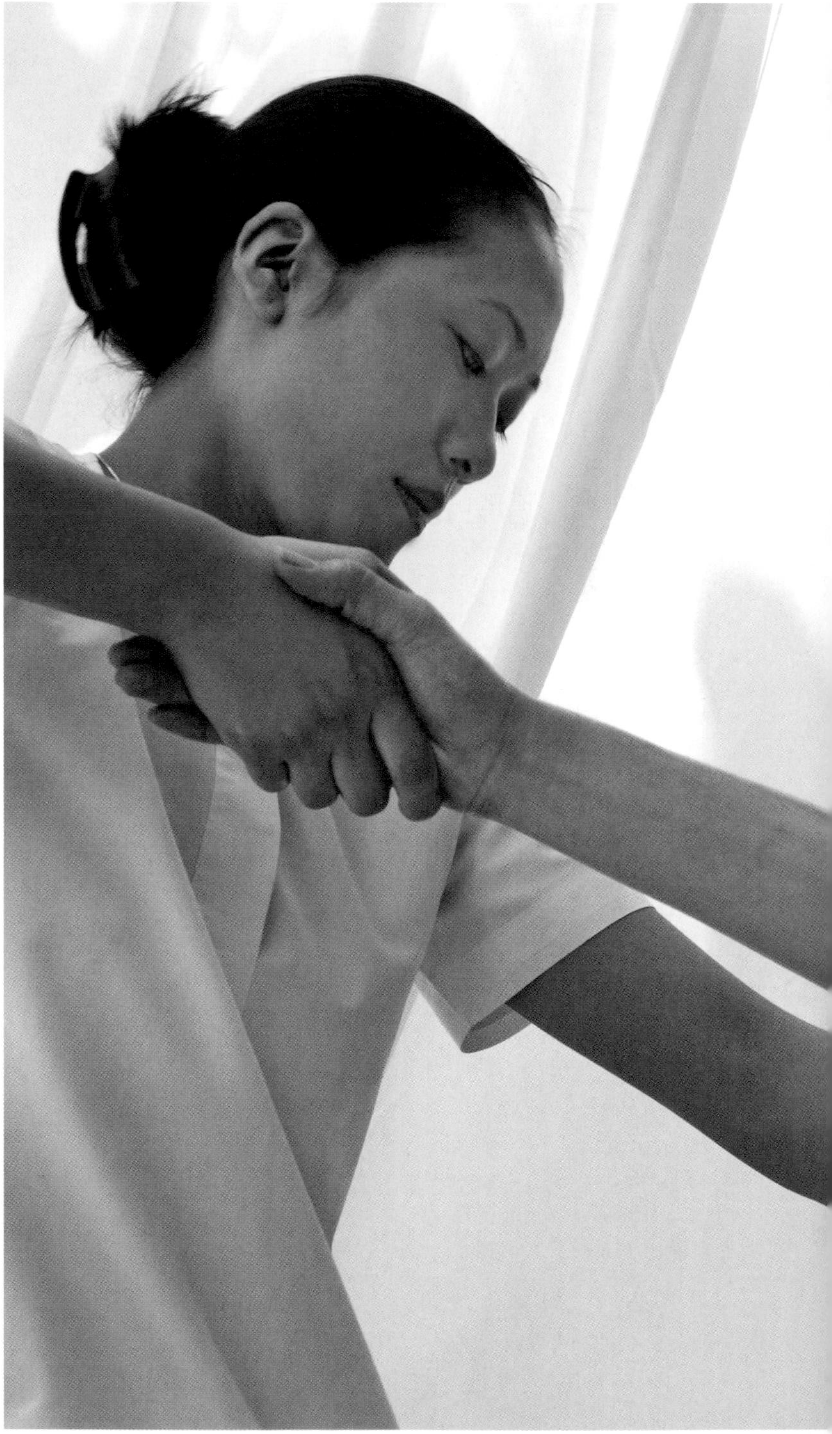

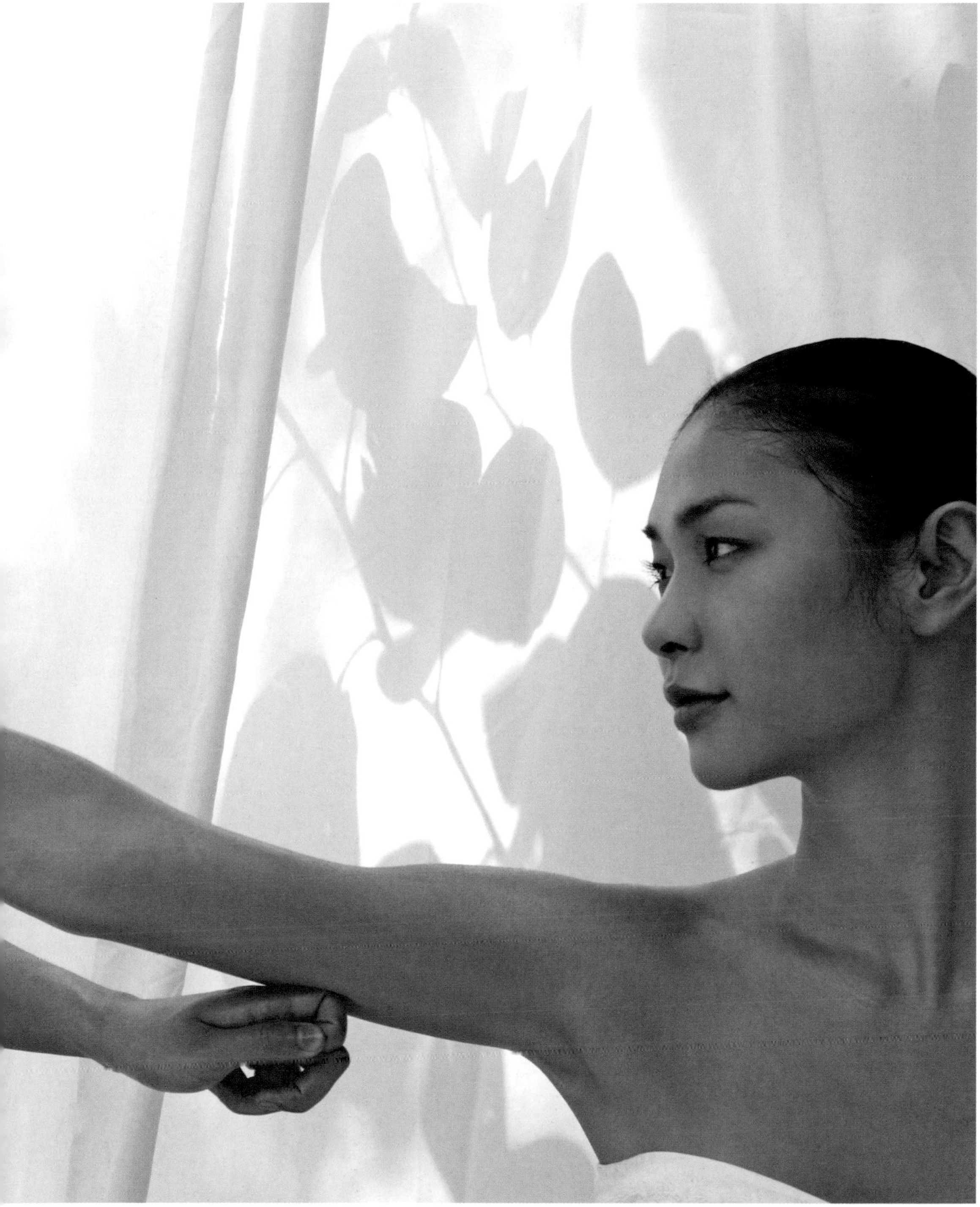

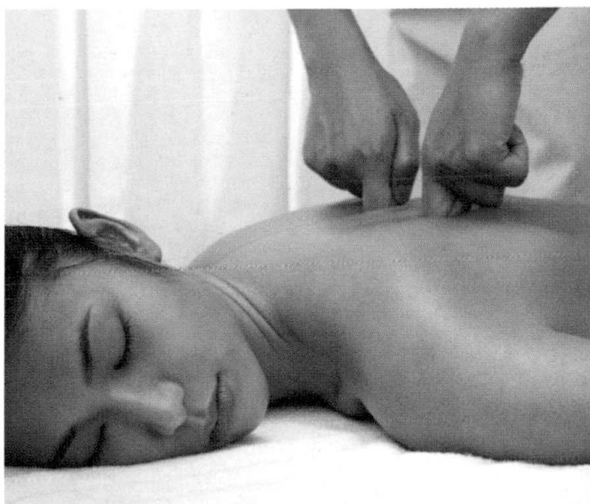

Therapists tend to use elbows and knuckles as well as the palm of the hand when targeting particular *marma* points. It's believed that pranic flow can become blocked, so pressure at such points helps release the vital force; at the same time pent-up emotions may be subconsciously released too. It's reported that clients often have intense reactions to this treatment, so it should not be undertaken lightly.

soba rig-pa

Traditional Tibetan Medicine

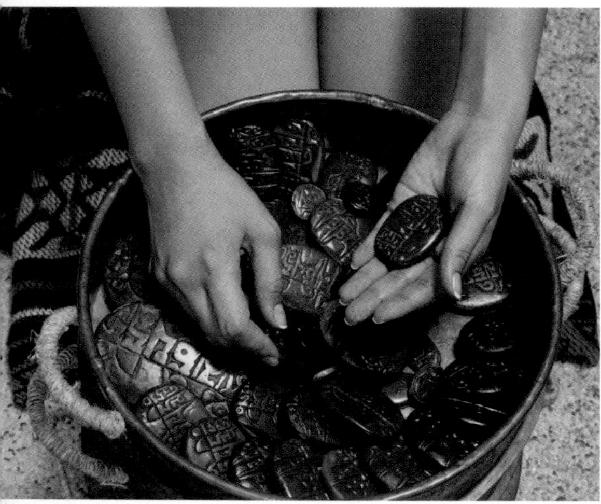

Tibetan medicine is a traditional system of medicine that has been practiced for over 2,500 years and is still practiced today both within Tibet and by Tibetans in exile. Called *Soba Rig-pa* or the "Science of Healing", it uses many natural ingredients including herbs, trees, rocks, resins, soils, precious metals and more. However, 95 percent of Tibetan medicine is based on herbs, and precious metals are used for the seven kinds of precious pill known as *rinchen rilpo*.

Soba Rig-pa's basic premise is that the body needs to be balanced to be well. When imbalances in what are called the three humors or *nyipa sum (rLung, mKhris-pa* and *Bad-kan)* occur, a person falls ill; symptoms may be physical, mental, spiritual or a combination of all three. In brief, *rLung* is the subtle flow of energy in the body; *mKhris-pa* is the hot nature or bile within the body; and *Bad-kan* is concerned with the body's cold nature signified by phlegm. Attachment, Aversion and Delusion are considered long-term causes of balance, whereas in the short-term, imbalances may be caused by time, temperature and season, the influence of spirits, improper diet and improper behavior.

After diagnosis, Tibetan doctors offer four types of prescription: behavioral suggestions, a medical prescription, diet advice, or surgery. As with other holistic systems of medicine, physical therapies are only part of a doctor's prescription. Based on the centuries-old Buddhist study of the mind, Tibetan medicine gives priority to factors of psychological and spiritual development as well.

Today, a limited number of spas offer a few Tibetan physical therapies that have been formulated over the centuries. A case in point is CHI spas at Shangri-La hotels found all over Asia: There, spa personnel have formulated some Himalayan therapies that are probably the closest you will get to an authentic Tibetan treatment outside a Tibetan clinic.

Healing Stone Massage

Described in Tibet's medical bible, the *Gui Shi*, massage with stones has all but died out in Tibet, only being practiced in the most remote and wild borderlands of the Tibetan plateau. As Tibetans are traditionally nomads, their therapies contain influences from many different sources, this profound practice being no exception. It was probably introduced to Tibet from Mongols that settled in the Hor region around Lake Kokonor; in its pure form, it uses heated stones that have been "cooked" in the bellies of sheep.

In the spa, the therapy combines the Mongolian concept of healing through stones; principles and techniques of Ayurveda that traveled up the Indian trade routes over Himalayan passes; pressure point techniques from Traditional Chinese Medicine; and Tibetan healing intent (imbuing the stones with awareness through visualization). The application of water-heated Himalayan river stones to key points on the body relaxes muscles, allowing manipulation of a greater intensity than

Left and right In Mongolia, stones and minerals are commonly used both internally and externally for various ailments. It is believed that when hot stones are applied to specific points on the body they help dispel blockages, enabling the smooth flow of *chi* or life force energy through the body. These stones have been carved with Sanskrit symbols by Buddhist monks and are used in the CHI spa hot stone massage at Shangri-La hotels.

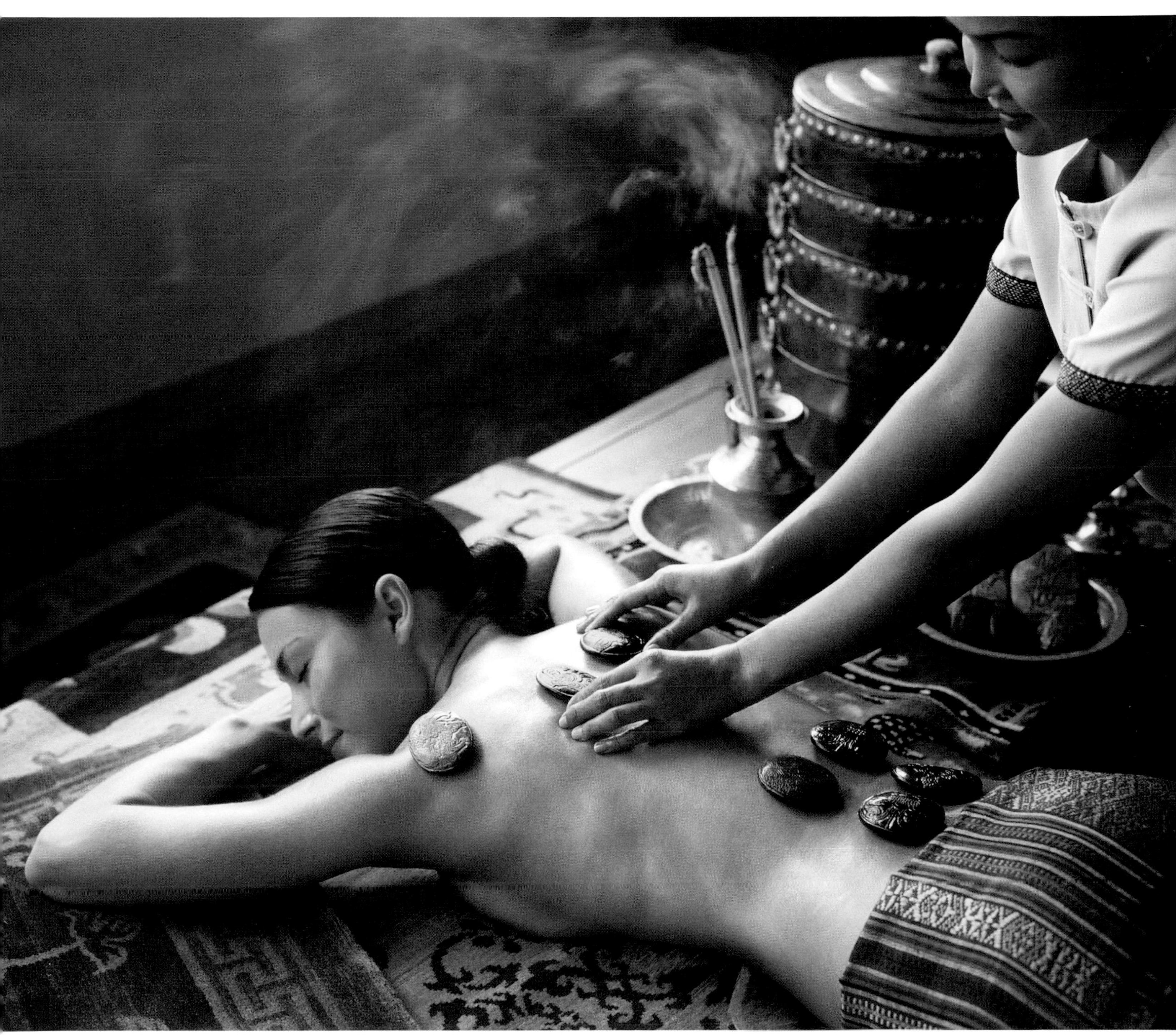

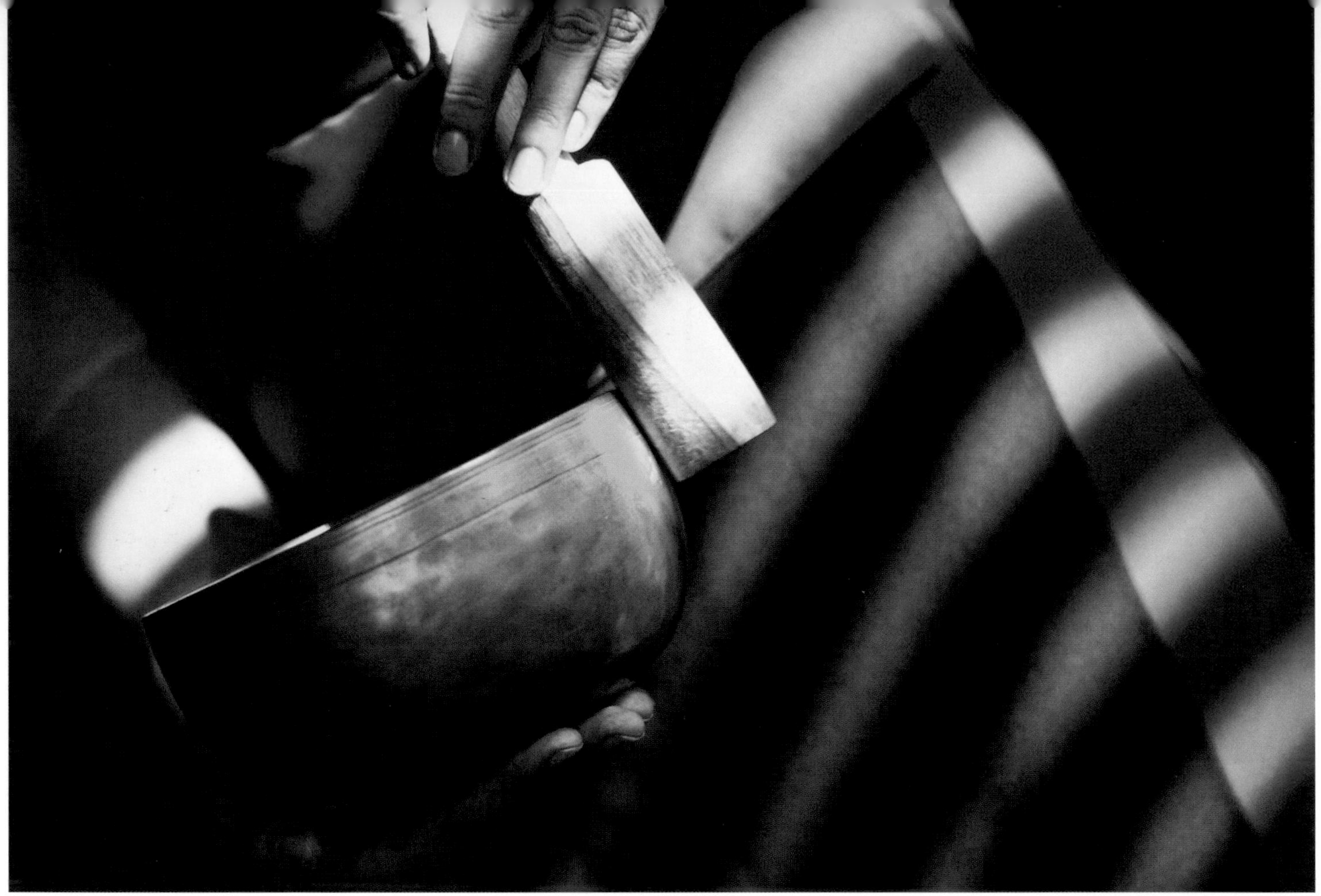

regular massage. Blood vessels expand, pushing blood and waste materials through the body. This has a strengthening and sedative effect on the nervous system, and relieves anxiety and stress. On a physical level, it provides relief to sore muscles and fosters deep muscle manipulation, all the time improving circulation and removing toxins from the body. On a mental level, it is nurturing and comforting.

Mountain Tsampa Rub

The second CHI treatment we focus on combines *tsampa* with ancient Tibetan massage techniques and transforms them into a powerful detoxifying and cleansing treatment. *Tsampa* is roast flour, most commonly of barley, and is the staple

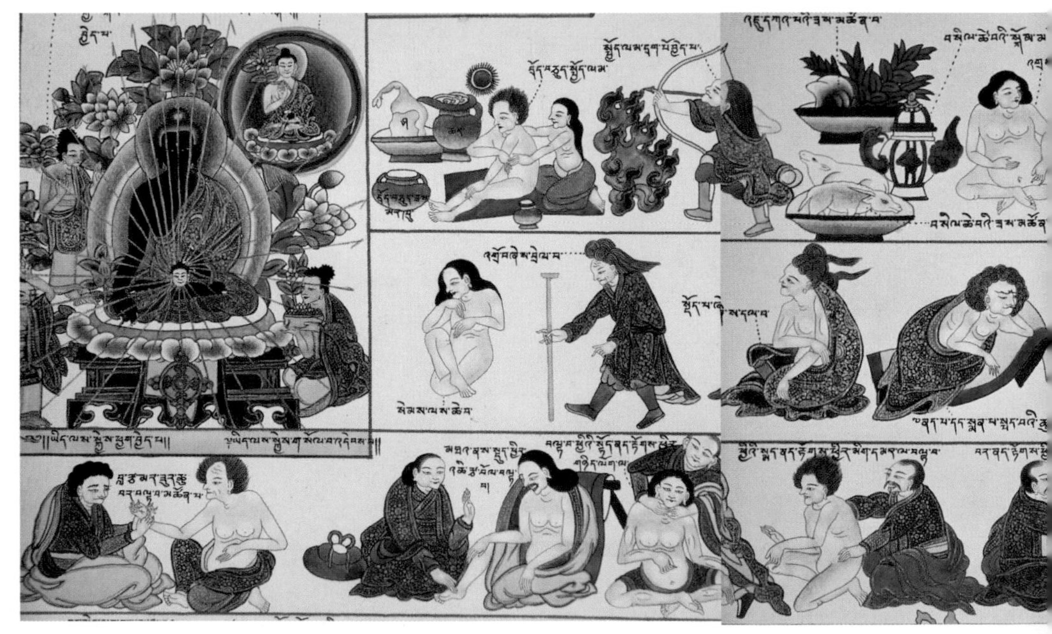

Left Tibetan singing bowls, often used in monasteries as aids for meditation, are rung before a treatment at CHI spas.
Below A *thangka* painting, one of a set of 79 illustrations of the Tibetan medical system, demonstrating diagnosis, treatments and cures.
Right Unlike Indian texts, this old Tibetan medical text has colorful illustrations depicting both healing and illness.
Below right A *tsampa* mix applied to the back is massaged in to drain toxins out from the lymphatic system.

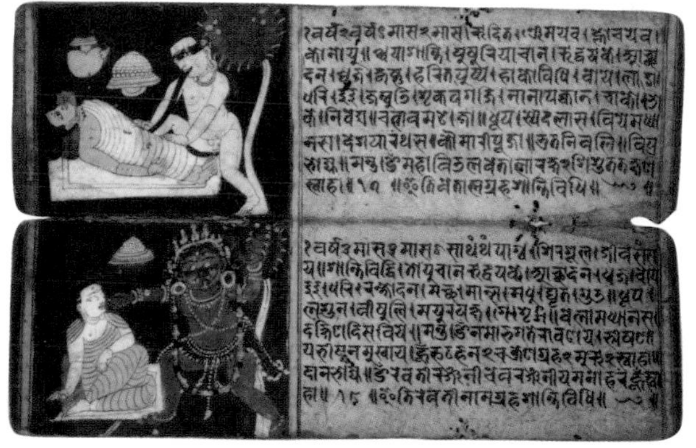

foodstuff of Tibetans. Most Tibetans used to live (and many still do) on the high Tibetan plateau, where harsh conditions, thin air and a definite lack of resources result in a scarcity of food. *Tsampa* mixed with butter tea (tea flavored with salty yak butter) has historically been a life saver, giving energy and sustenance year round. Here, the flour is used as the postscript to the treatment.

Unlike acupressure or the Chinese style of massage, Tibetan massage works on the "wind" channels of the body — those that deal with the circulation of energy, blood and lymph. Generally, massage techniques include stroking (long, longitudinal strokes or *effleurage)*, rubbing with vigorous circular motions to create friction, and kneading. The aim is to increase lymphatic drainage and blood circulation in order to aid muscle nutrition, reduce stiffness in joints, improve flexibility and heighten body awareness.

The initial part of this treatment comprises an invigorating massage combined with powerful lymph draining herbal oils to drain the lymph system; this helps to refresh and uplift the client, restoring energy and *chi*. As in Ayurveda, the herbs infused into the oils are just as important as the techniques used in application. Particular focus is given to specific energy points on the body to help the oils penetrate into the skin and awaken *chi*.

The second part of the treatment is considerably gentler and more relaxing. A blend of *tsampa* flour and powerful lymph draining herbs is applied all over the body to absorb excess oil and toxins that have come up to the surface of the skin. Rubbing the *tsampa* herb blend into the skin leaves the skin soft, gently exfoliated and free of inner toxins.

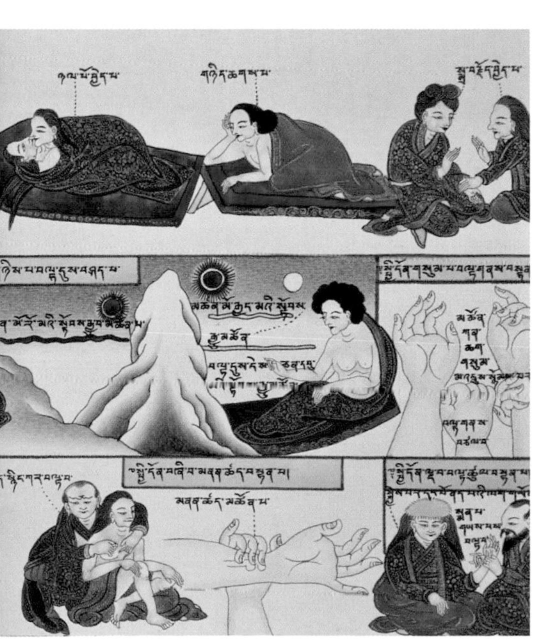

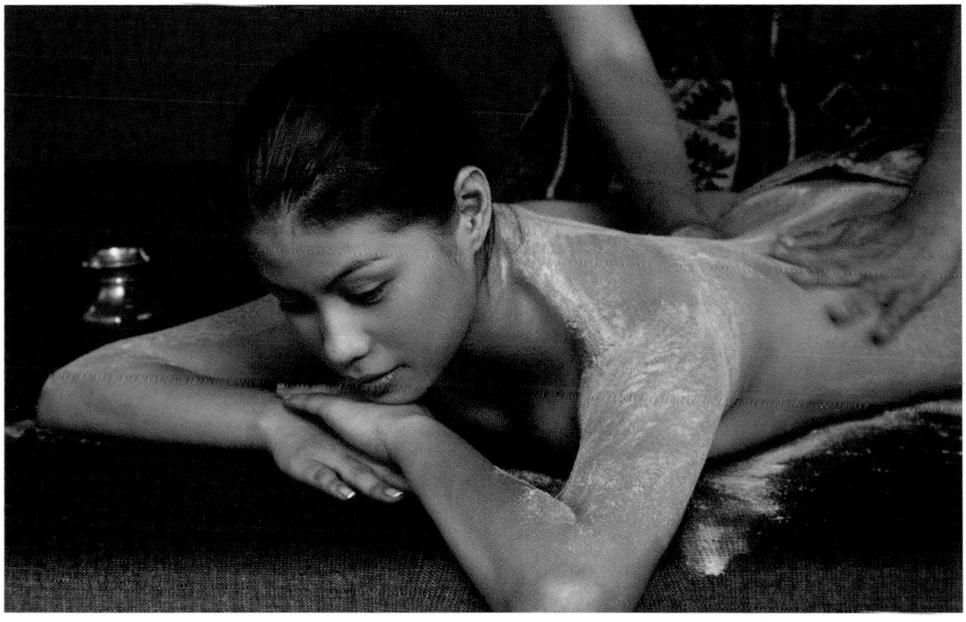

panchakarma

Ayurvedic Revitalization

Traditionally undertaken during the monsoon season when herbs have been newly harvested and skin is most receptive to oil, the purging *panchakarma* treatment is an annual event in many Indians' lives. According to the *Ashtanga Hridaya*, it "leads to clarity of intellect, power to the organs, elemental stability and glow to digestive fire" and it delays aging if it is properly carried out.

Offered at many Ayurvedic hospitals, homestays and retreats as a stand-alone rejuvenation and detoxification treatment, *panchakarma* is really one part of a group of therapies belonging to a class of cleansing procedures called *shodhana*. Clients are given an individual program of medication, diet and treatments after an intensive consultation with a physician, and are monitored throughout the two to six week program. However, regardless of the *panchakarma* prescription, there are always three basic procedures: *Purvakarma* or preparation, *pradhanakarma* or treatments and *paschatkarma*, post-treatment care.

At Kalari Kovilakom, an Ayurvedic retreat situated in a palace estate in the Annamalai foothills in Kerala, the preparatory procedures take from three days to a week: They are designed to help the body discard toxins present in the stomach and tissues and help facilitate their movement to the alimentary canal. "This stage often includes special internal medicines and *snehanan* or oleation therapy and *swedanam* or sweat therapy," explains Dr Jayan. "The latter may take the form of the application of warm oil over the body and the application of heated pouches of herbs on the body, but each patient is different, with different *dosha* imbalances, so the treatments always vary."

When the body and mind are deemed ready, *pradhanakarma* or the main treatment designed to each individual's needs, begins. As its name suggests (*panch* means "five" and *karma* means "action"), the process comprises five cleansing procedures, each designed to correct doshic imbalances. They are *vamanam* or induced vomiting, allegedly a painless, drug-induced emetic process; *virechanam* or induced purgation, whereby drugs that stimulate bowel movements are taken internally; *vasthi*, the use of medicated enemas (see pages 32–35); *nasyam* or nasal cleansing through the application of medical oils or powders (see right); and *rakthamoksham* or detoxification of the blood.

Clearly, this therapy is not for the faint-hearted, and the patient/doctor level of trust needs to be very high. This is why Kalari Kovilakom insists on a minimum stay of 14 days, so that doctors can truly assess and monitor a patient's needs.

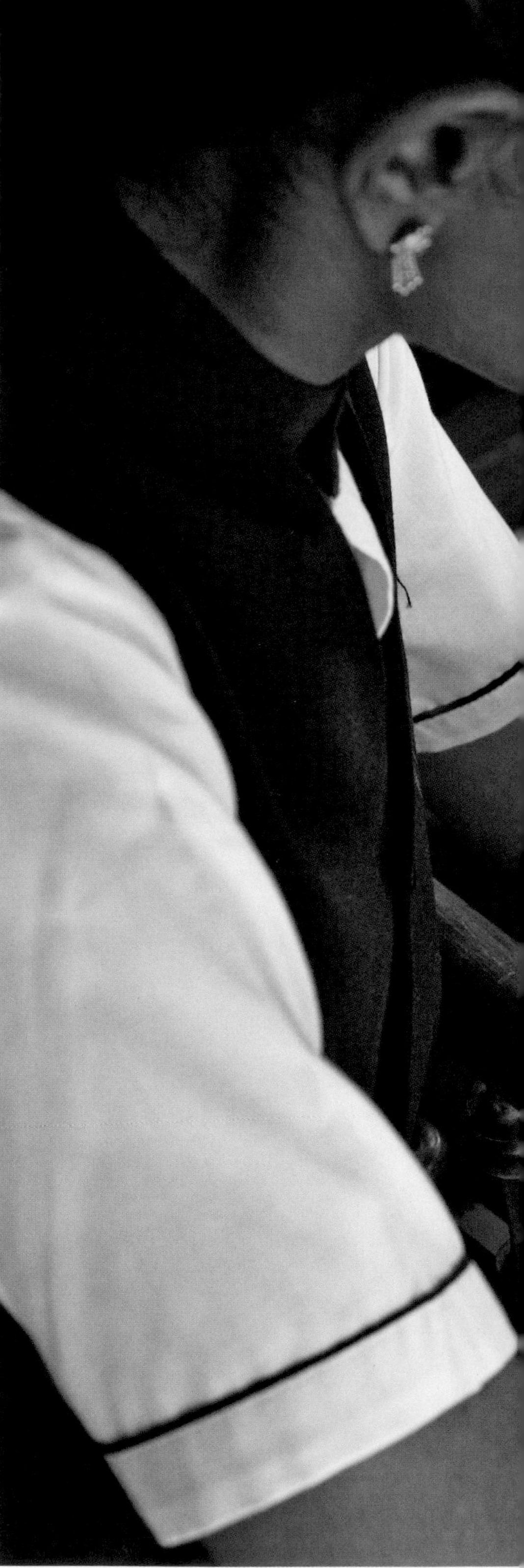

A *nasyam* session at Ayurmana illustrates how a therapist pours medication into the nostrils. Ghee, *choornam* or powders, or medicated oils are used.

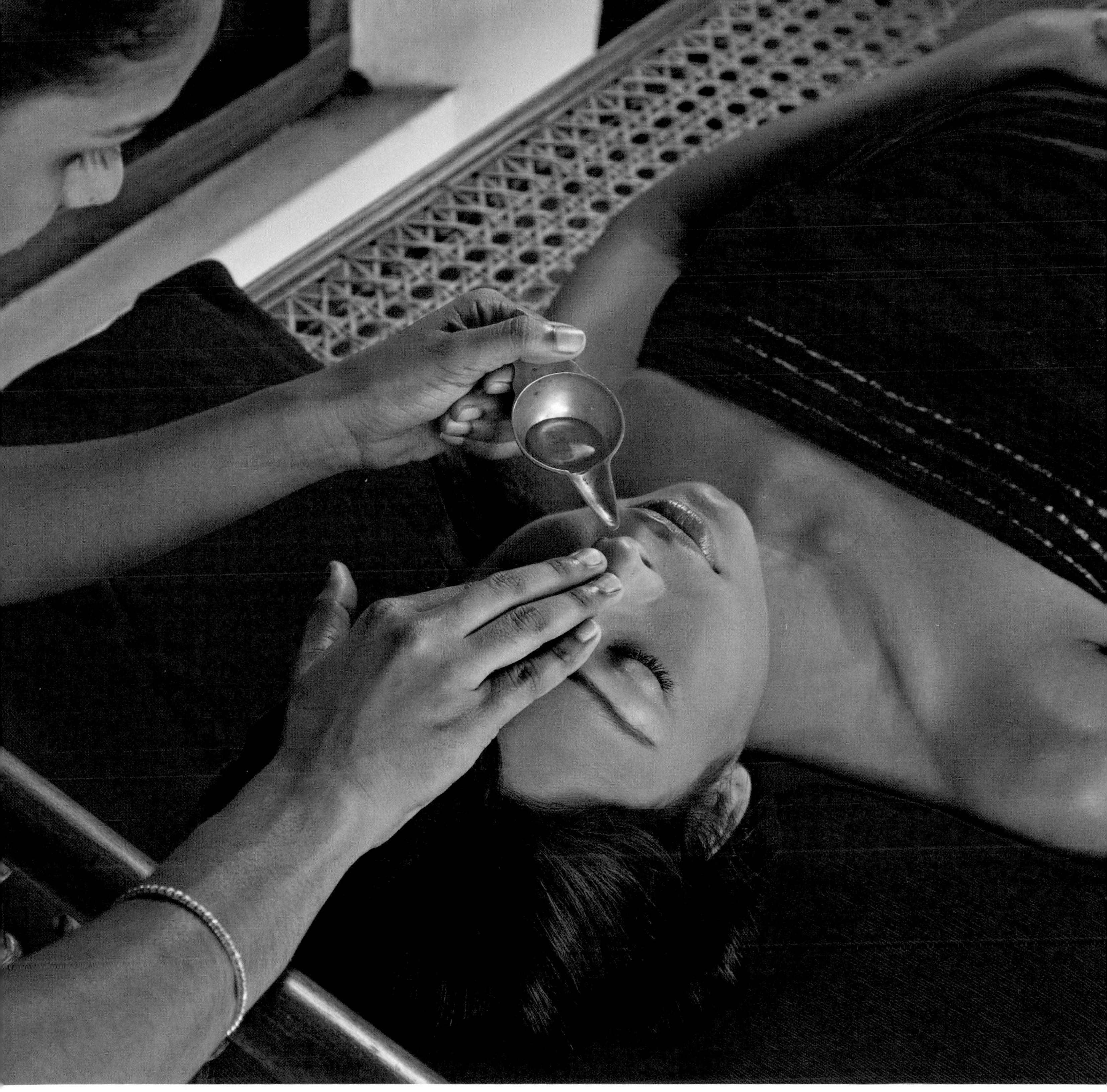

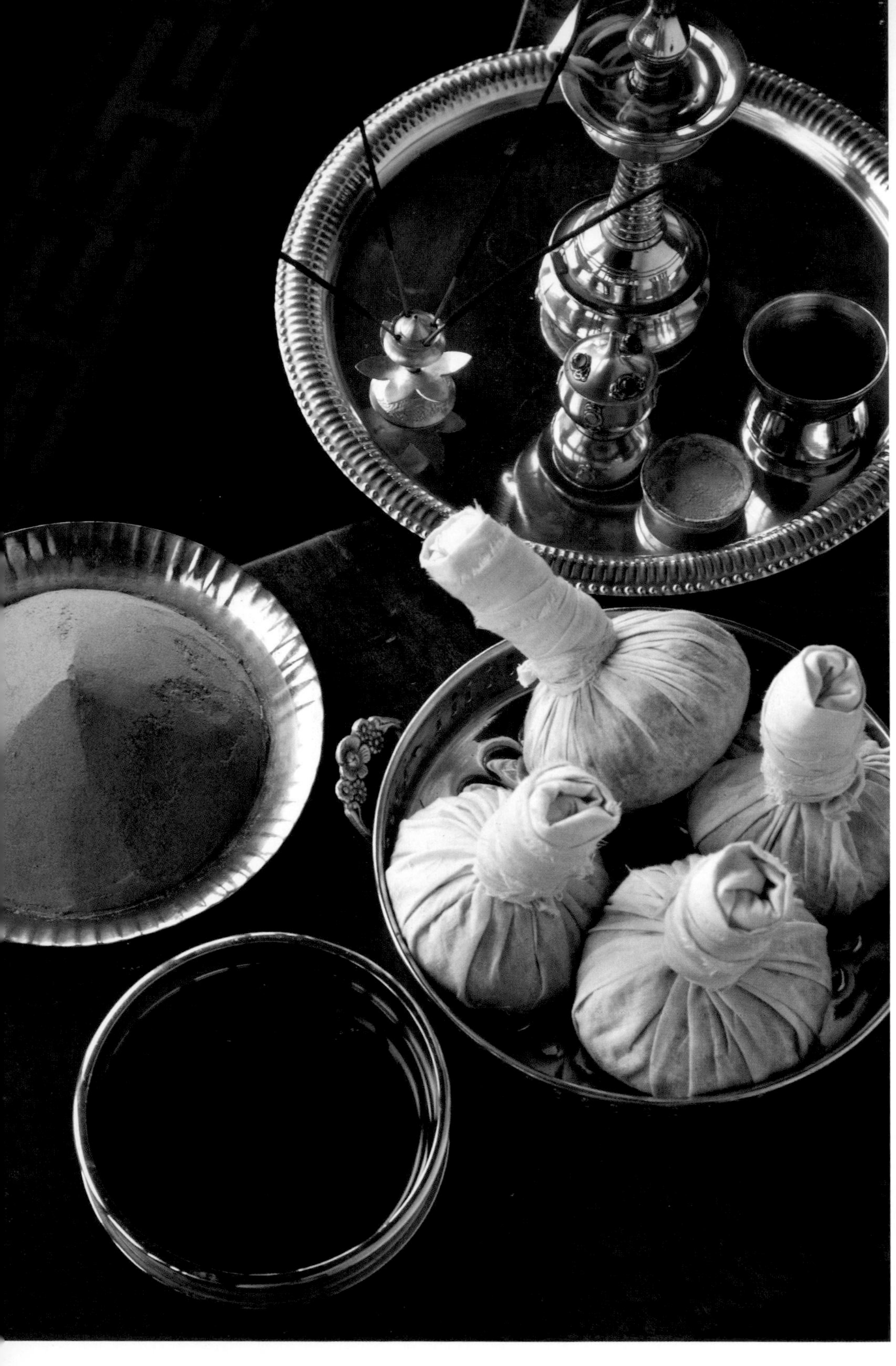

Dr Jayan explains that rarely are all five therapies prescribed. "For *pitta* imbalances, we prescribe purgation with oils or powders, *vata* imbalances go the herbal and oil enema route, and *kapha* imbalances are always prescribed *vamanam*. Here patients drink two liters of milk or sugar cane juice mixed with special herbal medicines to induce vomiting after 45 minutes." He goes on to say that *nasyam* is included if there are nasal, throat or brain problems and bloodletting is useful for skin problems. Hence, a patient may be prescribed only one of the five processes; sometimes two or three, and in rare cases, five.

Naturally, the strict routine and caring staff at Kalari Kovilakom go a long way to supporting guests on this somewhat gruesome journey; nevertheless, many first-timers to the process describe both physical symptoms of discomfort and mental anguish. It is believed, however, that a special diet and medication, sessions of meditation and yoga and an unchanging routine provide the support network needed. Similarly, post-treatment after the guest leaves the premises in the form of medication, contact with doctors, rest and diet is highly recommended.

Ayurveda, from time immemorial, has focused on anti-aging and rejuvenation programs to prevent disease and to maintain an optimum healthy state. In today's world, curative therapies are increasingly replacing preventative ones — and *panchakarma* (both curative and preventative) is one of the more extreme examples on the Ayurvedic menu. Nevertheless, devotees with the stamina and the will swear by it, and if the venue is carefully chosen, it may turn out to be a life-changing experience.

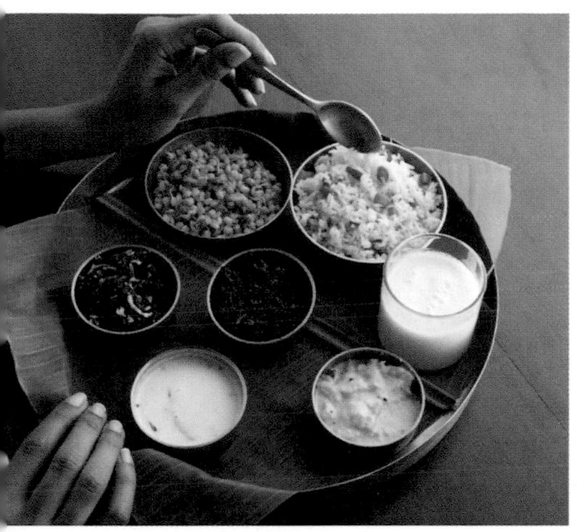

Left, right and below Proper diet is considered an important part of the healing process in *panchakarma*. At Kalari Kovilakom all food is prepared according to Ayurvedic principles with only copper, bell metal, earthenware, stone or brass vessels used in preparation, cooking and serving. Every patient has a special drink on hand 24 hours a day and meals are served in gleaming brass *katories* (cups) on a banana leaf covered *thali* tray.

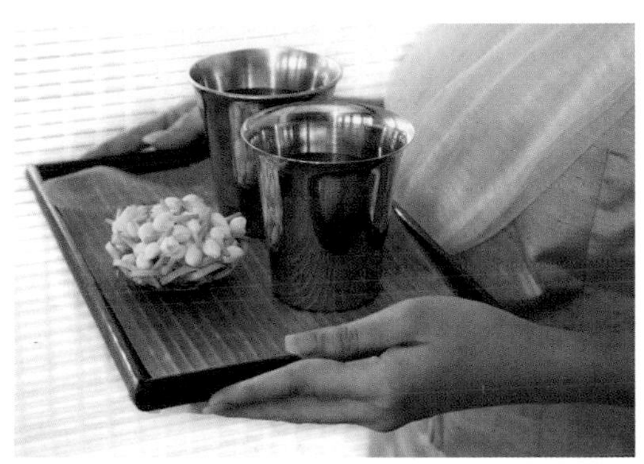

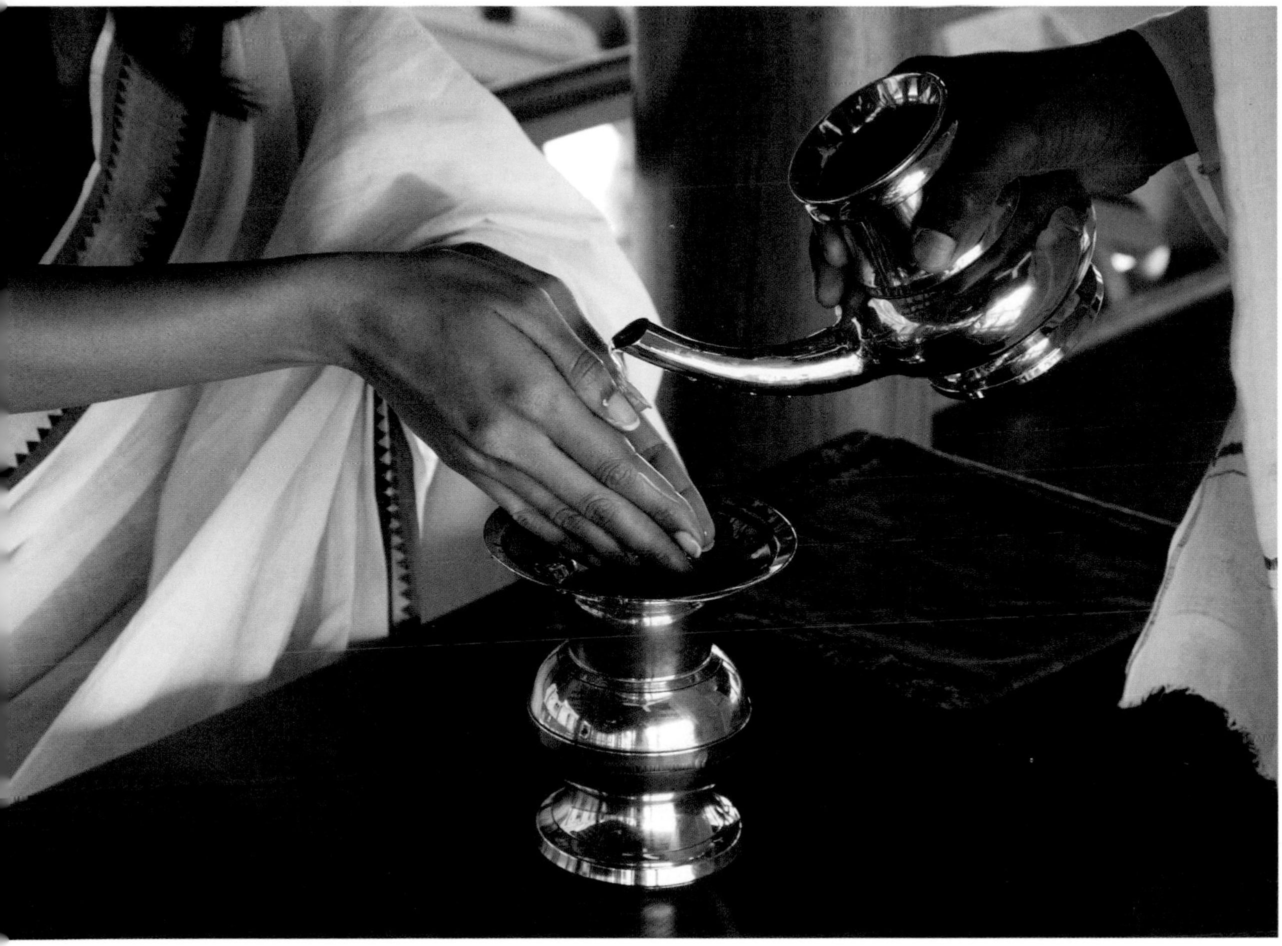

Opposite Ayurvedic powders and oils used in the *panchakarma* treatment at Kalari Kovilakom, a retreat in Kerala. The *kizhi* pouches are for the preparation stage, while the tray with the oil lamp is used to bless the patient before any therapy commences.

mud therapy

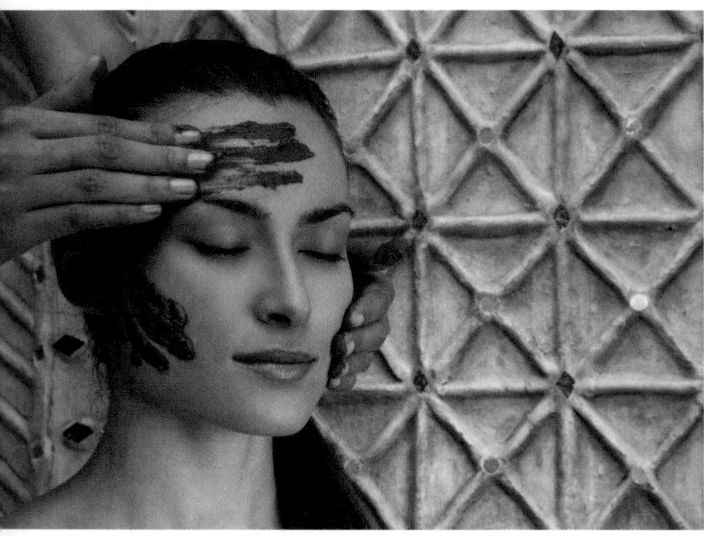

In India, mud therapy falls under the Naturopathy umbrella, as it employs one of the Five Great Elements or *Panchmahabhutas (panch* is "five", *maha* is "great", *bhuta* is "element"). Comprising Earth, Water, Fire, Air and Ether, mud therapy unsurprisingly utilizes Earth as its main healing ingredient. Mud absorbs, dissolves and eliminates toxins from beneath the skin's surface, opens the pores and improves peripheral blood circulation. As such, it is rejuvenating for the body and soothing for the skin.

Mud therapy is employed in the treatment of a variety of ailments such as digestive disorders, skin diseases and more. The world-famous *Multani mitti or* "mud from Multan", an area now in Pakistan, was one of the earliest substances to be used as a beauty mask. This lime-rich clay was mixed with rice bran and milk or curd and used as a face pack to draw out toxins and polluting free radicals. Indeed, it is still used as such today. Because of its high mineral content and moisturizing effect, it is a great nourisher and often acts as a conduit for healing ingredients to be absorbed into the system. Ayurvedic texts record that mud draws out heat and excess *pitta* through the skin; it also says that *Multani mitti* can be used by all three *doshas*.

At Soukya, the integrated wellness center near Bangalore where Naturopathy is combined with other modalities to create individual therapeutic programs, mud is used in three ways: as a localized application, as a pack and as a full mud bath. Mud is harvested from the many ant hills found on site; as the ants have taken the mud from deep down, it's incredibly pure without any surface pollutants. Therapists further prepare it by sieving it, washing it properly, and sterilizing it by drying it in sunlight. It is then stored carefully in airtight containers.

"Mud is healing in itself," explains the resident naturopath Dr Usha Devi. "It has the property of retaining temperature for a long time, so depending on the ailment, can be applied either hot or cold." Hot mud is used for joint conditions such as arthritis and to reduce oedema or water retention in localized areas of the body, and cold mud helps in the treatment of skin diseases, such as psoriasis for example.

Sometimes, herbs may be added such as disinfecting neem and turmeric if there is a possibility of infection and castor oil may be added to an abdominal pack in liver conditions. It helps stimulate the circulation of blood towards the liver, thereby aiding in the detoxification process.

Whichever mud therapy is assigned, the feeling is nurturing and strengthening. The tightening experienced when the mud dries on the skin is pleasant — be it hot or cold — and as it is straight from nature, you can be sure it is doing good work. The full mud bath is particularly invigorating: being slathered in soft, creamy mud, then having it washed off afterwards is a self-indulgent treat. The skin feels soft, smooth, tight and tingly afterwards — and there is no need for extra moisturizing.

Left Used on the face, mud draws out toxins very quickly, so it makes for an effective face mask. It may also be used on the eyes (but only in a pack) to strengthen the optic nerve and muscles, relax the eyes, and impart a cooling and de-stressing effect on the entire eye area.
Right Application of mud from top to toe may sound a bit messy (gross even), but it is an invigorating experience especially if the body is wrapped in a blanket after application. Micro elements from the mud are absorbed into the body and toxins expelled leaving skin and internal organs refreshed.

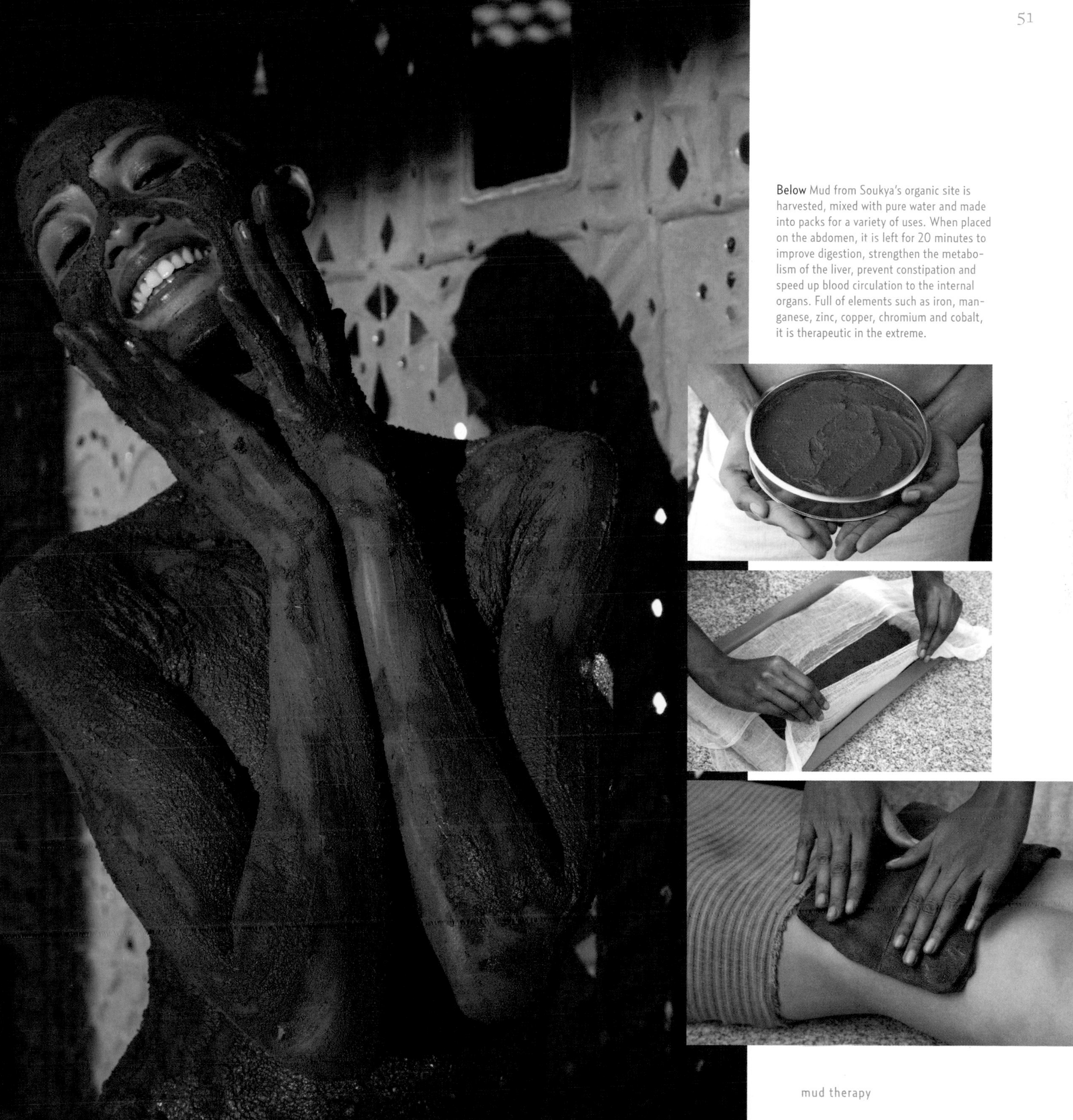

Below Mud from Soukya's organic site is harvested, mixed with pure water and made into packs for a variety of uses. When placed on the abdomen, it is left for 20 minutes to improve digestion, strengthen the metabolism of the liver, prevent constipation and speed up blood circulation to the internal organs. Full of elements such as iron, manganese, zinc, copper, chromium and cobalt, it is therapeutic in the extreme.

ksheera dhooma

Medicated Milk Steam

A particular Ayurvedic method unique to Kerala, *ksheera dhooma* is prescribed for patients with facial palsy, certain nervous disorders, difficulty in voice and speech, headaches and trigeminal neuralgia (the trigeminal nerve is a cranial nerve that supplies the face). The word *ksheera* translates as "milk" and *dhooma* indicates a "fomentation by vapor". Generally given to the face, although the steam may be directed to other parts of the body suffering from different conditions, it consists of a steaming with medicated milk. It is considered a treatment for *vata* related disorders.

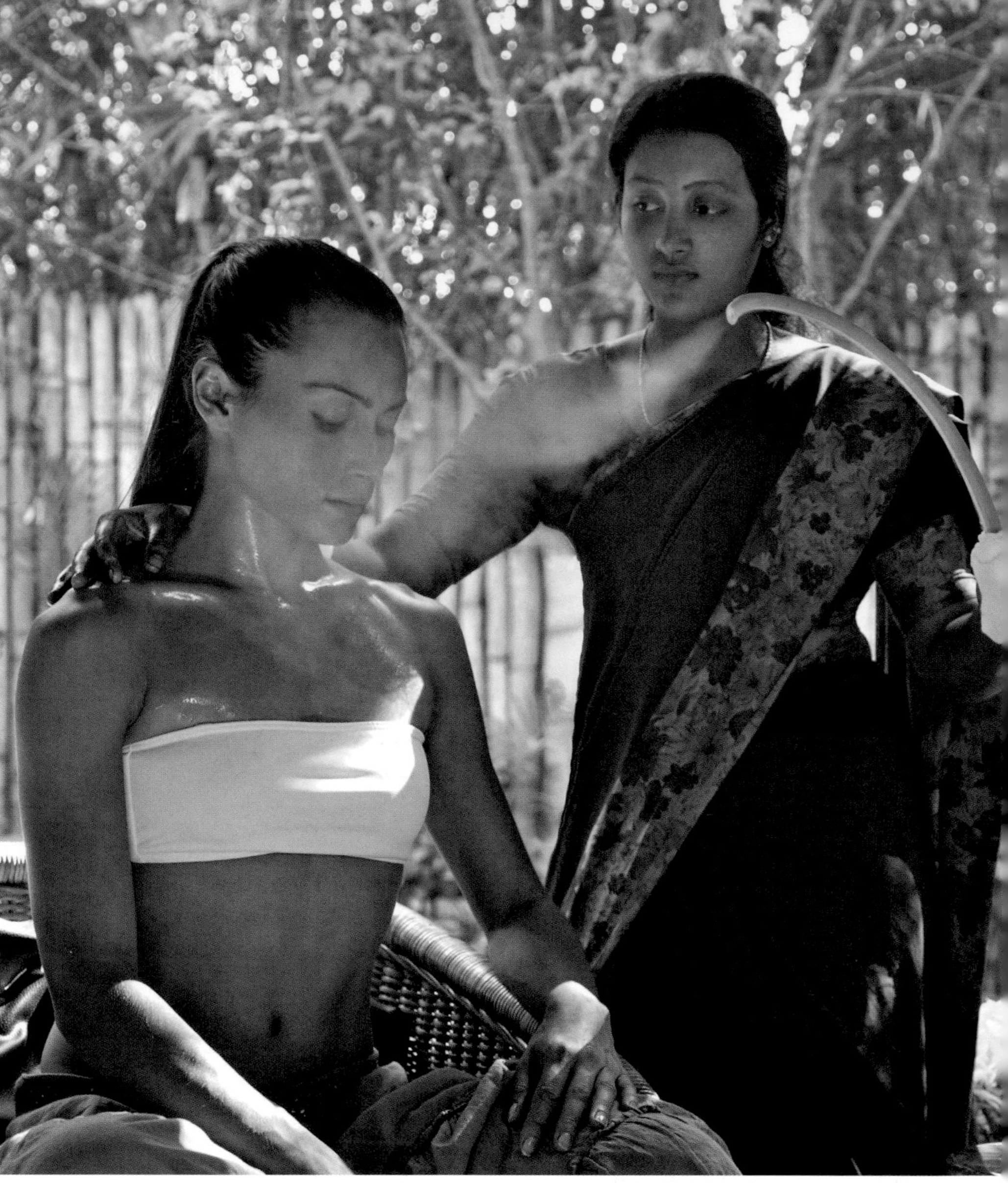

A therapist directs steam from boiling medicated milk on to the face of a patient at the integrated wellness center called Soukya. Known as a *swedan* (fomentation) therapy, *ksheera dhooma* is traditionally prescribed for people with *vata* related disorders (any muscle, ligament, joint or nerve-related disorder).

First of all, a selection of herbs is boiled up with cow's milk, then the steam issuing from the mix is passed through a tube to the affected area of the body (this has first been oiled with medicated herbal oil chosen according to the body's constitution and condition). The steam makes what is known in Ayurvedic circles as a fomentation on the face, thereby allowing medicinal properties to be absorbed. The idea is to stimulate nerve endings and open up the micro-channels just below the skin's surface.

At Soukya International Holistic Health Center, the medicated milk is steamed through a papaya stalk onto the chosen area. This allows the properties of the herbs and the milk to mix with papain, the active enzyme in papaya, before it reaches its destination. Papain is helpful in loosening and dissolving the top layer of dead skin cells, so, in this case, it helps prepare the skin for the absorption of the medicated herbs. The treatment is prescribed once a day for three, five or seven days consecutively and may be offered in combination with other treatments. It's a good example of a traditional therapy offered in modern surrounds.

netra tarpanam

Vasthi Therapy for the Eyes

At an Ayurveda clinic, *netra tarpanam* is seen as an oral eye care treatment to help with eye strain, dryness of eyes, poor sight and other eye-related conditions. It is believed to strengthen the muscles round the eyes, cool the eyes, oleate the area round the eyes and may even help with myopia. As with all Ayurvedic prescriptions, at least a two-week course is suggested, and during the course of the treatment the patient should not be exposed to harsh light.

The treatment uses the medium of ghee or *gritham*, a type of clarified butter that is used all over India in cooking. "Ghee has what we call *samskarika anuvarthana* in Sanskrit," explains Ayurvedic doctor, Dr Yogesh, "this means it has the specific quality of being able to absorb properties of herbal products and transfer them into the skin." Depending on the condition, *triphala gritham*, good for the eyesight, or *jeevanthyadhi gritham*, a ghee that helps develop immunity, may be used.

To keep the ghee in place over the eye socket, a dough of black or green gram flour paste (gram powder mixed with water) is made and stuck around both eye cavities. A small amount of ghee melted to room temperature is then poured into the watertight enclosure, so that it fills the contained area and makes the eyelashes sink shut. The ghee is kept on the eyes for 20 minutes, during which time the patient is encouraged to move the eyes around.

It is a slightly fiddly process, and may not be for everybody. Some people experience a burning sensation when the medicated ghee is poured in, and having to hold still for a long time isn't to every body's liking.

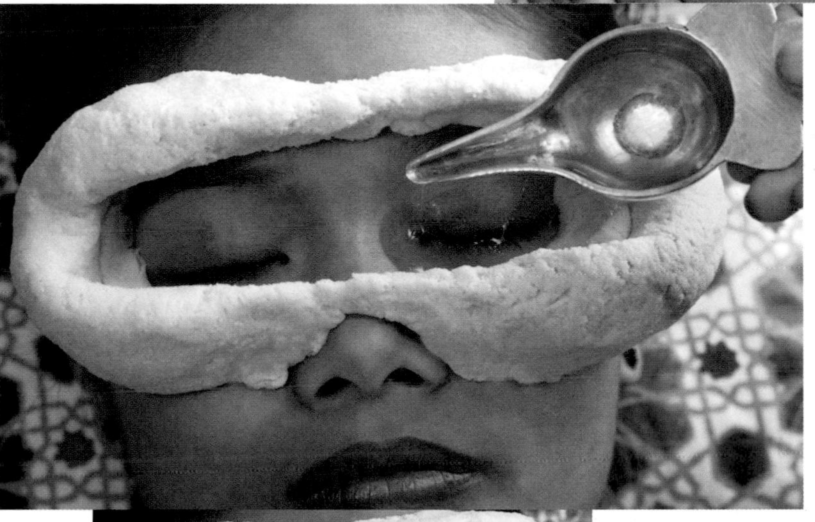

Strictly speaking, *netra tarpanam* is a *vasthi* therapy (see pages 32–35), as medicated ghee is kept trapped on a topical area in a watertight "reservoir" of dough. Whilst the ghee rests in its place, eyes should be rolled around, opened and closed, thereby allowing the ghee's properties to be fully absorbed.

kizhi therapy

The Hot Herbal Pouch

In Ayurveda, the herbal poultice is a time-honored tradition of healing with heat. Packed with goodness, warmed pouches of herbs, plants, roots, and more, have been applied to sore, sprained or sad bodies for centuries. Classified as a *swedanam* (Sanskrit for sweat therapy) in the Vedic texts, the herbal poultice is both detoxifying and healing. Specially selected ingredients are tied tightly in natural cloth, steamed for a few minutes, then dipped in medicated herbal oil and applied to the body. On application, the heat induces sweating, thereby helping to bring toxins to the surface of the skin; then, once the pores are open, skin absorbs the properties of the herbs for healing.

The *kizhi* (Mahalayam word for bundle) has proved so popular over the centuries, its fame has spread to other cultures too. Many South East Asian herbal healthcare practices rely on the herbal poultice to relieve sore muscles and joint pains, while in India, hospitals, homestays, spas, wellness centers and salons offer various forms both as a stand-alone treatment or in conjunction with another therapy such as massage. The content, method of application and usage varies widely.

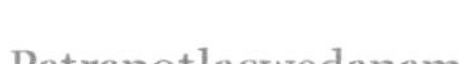

Patrapotlaswedanam
The Sanskrit name for this ancient Ayurvedic treatment is taken from *patra* meaning "leaves", *potla* translating as "pouch" and *swedanam* meaning "fomentation" or "sweat therapy". The integrated medical center called Soukya, just outside Bangalore, is known for its extensive herb gardens — so their *potla* makes full use of plants grown on site.

Leaves from the castor oil plant (*Ricinus communis*), rich in oil, are combined with *Datura alba* leaves (this plant is widely used by Ayurvedic and Siddha practitioners in oil-based preparations for dressings on wounds), skin tonifying *nirgundi* or *Vitex nigundo* leaves, and leaves from the *moringo* or drumstick tree. These latter leaves are a well-known natural antibiotic. In fact, all

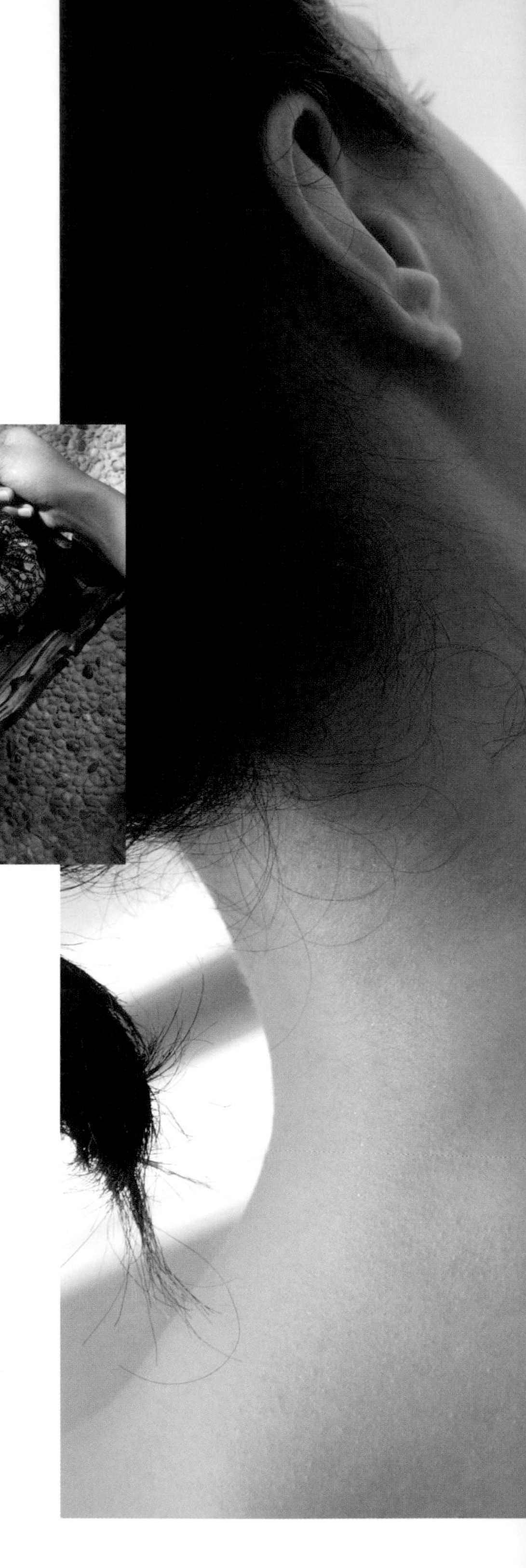

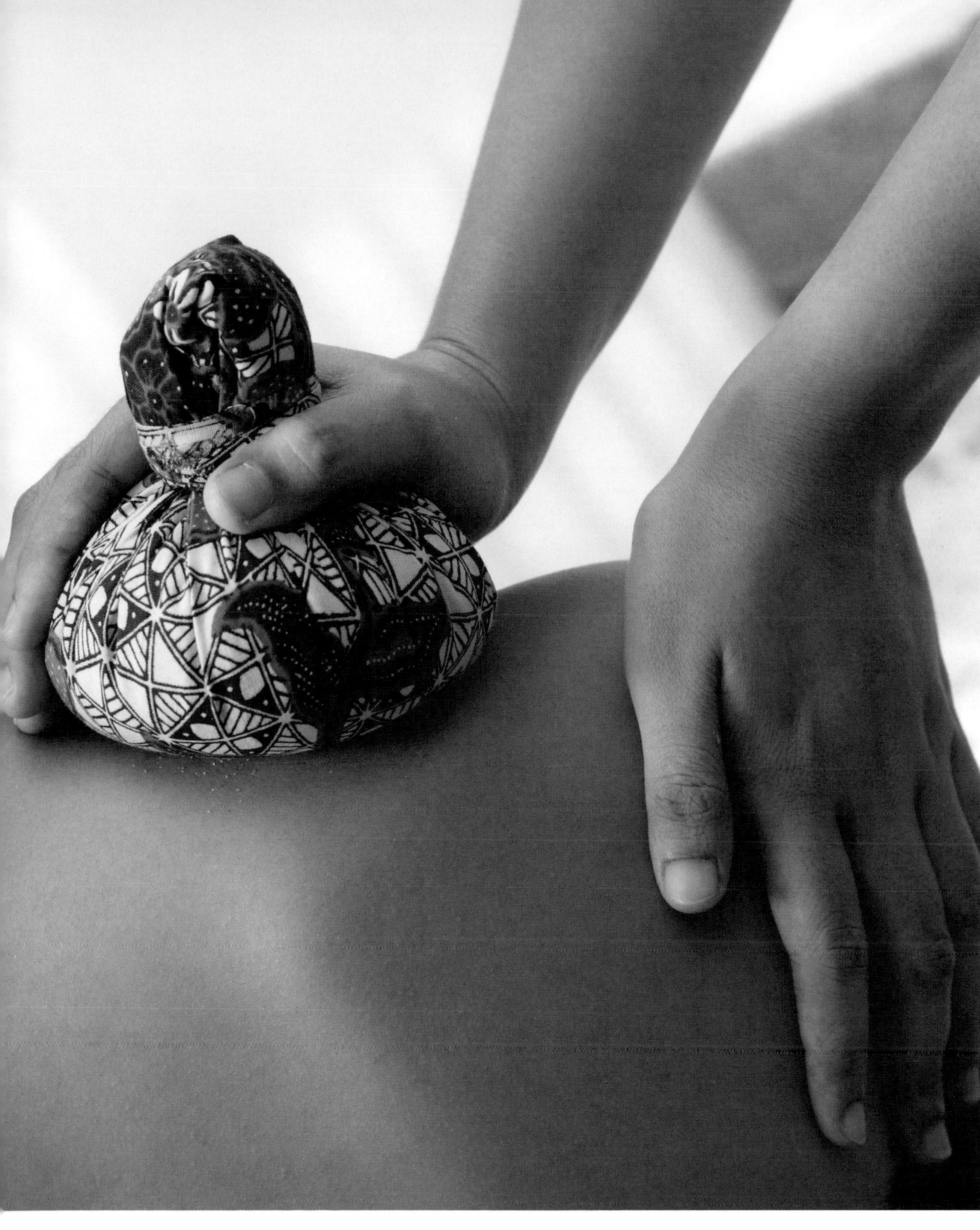

Sand, like clay and mud, has the ability to retain heat or cold, so is an ideal filler for a heated compress. When dipped in warm, medicated oil, these bundles of goodness spread warmth and healing deep into tense or knotted muscles. At the tranquil Spa Village in the Pangkor Island Resort in Malaysia, pretty batik cottons are used to further the pouch's appeal.

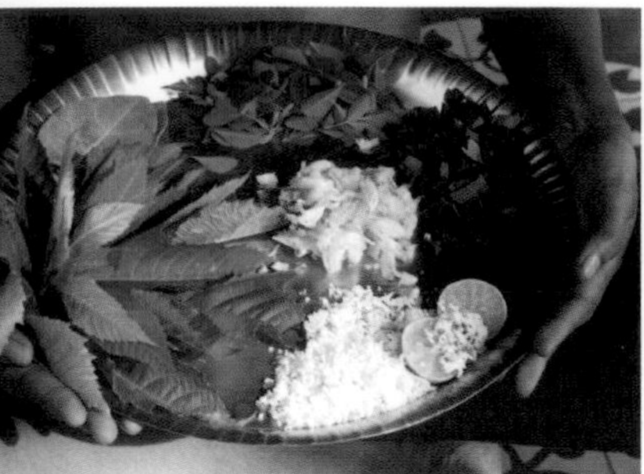
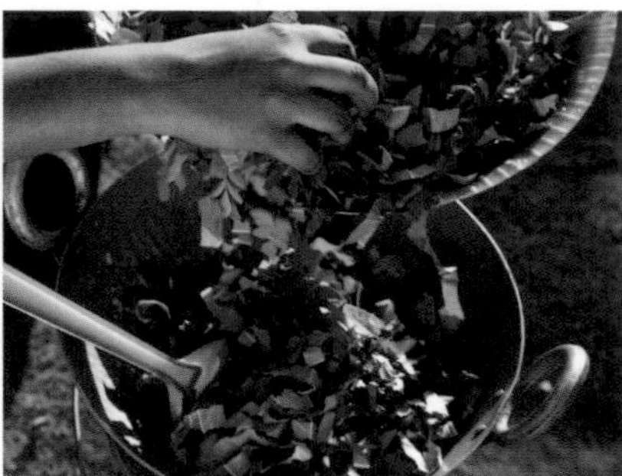
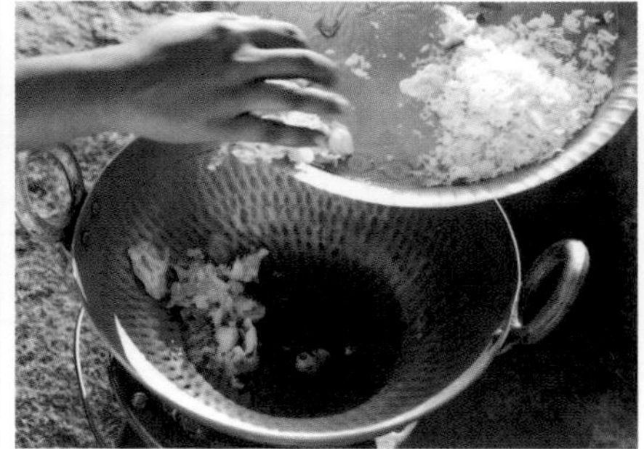
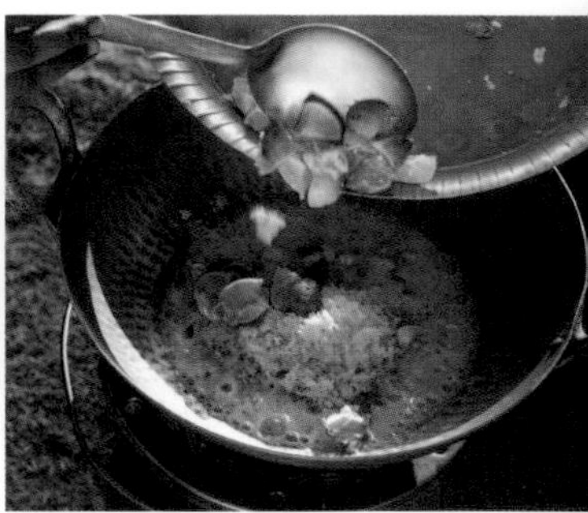

these leaves contain anti-inflammatory and pain-reducing properties, so are useful in arthritic conditions. To prepare the *potla*, they are washed, torn up and mixed with crushed garlic, lime and shredded coconut flesh, then fried with medicated oil in a wok, before being knotted up into small pouches.

At Soukya, patients who have been prescribed this therapy are on a course of seven to 21 days, and the pouch is combined with other therapies. It may be given to people with sciatica, disc prolapse or lower back pain, and is usually applied after an external massage with medicated oil. Two therapists administer the *potla*: one warms two of the pouches in medicated oil, while the other massages the other two on to affected areas. Movements include gentle thudding and rubbing away from the heart.

Navara Kizhi

Definitely worth a try is the intriguingly named Navara *kizhi*, a Keralan treatment offered at many spas and clinics throughout India. At Oberoi Spa at Udaivilas, Navara rice (a type of dehusked, red rice) is mixed with milk and a decoction of *bala* root (*Sida cordifolia*) and boiled for half an hour until it achieves a gruel-like consistency. It is then wrapped into a loosely spun cotton cloth that allows the mixture to come through easily, and applied on to the body. The excess liquid is kept in a reserve pan on a warmer, so that the pouches may be periodically re-warmed.

Bala root is a powerful cell nourishing and regenerating herb, and is used in many Ayurvedic treatments to maintain youth and vitality. It means "youth" in Sanskrit, and is considered analgesic, diuretic and stimulating as well. When mixed with Navara rice and milk, the properties "go quite deep", according to Ayurvedic doctor, Dr Yogesh, who recommends the treatment to develop muscles and improve muscle tone. "The pouch nourishes the skin, alleviates *vata* problems, improves blood circulation, reduces stiffness and strengthens both the quantity and quality of the muscles," he says.

Variations on the Navara *kizhi* include *podi kizhi (podi* means "powder"; *triphala* or *dashmool* are often used); *dhanya kizhi (dhanyam* translates as "grains", so a combination of processed grains is used here; *naranga kizhi* using a cloth pouch filled with lemon and herbs dipped in medicated oils; and *elakizhi (ela* means "leaves". All are designed to act as a potent anti-rheumatic, so are helpful for stiffness in the joints.

The spa at Amanbagh uses *dashmool* powder (*das* means ten, *mool* translates as roots) in its specialized *kizhi* treatment. Tied securely in immaculate linen pouches, the pretty little bundles are dipped into warmed, medicated sesame first boiled with handpicked *aak* leaves (*Calotropis gigantea*) before application. *Aak* is a plant in the milkweed family that grows profusely in the immediate locality; known as swallow-wort, *aak* is useful in the treatment of paralysis, swellings and fever, and it is anti-inflammatory when applied externally.

The Sand Bundle

At the spa at Rajvilas and Spa Village spas in South East Asia, fomentation with small linen pouches filled with sand are the norm. The sand bundle is classified under *ushema swedanam* therapies, which translates as "to warm up (bundles) to sweat".

At Rajvilas, sulphur sand from Simla (it can hold its temperature for a long time) is tied in small linen pouches, which are then dipped in warm medicated oil chosen according to one's *dosha* and pounded on the body. Accompanied by massage, the therapy is soothing for inflammatory conditions, stiffness of joints and aching muscles; it also promotes general wellbeing. The heat speeds up blood circulation and promotes sweating, which in turn helps to eliminate toxins from the body.

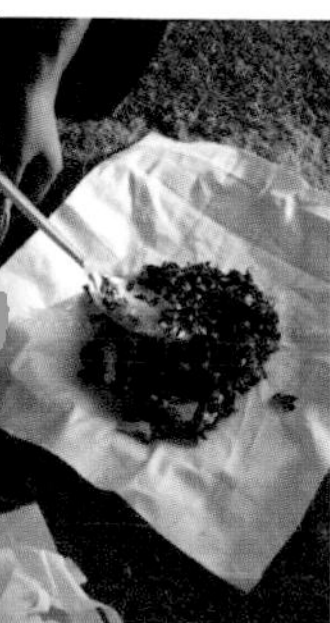

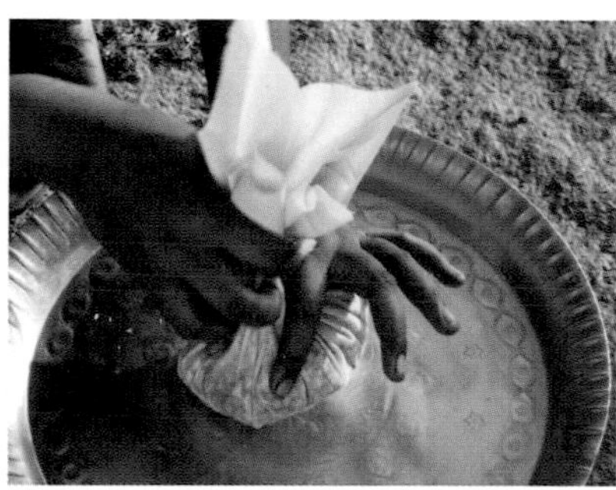

Left Plucked from the organic garden, Soukya's leaves are washed and chopped, then mixed with lime, coconut and garlic and fried in a wok with medicated oil chosen according to a patient's health status and *dosha* imbalance. After frying for 10 to 15 minutes, the ingredients are transferred into soft cotton pouches, before being administered, wonderfully warmed in oil, on problem areas.
Below The gorgeous property in Udaipur known as Udaivilas not only boasts tranquil surrounds on Lake Pichola, it offers numerous sites for therapy. Built to resemble a Mewari palace, scallop-edged arches, *jaali* windows, cool sandstone and marble decorations, as well as abundant gardens, offer a delightful backdrop to a spa suite.

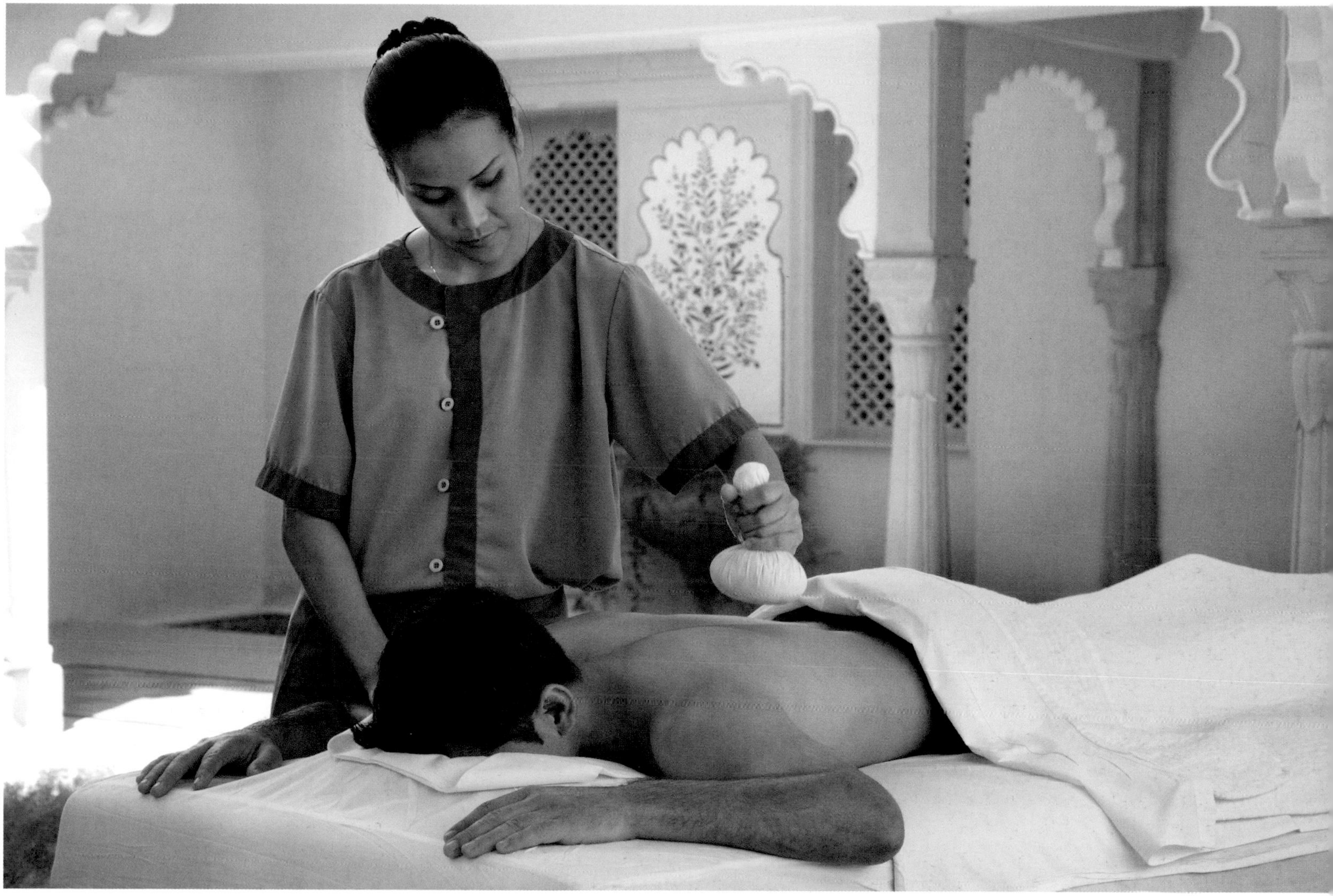

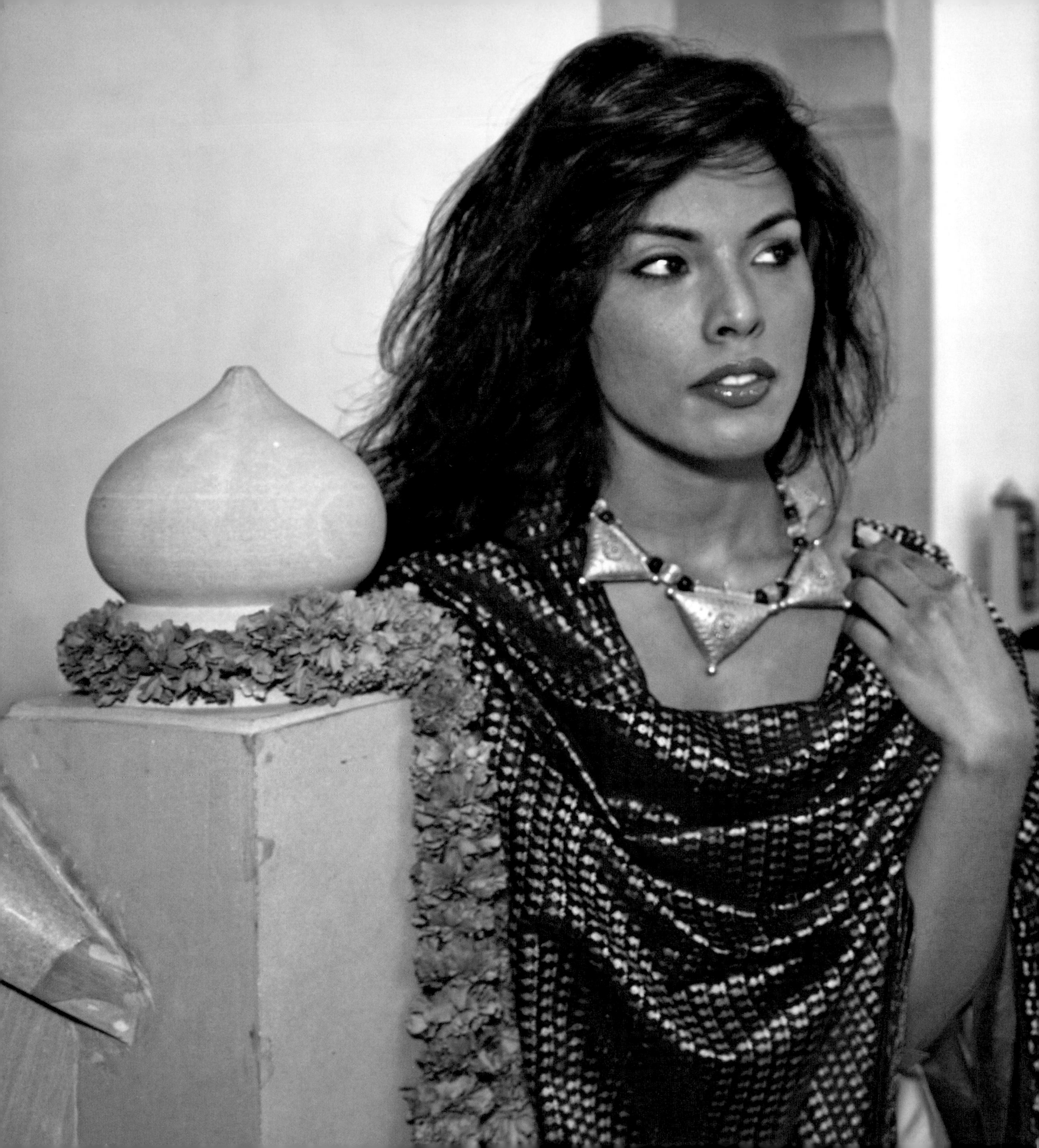

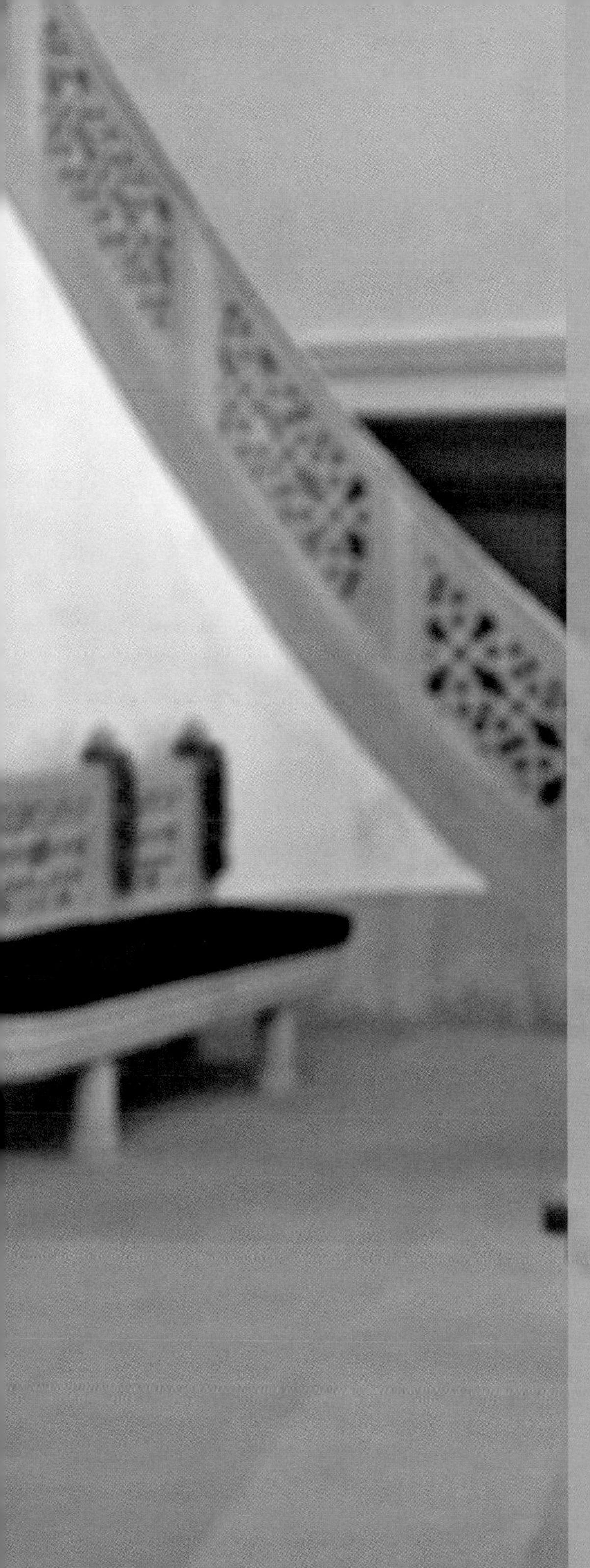

beauty

Ancient beauty-enhancing rituals are experiencing a renaissance globally, as people look towards "natural" rather than "chemical" solutions to the symptoms of aging. India is well placed to cater to such needs, as it is home to a rich selection of hair, skin and body treatments, all of which work both internally and externally to create a glowing complexion, soft skin and lustrous locks. In addition, we consider some wonderful de-toxing and beautifying baths and some inspiring therapies that employ gems, crystals, metals and minerals for healing.

ayurvedic facial care

Indian women have been harnessing herbs and plants for skin care for centuries. Numerous Sanskrit texts outline facial and other beauty treatments, and evidence of natural cosmetics dates back to at least 3,000 BC in excavations of the Indus Valley civilization in present-day Pakistan. Instructions for extracts of flowers, leaves, barks and herbs for both medicinal and cosmetic purposes are plentiful in the Vedas — and the flawlessness of Indian women's skin is captured in countless paintings from the past.

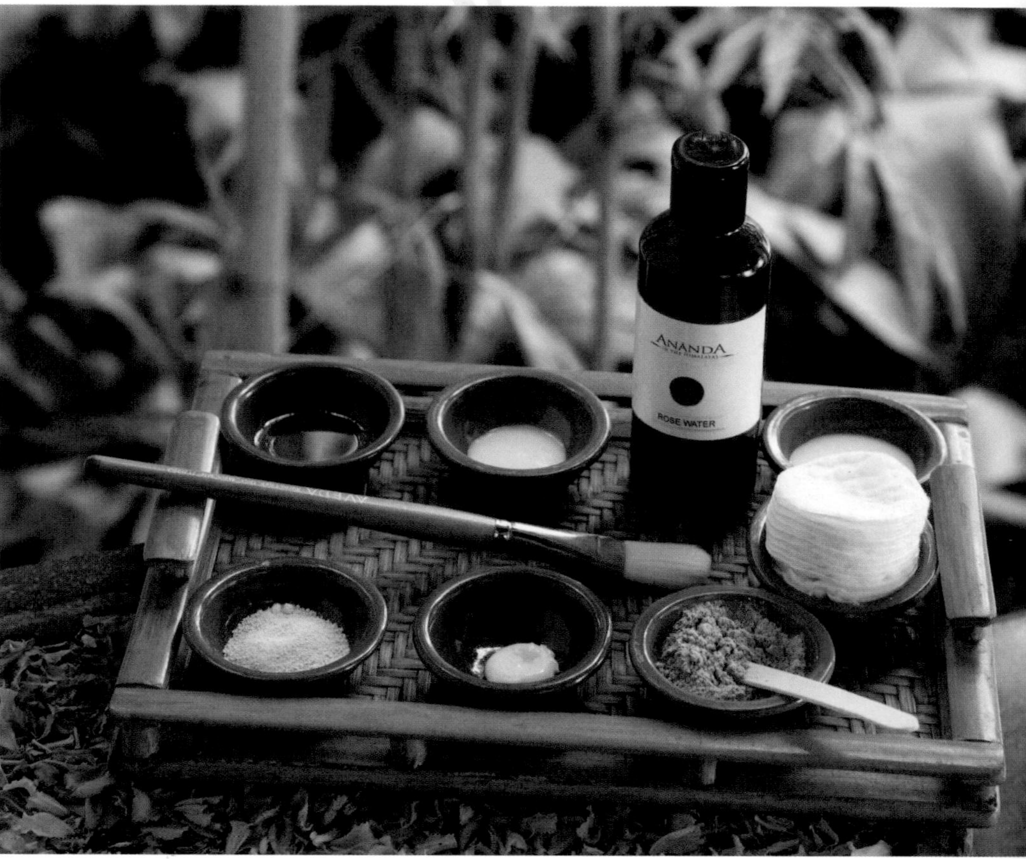

Some of the more common Indian beauty products that have found a worldwide market include *kajal* or kohl eyeliner and *mehndi* (henna), as well as various perfumes and oils. *Kajal* found fame with the Moghul Empress Nur Jehan; it is traditionally made from *triphala*, almond, camphor and cabbage, all burnt in the oil of rose, and has been exported for decades. Oils of sandalwood, musk and rose have been traded along with India's cotton and spices for centuries, and the Rajput combination of rose and milk for facial scenting and cleansing is well documented. More recently, as people have become aware of the potential pitfalls of chemical and synthetic skin, hair and beauty products, Indian herbal recipes have become increasingly popular in global markets.

In addition to formulating, manufacturing and selling facial products, India is starting to capitalize on some of its ancient beauty treatments too. Threading, the ancient art of facial hair extraction, is finding favor in London and New York day spas, and henna hair treatments are increasingly promoted in high-end hair salons. *Marma* massage on the vital energy points of the face is a therapy offered in many South East Asian spas and the Indian head massage is widely used as a "filler" whilst a client is resting with a face mask, for example. These, along with some of the more medicinal Ayurvedic treatments, are ones to watch out for.

According to Ayurvedic texts, the secret to lasting beauty is *ojas* or the subtle quality of vigor or vitality that is the superfine essence of the seven *dhatus* or tissues of the body. If *ojas* is strong and healthy, one has

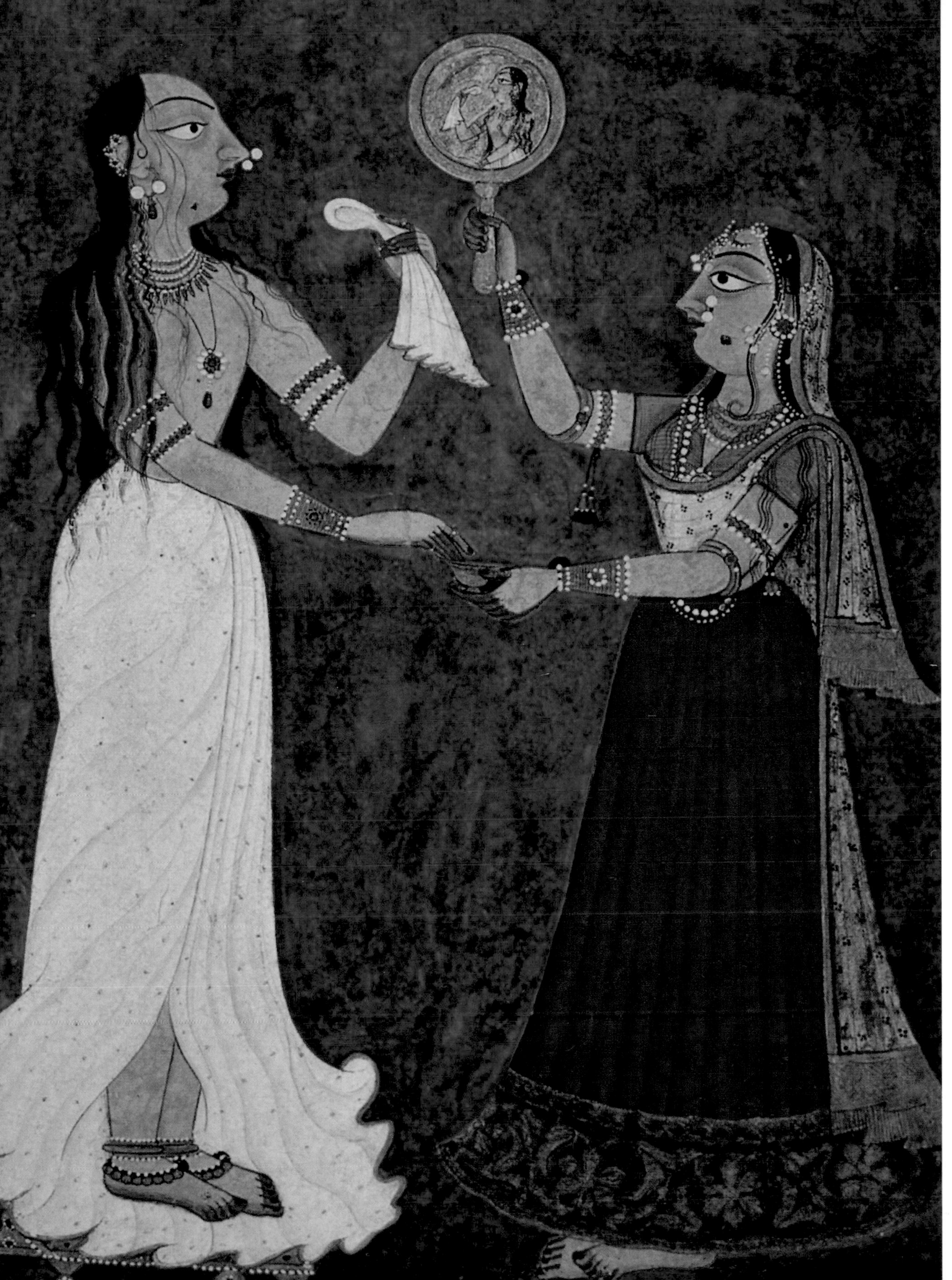

Opposite Many spas, salons and Ayurvedic centers in India are now manufacturing their own herbal products for sale both domestically and overseas. The ingredients for the Ananda facial are artfully arranged here on a tray. Preceded by a back massage, it comprises a cleanse, exfoliate, tone, facial massage, clay mask and moisturize.
Left A Rajasthani miniature painting depicts a maid helping her mistress with her toilette (Mankot, *circa* 1720).

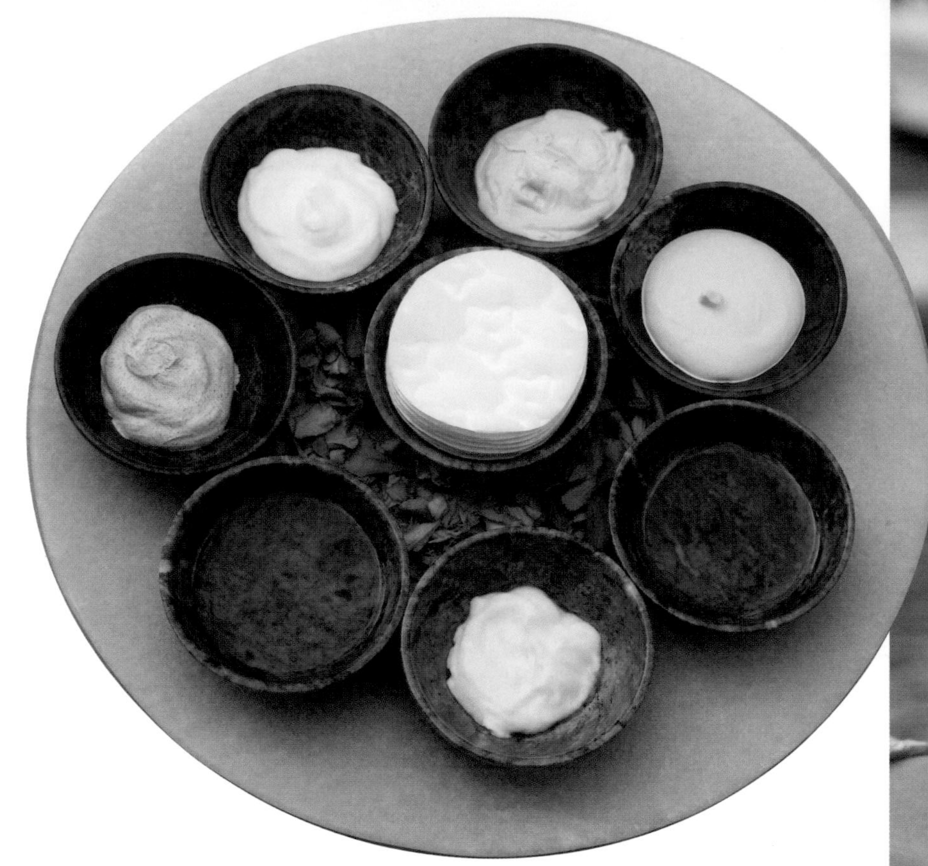

a radiant inner self; this, in turn, manifests itself in one's outer physical appearance. Of course, a facial treatment will help also, and it's important to note that many Ayurvedic facial treatments, offered at numerous spas and salons throughout India, are designed for both outer beauty and inner detoxification. Often called *mukhalepam* (*mukha* is "face", *lepam* translates as "pack"), they condition and nourish the skin, open blocked pores, eliminate toxins internally and cleanse the face to improve skin texture.

Traditionally, Ayurvedic skin care recipes were formulated according to the healing ingredients that women had to hand in their immediate vicinity. They took into account the condition or *vikruti* of a person's skin, and were made in the kitchen and used immediately. Cleansing, nourishing and protecting are the three key components in Ayurvedic skin care and a full treatment is composed of eight steps: A thorough cleanse with an *ubtan* paste; an oleation massage on the reflex points and energy meridians on the face; a herbal steam or compress to bring out impurities; a gentle scrub to stimulate circulation and cleanse the pores; a mask or pack to deep cleanse, tauten and/or nourish the skin; a toning and rejuvenating refresher to refine pores and tone the skin; a deep moisturizer to protect the skin from the elements and bacteria; and a gentle spray mist to assist absorption of the moisturizer and bring vitality to the entire complexion.

Although it would be too tedious to outline all the invigorating facials you may have the luck to come across in India, a few deserve special mention for the quality of their products and the skill of the therapists. Aman spas should be sought out in New Delhi and Rajasthan (see opposite) as much for their superb surrounds as their specialist treatments and Shahnaz Husain, the herbal beauty tour de force, is another name to watch out for. Another must is the Ayurvedic facial at Soukya that works on both the inner and outer levels in order to develop *ojas*. It goes without saying that all sections are performed with Ayurvedic herbs chosen according to one's constitution and present state of health, combined with fresh fruits and vegetables selected according to skin types. Milk, curd, mint, honey, turmeric and sandal form its basis. The handpicked ingredients supply much-needed vitamins and minerals, while packs even out color tone, soothe and moisturize the skin, and leave the face soft and supple.

Above and right Aman spas' "Royal Beauty" or *Shahi Nikhar* is a complete facial treatment fit for a Maharani. Featuring such Indian exotics as honey, milk and rose, passionflower, geranium, cassia flower and chamomile, it smells as good as it feels. Designed to cleanse and soften skin, it also boosts cell renewal and draws out pollutants from the complexion.

Steam ensures that the ingredients are absorbed into the deepest layer of the skin, stimulating it and ensuring healthy new cell growth.

The Park Hotels' line of day spas called Aura also offer a number of super-fresh, natural facial sequences. Harnessing the power of rare combinations of natural herbs, fruits, flowers and spices, each is individually designed for different complexions. Those with dry skin would

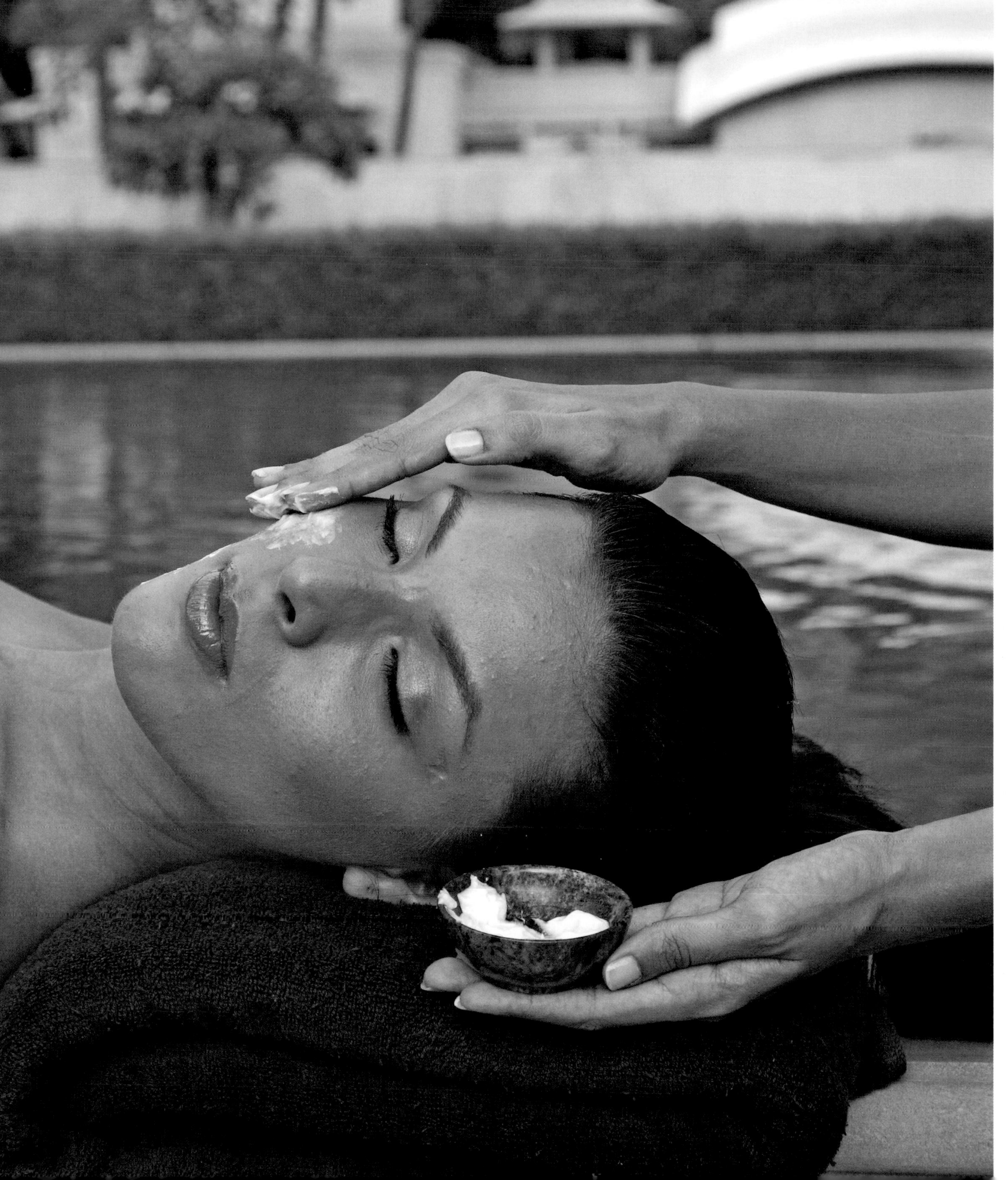

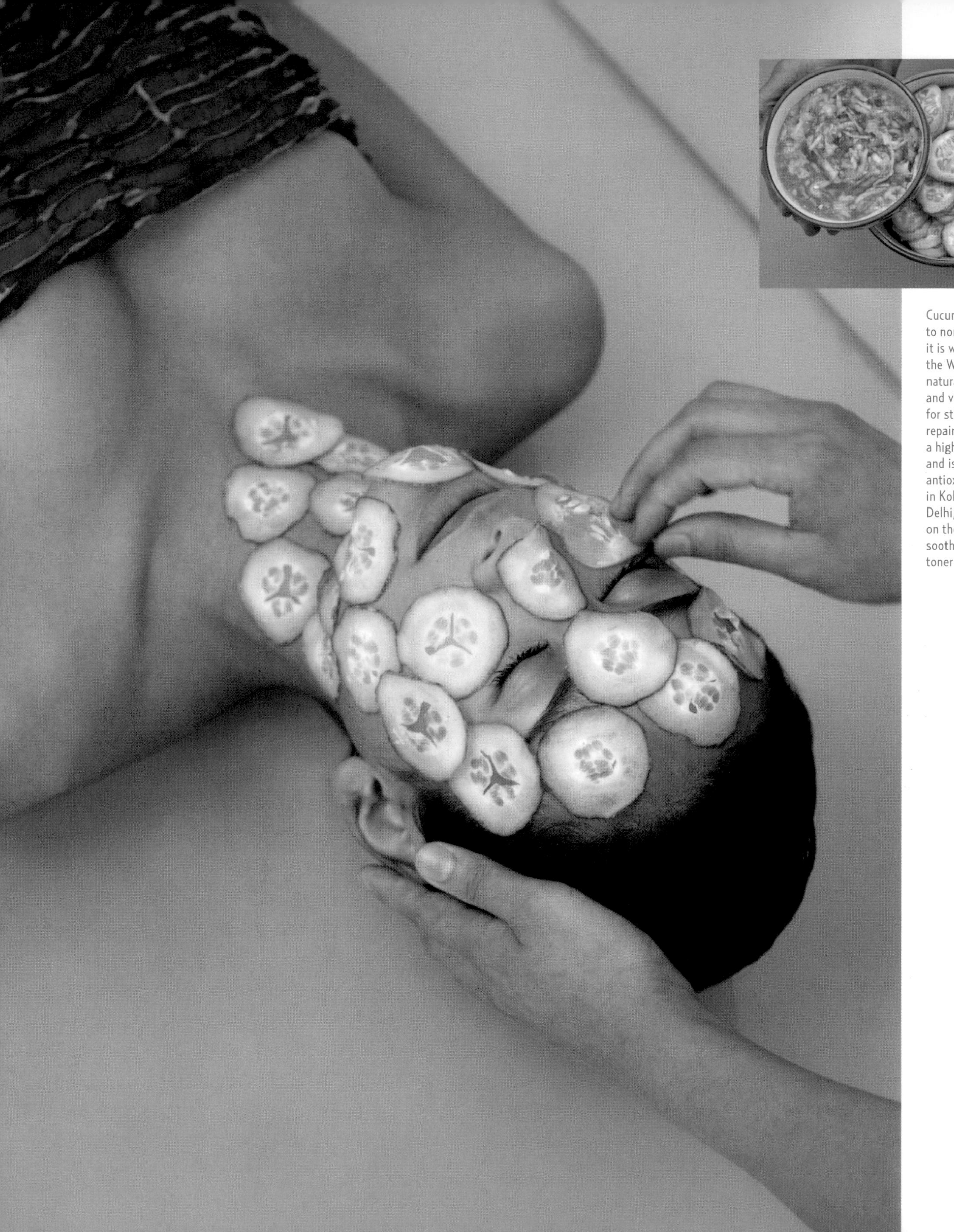

Cucumber traces its roots to northern India, although it is widely available in the West. It contains natural salts, enzymes and vitamins essential for strong cell growth and repair; in addition, it has a high mineral content and is a natural source of antioxidants. At Aura spas in Kolkata, Chennai and New Delhi, cucumber is used on the skin as a sunburn soother, as well as a facial toner and moisturizer.

be well advised to try the saffron and almond number: a gentle anti-aging treatment, it uses pure *rawa* (semolina) for exfoliation and then gives skin a blast with a saffron and almond mask. Saffron is a powerful ingredient for boosting skin longevity and almonds are high in vitamin E, a crucial component in skin softening. The result is the minimizing of fine lines and a refreshed, clearer complexion.

The fresh apple facial, on the other hand, is recommended for oily to normal skins. Kashmiri women, renowned for their clear, fair complexions, have applied mashed apple and apricots, mixed with honey, to their faces for centuries. At Aura, slices of apple, rich in antioxidants and creamed with humectant honey, are rubbed on to the face to rehydrate and revitalize. With its fresh, fruity aroma and the gentle nurturing movements of well-trained therapists, this facial fires skin with an inner glow.

The Kumarakom *mukhalepam* is another one to look out for: it is excellent for dry, oily and combination skins and for people with different *doshas*. Made entirely from ingredients fresh from the market, it is a wonderfully natural sequence. Utilizing a wheat powder and juice combo to tighten skin; an aloe vera massage; a moisturizing cucumber freshener; a scrub from orange peel, ground strawberry, guava and apple seeds to exfoliate; a crushed papaya polish; a pack of *Multani mitti* powder mixed with lots of fresh produce and juice, it is good enough to eat!

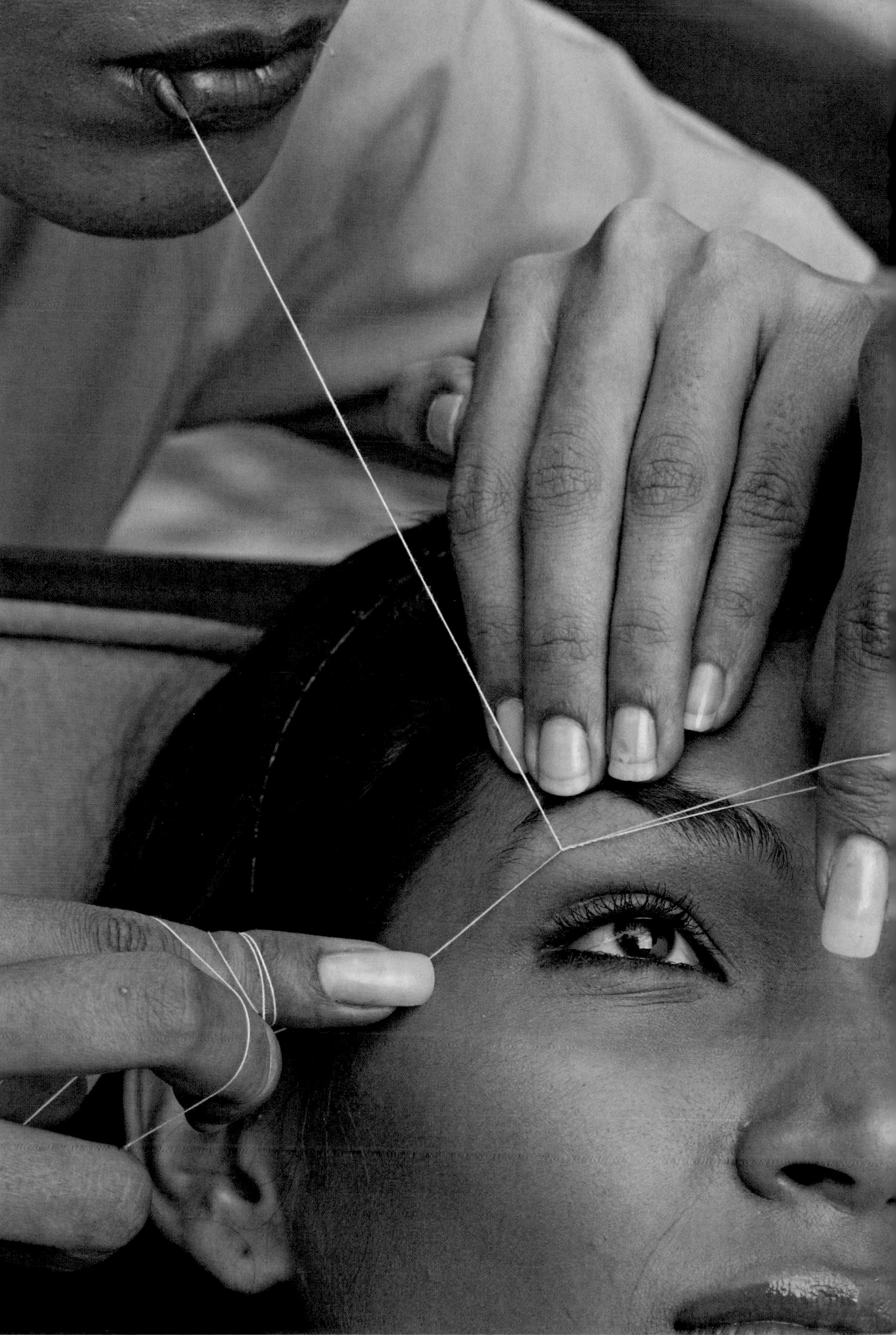

Inexpensive, fast and neat, threading works well to remove facial hair and stray eyebrow hairs. Using teeth and hands, the practitioner utilizes a loop of cotton to trap a series of unwanted hairs and pull them from the skin. As with tweezers, results last from two to four weeks.

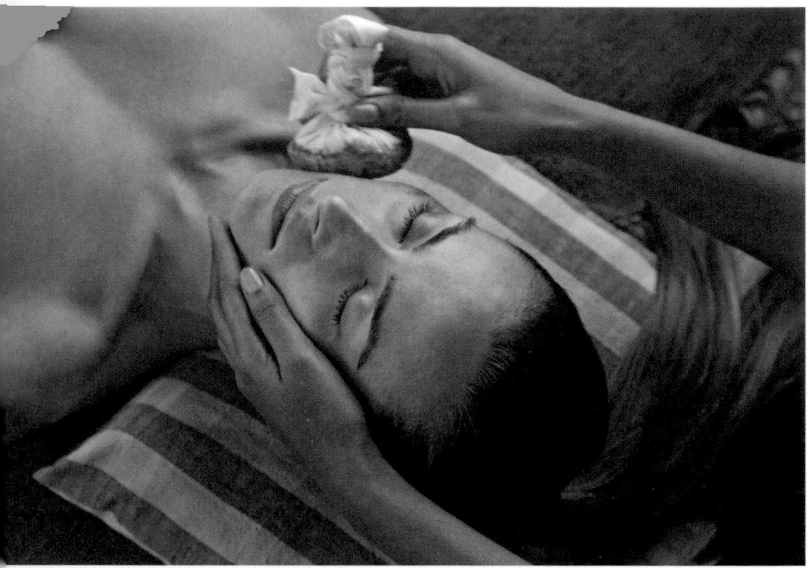

The energizing facial treatment ingredients at Soukya (see **below**): While the properties fom Soukya's delicate warmed herbal pouches penetrate into the skin (see **left**), a gentle massage increases peripheral circulation and oxygenates the facial cells. Turmeric, a staple in Indian cuisine, doubles up as a beauty product (see **right**). When combined with *rawa* (semolina) and cleansing red sandal powder, it effectively exfoliates dead skin cells.

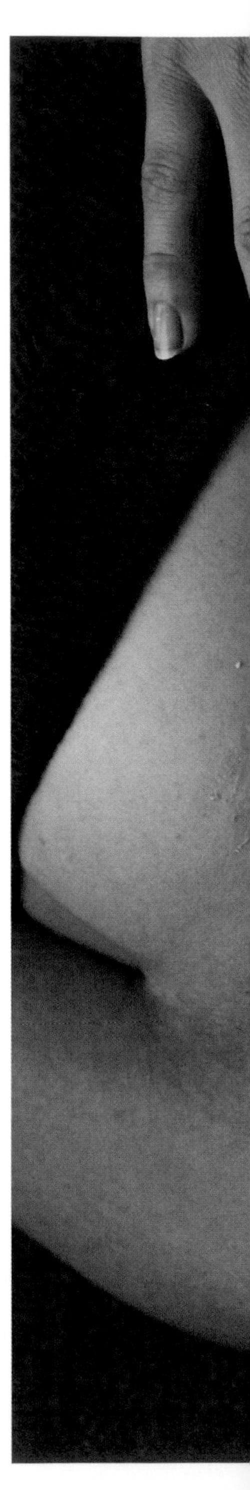

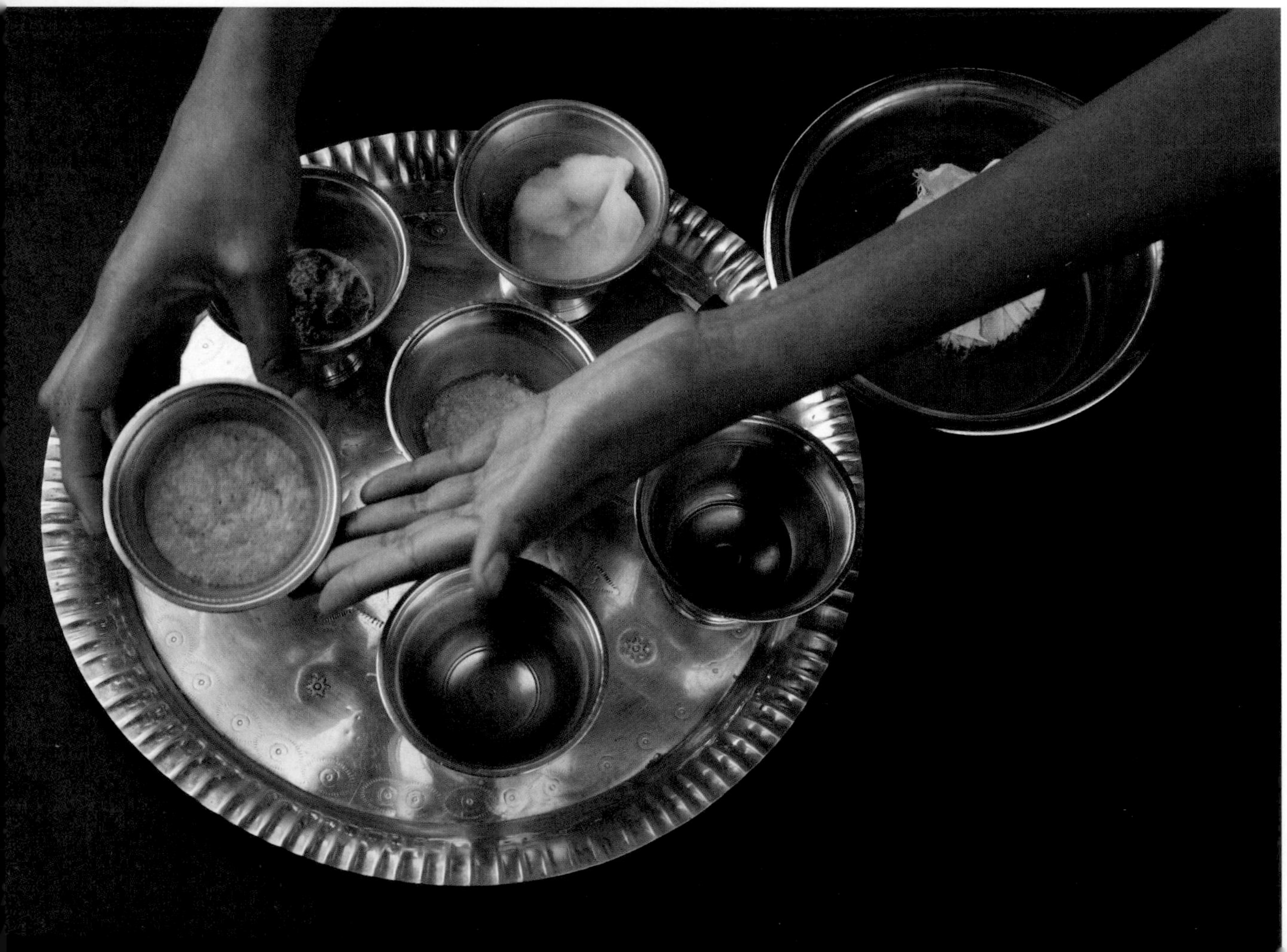

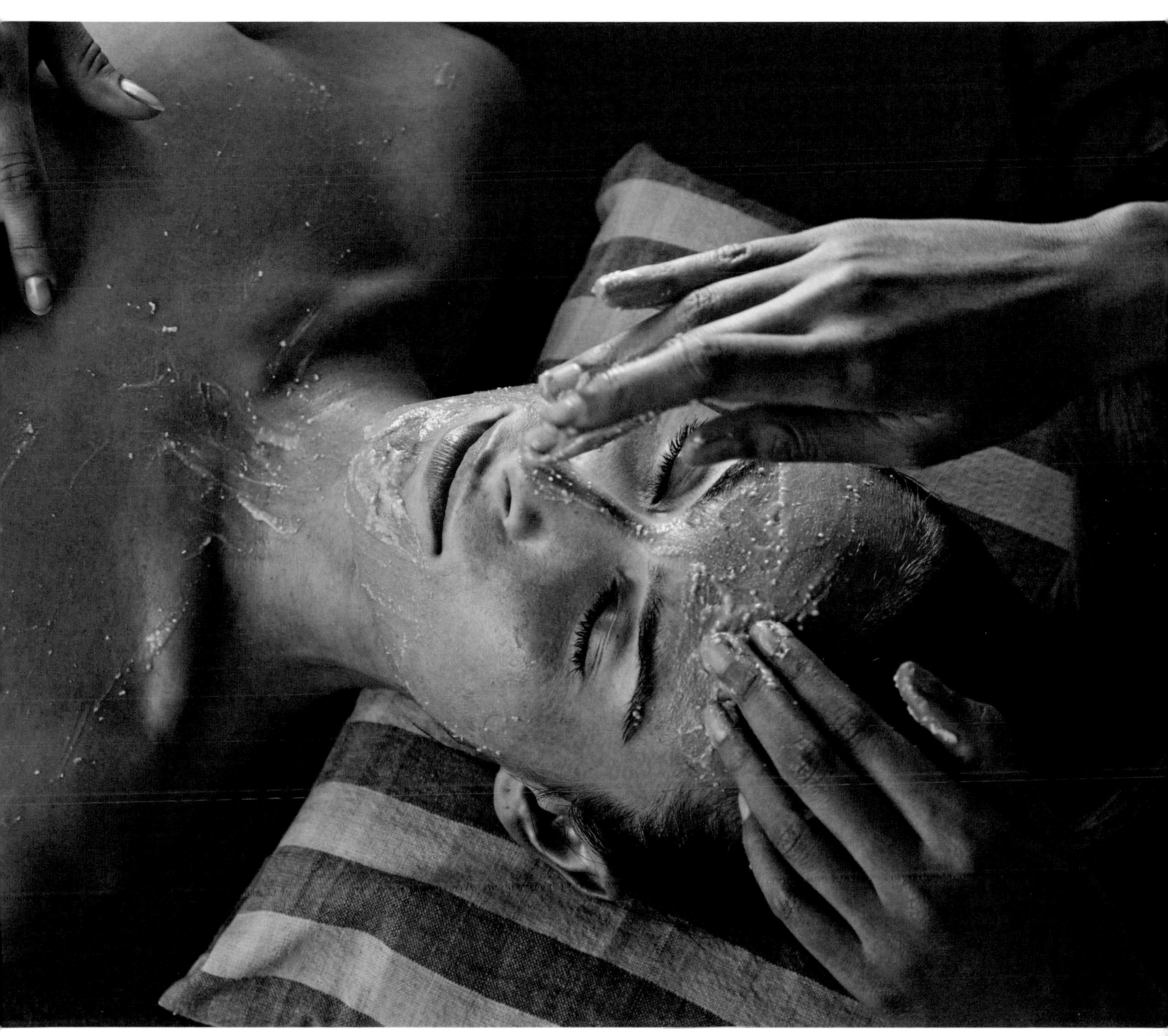

hand care

Ayurvedic texts emphasize the importance of self-care, declaring that the body has the means to heal itself. As such, there are numerous guidelines in the major medical treatises for maintenance of healthy skin, organs, digestive system and more. If *ojas* is strong and the life force is flowing freely, a person looks dynamic, vigorous and well cared for. A toxin-free internal system is reflected externally with glowing skin, bright eyes and healthy limbs. Similarly, such a person is mentally assertive, emotionally caring and spiritually pure.

On the other hand, if there are internal health problems, these may be detectable externally. In many cases, they are reflected in the state of one's finger nails. As nails are a by-product (*mala*) of bones (*asthi dhatu*), they often reflect problems within the body tissues (*dhatu*). For example, a liver condition called Wilson's Disease is easily spotted by the formation of exaggerated large whitish areas on the nails. White spots on the nails show a calcium or zinc deficiency, while brown lines running down the nail indicate possible inflammatory bowel disease. Brittle nails can warn of low iron or Vitamin A, kidney malfunction or poor circulation. Ridges across the nails often accompany acute infections.

Ayurvedic doctors suggest regular nail inspection, and daily or weekly hand and nail care. Hands are a vulnerable part of the body and are subject to premature aging, so need daily care. A hand massage is an excellent way to stimulate *marma* points and energy meridians, thus releasing toxins and invigorating *ojas*. As with the face, certain points on the hands are associated with various organs and systems within the body, so a hand massage is not only locally stimulating. For example, pressing gently into the center of the palm stimulates the kidney area, while a massage between the thumb and index finger helps with digestion.

Many spas and clinics in India offer hand massage, often as a prelude or to accompany another treatment. Comprising part of a

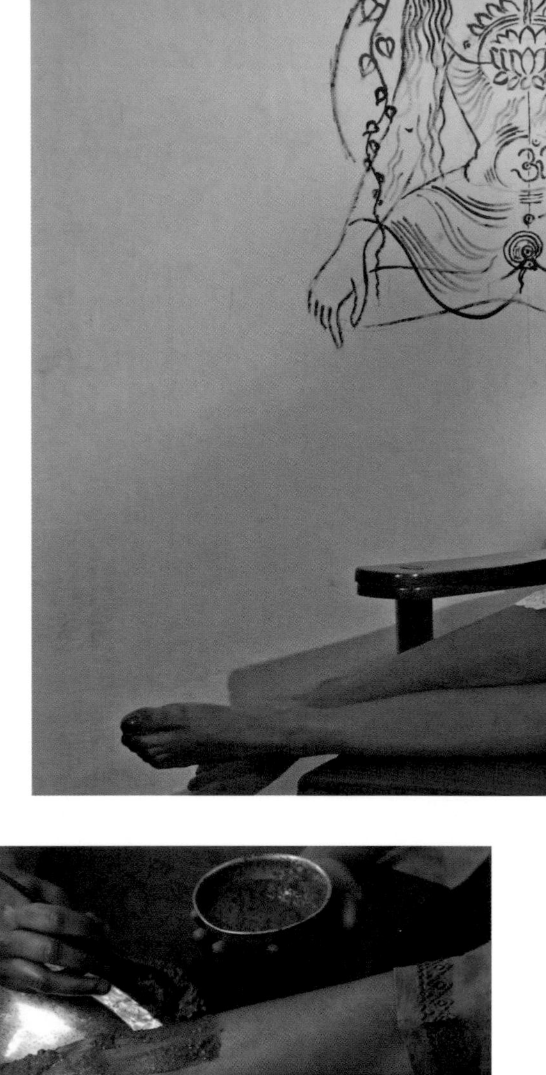

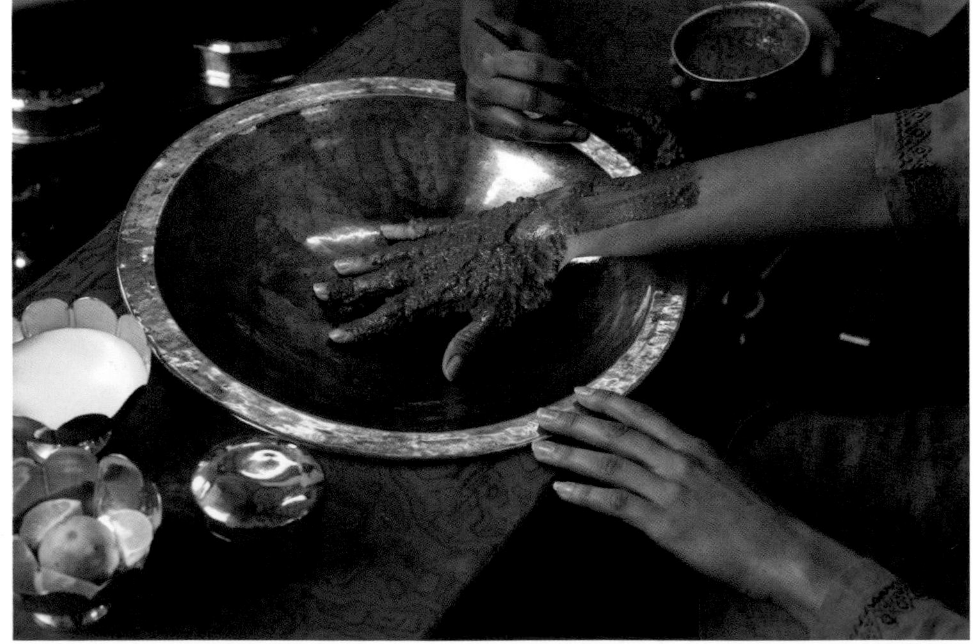

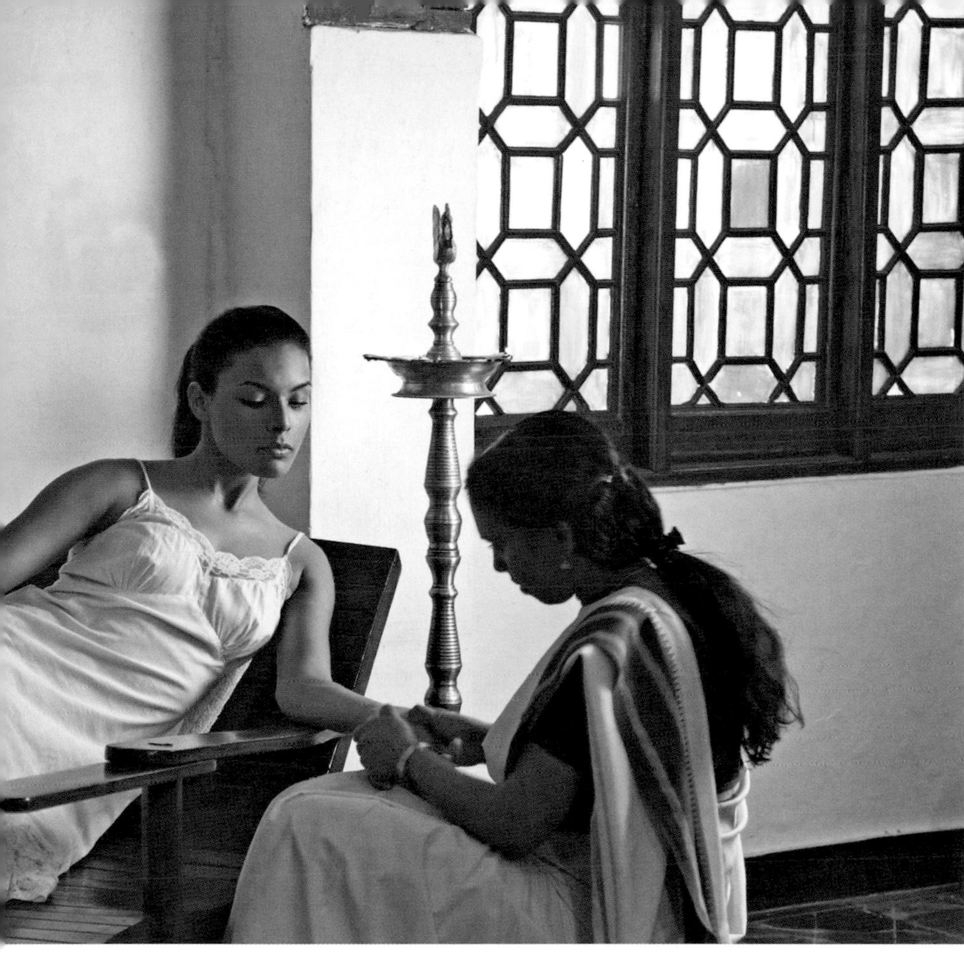

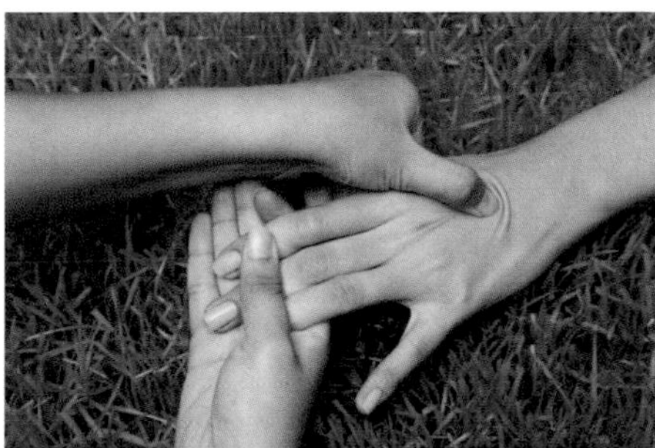

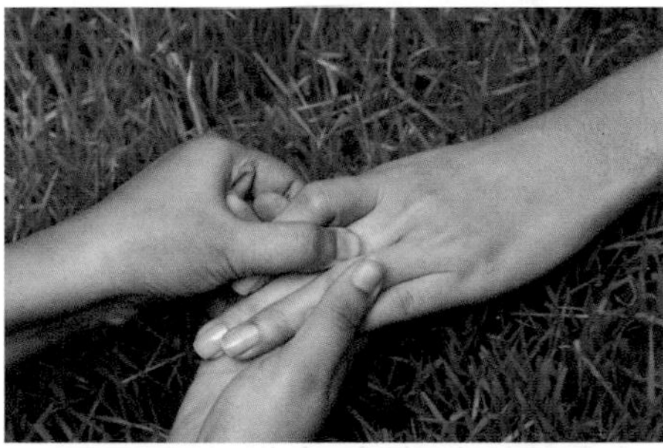

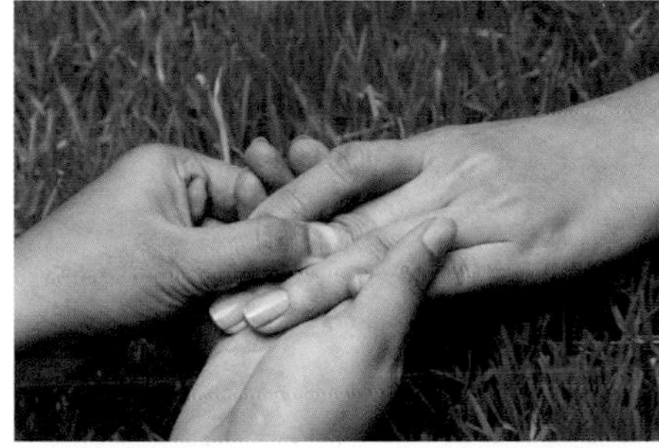

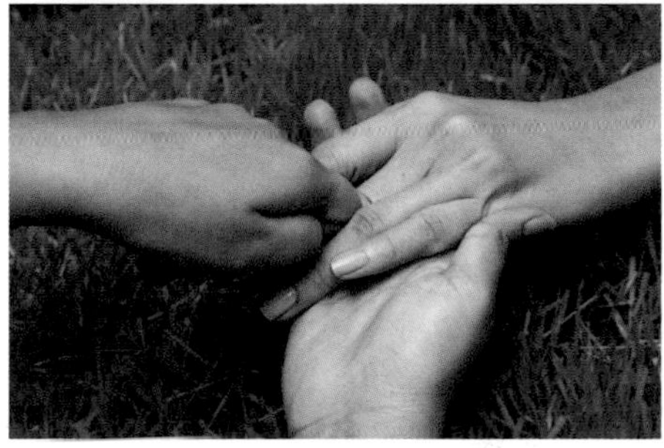

karashubakari ("manicure" in Sanskrit), it can be particularly pleasant. Many of these manicures utilize homemade herbal pastes, scrubs and tonics and combine them with mainstream hand and nail care such as cutting and filing nails, cuticle care and the application of nail polish. Of particular note is the pampering manicure at the Indus Valley Ayurvedic Center: in this sequence, milk (high in lactic acid) is used to soften hands; a disinfecting neem paste makes for a tingling purifier; herbal medicated oil according to one's *dosha* is the base for a vigorous hand massage; gelatine and lemon removes dead surface cells while lemon juice and sugar exfoliates; and a herbal pack made from *Multani mitti*, milk and rosewater tightens the skin. At over 90 minutes, it is a ritual to relish.

Above In Indian salons, a manicure often includes a hand massage that extends all the way up the arms. At the spa at Neemrana Fort Palace, a therapist locates pressure points on the wrist — for deep cleansing as well as relaxation.
Left A rich jade color, this neem paste is part of the relaxing herbal manicure given in the comfortable Shringar Herbal Beauty Salon at the Indus Valley Ayurvedic Center.
Right Certain Aura spas' therapists are trained in the art of a very particular hand massage technique. Designed to release emotions, it can be quite a powerful experience. Using thumbs and knuckles, the therapist pushes up from the tip of each finger to release energy — and the same techniques are also employed elsewhere on the body for a similar effect.

foot care

In India, when entering a home it is traditional to step across the threshold with the right foot first. Shoes are often taken off, as they are when entering a temple or mosque (here feet are often washed too), and touching the feet of an elder is considered a mark of respect. As in other parts of Asia, feet are full of symbolism.

According to Ayurvedic lore, an imbalance of *vata* lies at the heart of all foot problems. As is usual, most physicians recommend prevention rather than cure, stressing that regular foot care, proper posture and sensible footwear also go a long way towards ameliorating existing problems. Alternating hot and cold footbaths help with aching feet and poor circulation, while regular foot hygiene and exercise allow you to put your best foot forward at all times. In the same way that a footbath was traditionally offered to visitors after a long journey, today it often sets the tone at a spa. Given before a treatment, it benefits more than just the feet as it revitalizes the nervous system, improves circulation and provides a feeling of general wellbeing.

The *Charaka Samita* notes that the application of oil is the best remedy for tired or neglected feet. It is said to alleviate coarse and rough skin and reduce stiffness, fatigue and numbness. Furthermore, after a *padhabyangha* massage (foot massage with oil), localized veins and ligaments are strengthened and feet become firm and strong. In addition, vision is supposed to be enhanced, as nerves in the soles of the feet are associated with the eyes.

Padhabyangham tends to concentrate on the pressure points located on the soles of the feet, as it is believed that these are connected by energy channels to internal organs. Sesame or cooling coconut oil is favored, and if the oil is enlivened with essential oils such as peppermint, *tulsi* or black pepper, feet are also given an antiseptic and tension-relieving boost. It is said that a strong rotating, kneading foot massage before bed results in a tranquil night's sleep.

At many spas both in India and elsewhere, foot reflexology or foot massage is a staple on the menu. Often given whilst a client

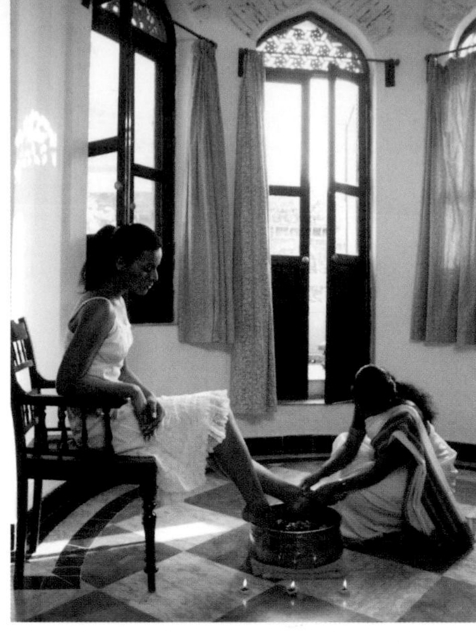

Above and left "As the snake doesn't approach the eagle, so disease doesn't affect the person who massages his feet before sleeping" goes an old Indian saying. As such, foot massage to the *marma* points on the feet is a family activity, often given by children to elders. Invigorating and enlivening, it is good not only for the feet, but for the entire body.

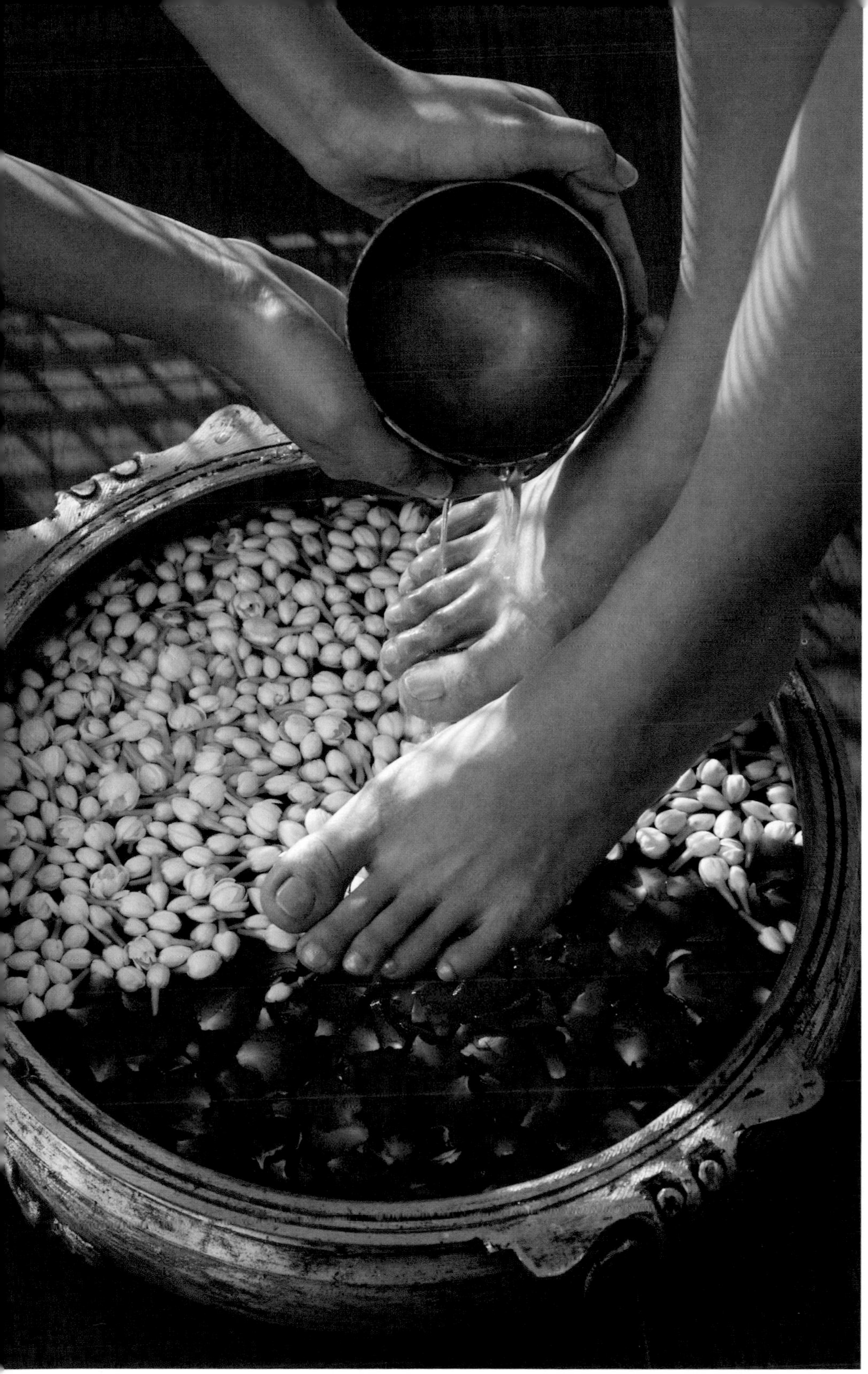

lies cocooned in a body wrap or as one part of a foot ritual, there is something wickedly sensual about having your feet nurtured in such a manner. Another option is to walk along an uneven path in bare feet (as recommended at Soukya and Kalari Kovilakom): a couple of circumambulations around such a path sends messages from the trigger points on the soles of the feet through the meridian channels to the internal organs. Your body will benefit, even if your feet feel a little painful.

In the same way that soap was eschewed for an *ubtan* scrub to cleanse and purify the body, Ayurvedic physicians and beauty therapists recommend cleaning the feet with a scrub. Not only does this exfoliate dead skin cells, it helps prevent foot odor and fungal and bacterial infections. For a very Indian sensation, try the Masala spice scrub at Taj spas: a boost for the circulation, it promotes deep cleansing. Another winner is the organic thyme and peppermint scrub at Quan spa in Mumbai: when followed by a *marma* massage with *parijat* oil, it leaves the whole body profoundly relaxed.

Left and below The floral footbath is a staple at Indian spas, as it is elsewhere around the globe. Jasmine, rose, frangipani and chrysanthemum blooms are all popular.

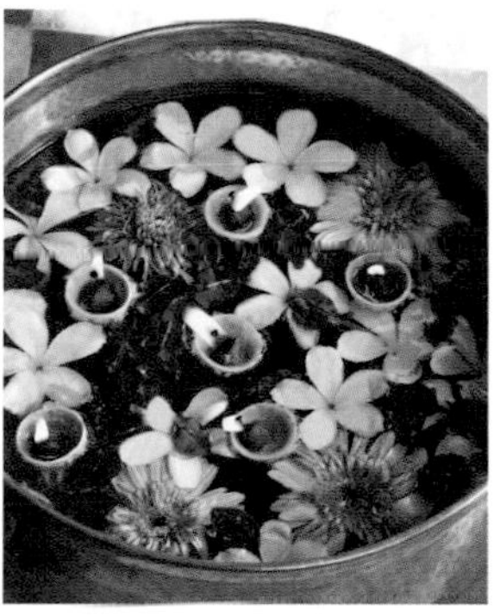

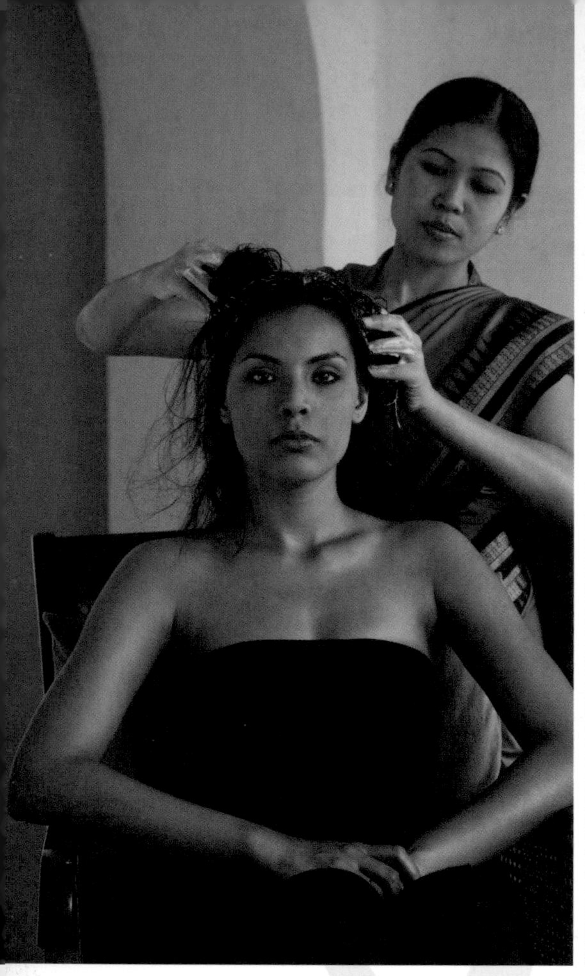
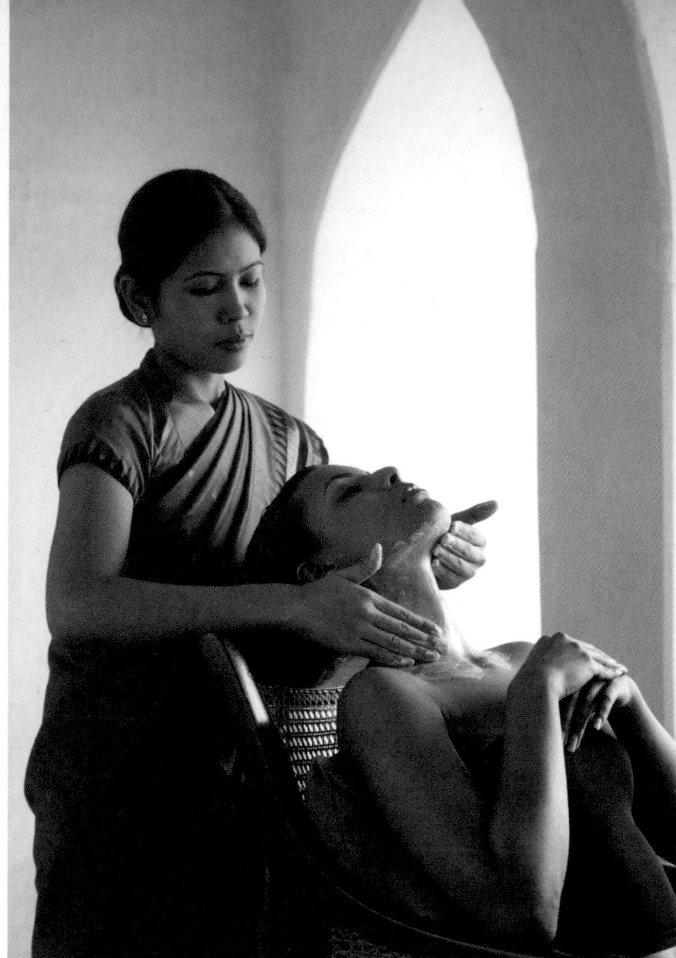
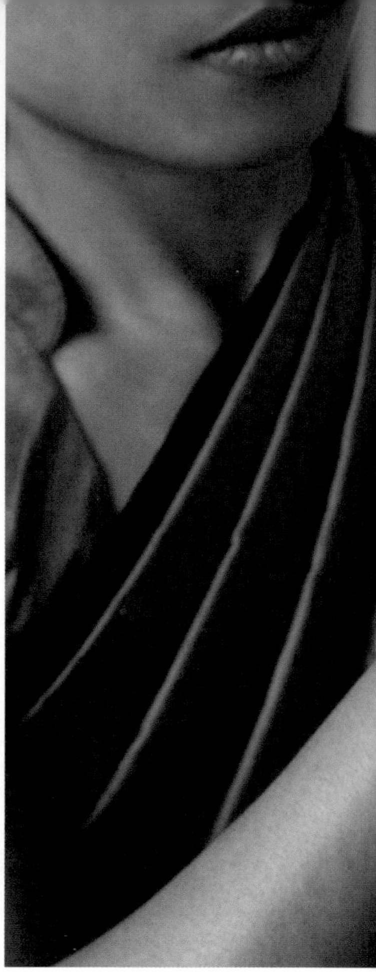

hair care

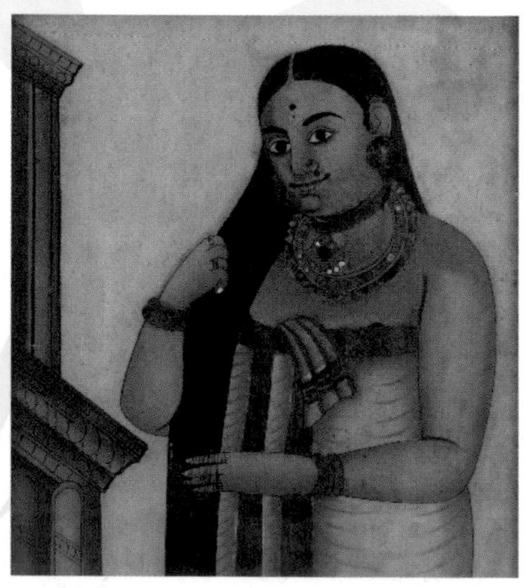

Indian women are renowned for their dark, thick and lustrous locks. Ancient texts contain numerous references to treatments, rinses, lotions, infusions and pastes for beautifying, strengthening and improving hair health, emphasizing how Indians have always prized hair as an integral part of beauty.

In Indian paintings, women are depicted with long hair or ornamented hairstyles, and the pantheon of Hindu goddesses always wear elaborate headgear. Similarly, Indian brides take great pride in their hairstyles, with different areas favoring different styles. The Punjabi bride wears a red *parandi* (a type of silk tassel) in her hair, while Bengali and Maharashtran brides opt for buns decorated with white flowers. Further south in Tamil Nadu, white, orange and pink blossoms are woven around a central plait, while Keralan brides sport a veil of jasmine buds tied to form a net.

In the *Kumarasambhavam*, the famous Sanskrit epic poem by the poet Kalidasa,

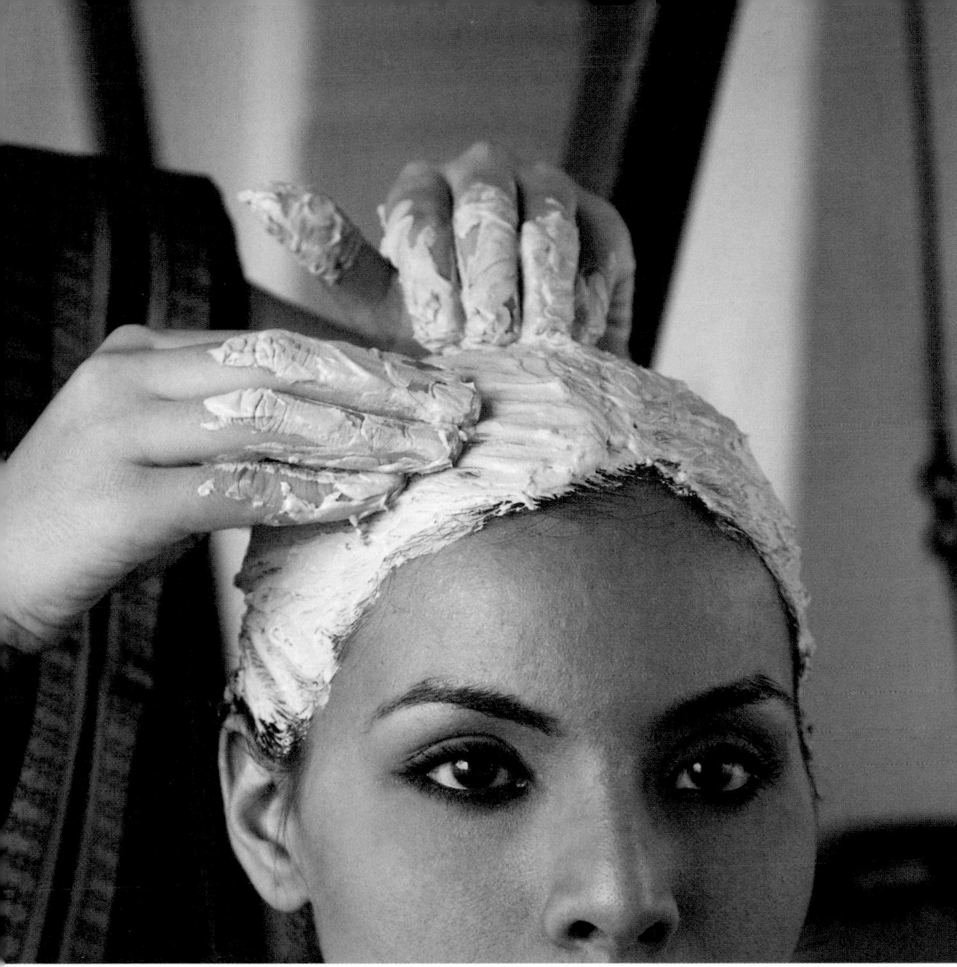

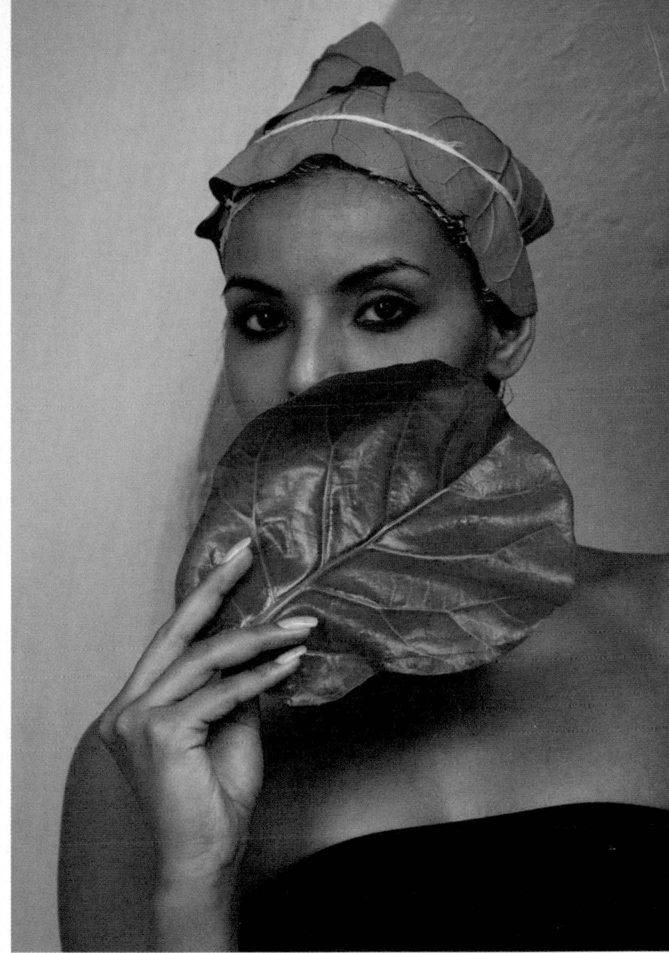

Left below Indian women traditionally sport long tresses as this Keralan portrait on glass illustrates. Often depicting everyday household activities, such paintings were probably introduced to India by the British in the 18th century. Subject matter included religious themes, portraiture, folk art, and more. Their usage was purely decorative.

Above left to right The four steps at Neemrana Fort Palace's sublime *sirolepam* treatment includes a head massage that extends to the face, neck and shoulder areas, a mud and yogurt pack that penetrates deeply into the epidermal layer of the scalp, a shampoo and a final conditioner. Traditionally, hair packs were covered with leaf wraps.

the hair preparations for the goddess Parvati's wedding to Shiva are described in detail: first her maids dried and scented her hair with incense, then they plaited it into a graceful braid, and finally decorated it with inlaid flowers and a garland of *madhuka* flowers woven with *durva* grass.

Scenting the hair with smoke or incense *(dhoop)* while it dries is a tradition that has been practiced by Indian womenfolk for centuries. Burning charcoal, mixed with *sallaki* or frankincense (a powder made from the gum of the *Boswellia serrata* tree), is placed on an earthen or brass tray and wafted beneath long tresses. The ancient equivalent of a hair dryer, it helps with drying after washing, imparts fragrance to the hair and prevents fungal infections, dandruff and other hair problems.

Shampoos were traditionally made from herbal powders, both Ayurvedic and otherwise, and many are still in use today. Popular herbs for cleansing are the highly scented orris root powder, thickening arrowroot powder, purifying *amla*, neem and sandalwood for their antiseptic properties, and *reetha* or soap nut. *Shikakai,* literally "fruit for hair" is another traditional shampoo in the form of a paste: made from *Acacia concinna* bark that contains high levels of saponins or foaming agents, it is a mild cleanser. Whilst the lather is rather weak, it has a naturally low pH, so does not strip hair of its natural oils. It also acts as a de-tangler and is a useful anti-dandruff tool.

Another ancient custom for healthy hair and scalp often given on a daily basis is an Indian head massage (see page 26). Less time intensive is a quick application of

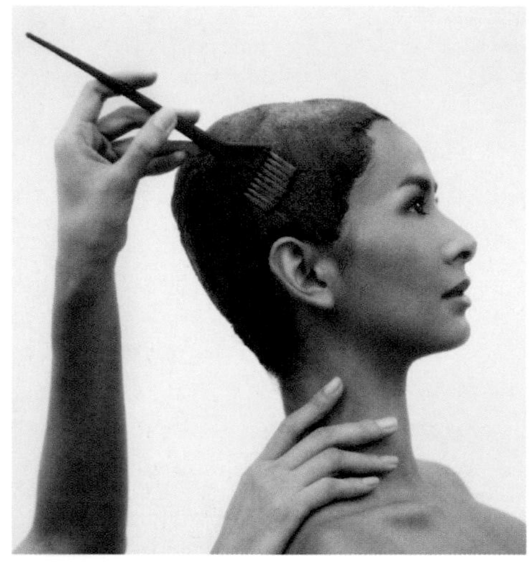

Above Regenerating for hair and stimulating for the scalp, a henna conditioning treatment is a staple at many Indian beauty salons. After application, the paste rests on the head for half an hour, then is washed off with lukewarm water.

hair oil: there are literally hundreds of such oils on the market as Indians believe that they help hair grow luxuriantly thick, soft and glossy. In addition, they are supposed to soothe and invigorate the sense organs and even remove wrinkles from the face! Popular hair oils contain *bhringaraj*, *brahmi* and *amla*, often combined with other strengthening, conditioning and antiseptic herbs and plants.

A plant much used in Indian hair care is *mehndi* or henna (*Lawsonia inermis*). Antiseptic and nutritious, it is a popular hair conditioner and gives grey hair a red-orange tint. It has the ability to coat the hair shaft, thereby protecting and thickening hair. "One of India's age-old beauty secrets is a henna conditioner," says herbal beauty advocate, Shahnaz Husain, "Made from henna paste, mixed with lemon juice, egg and yogurt, it cleanses and conditions hair, promotes new hair growth and restores

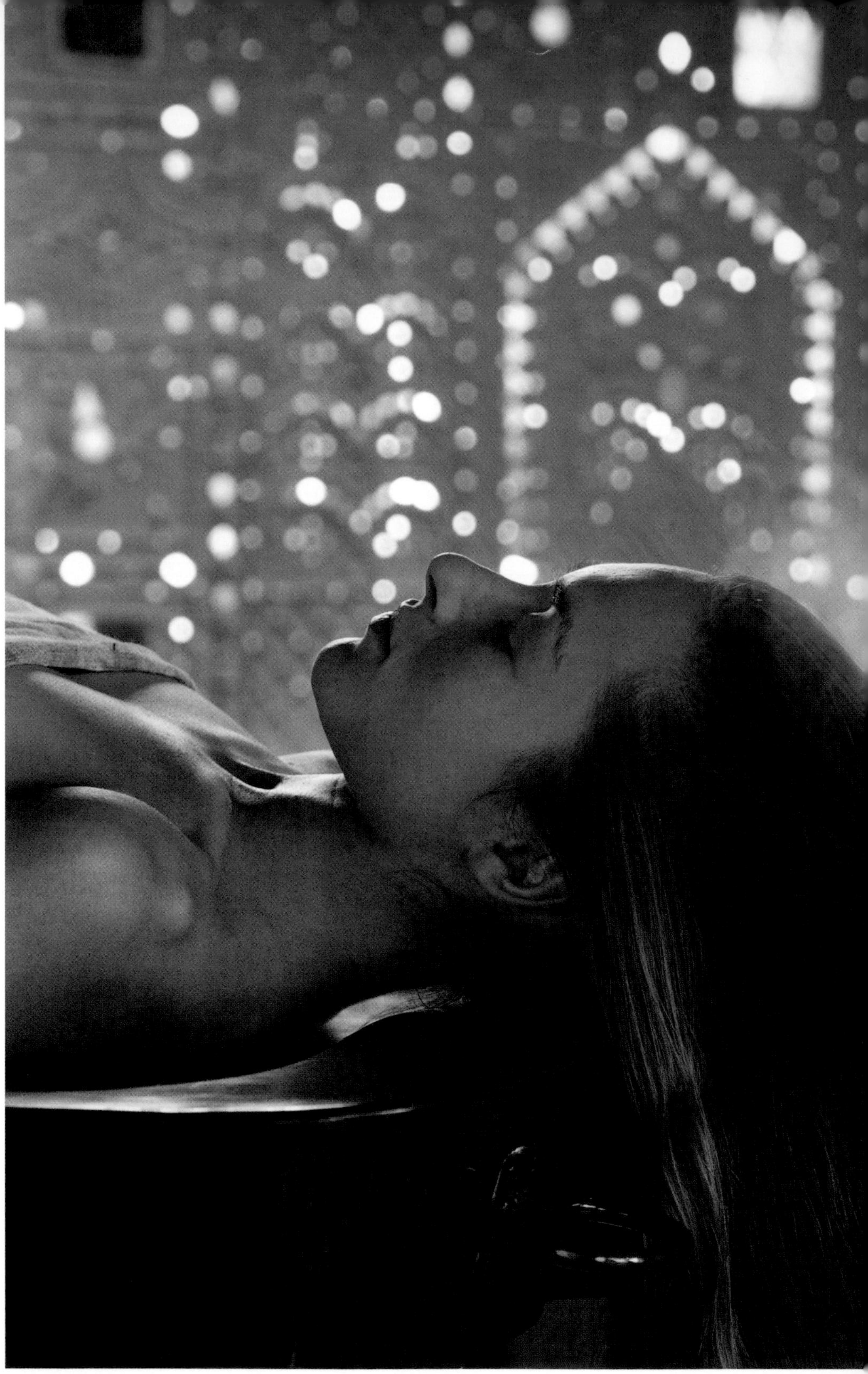

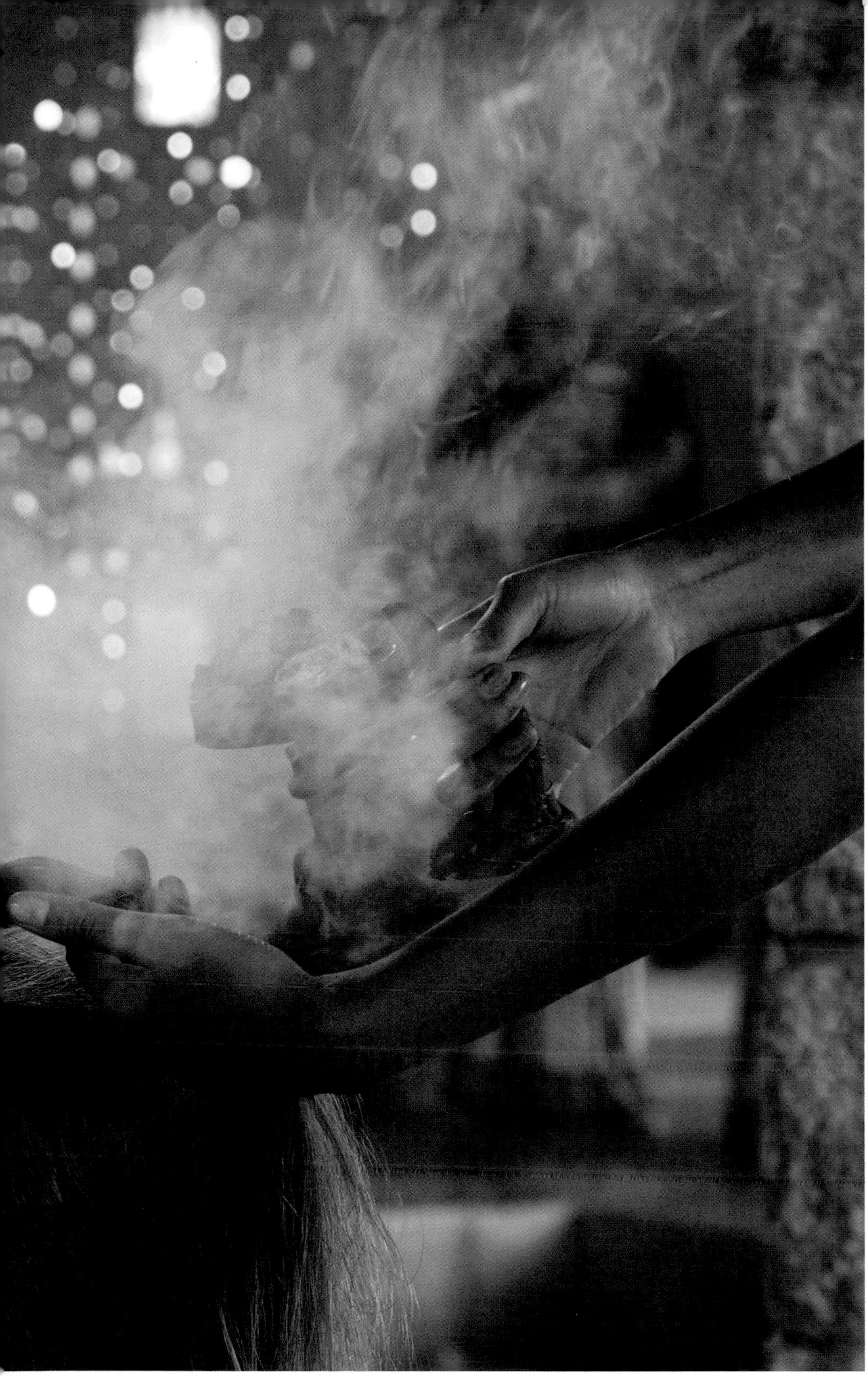

Left The resin of the *Boswellia serrata* tree is collected in a manner similar to rubber tapping; the harvested gum is then ground into a powder and used in a charcoal burner to scent the hair. More commonly known as frankincense, the powder is also used in religious rites and perfumery.

good health to the scalp." She goes on to add that, unlike chemical detergents, it doesn't destroy the natural acid nature of the scalp and leaves hair shiny and supple. Essential oil of henna is also very cooling on the head.

A variety of hair cleansing and conditioning routines are available at Shahnaz Husain salons and day spas — and over-the-counter conditioners, rinses and tonics are plentiful in her 100 percent herbal range. Many other Indian spas offer the sublime head massage, often as part of a face or body ritual, and a wonderful treat for dry, dehydrated and sensitive scalp and hair is the Ananda's aromatic hot oil treatment with pure essence of lavender, geranium and rosemary.

For a four-pronged treat, Neemrana Spa's heavenly *sirolepam* is a must: Taken from the words, *siro* meaning "head" and *lepam* translating as "pack", the treatment (see photos on previous page) includes a head, neck, face and shoulder massage along with a head pack to stimulate hair growth and revitalize the brain.

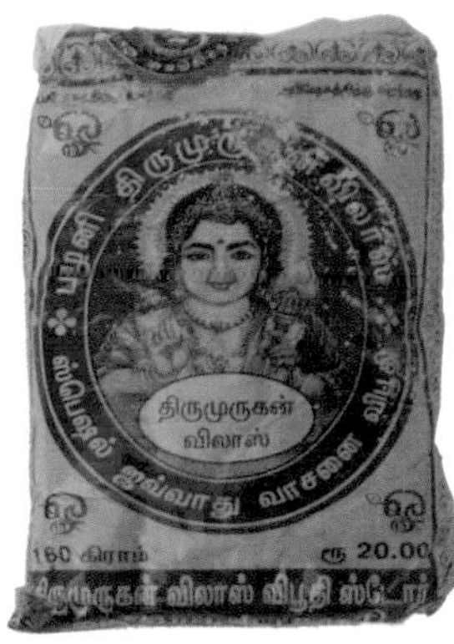

the art of mehndi

The application of *mehndi* (henna) as a colorant on hair, hands and nails is a time-honored tradition in India. With its origins in Egypt, *mehndi* was also extensively used in the Middle East, probably as a cooling device. Coming from the *Lawsonia inermis* shrub, it is known as *madayantika* in Sanskrit. The small leaves, crushed into a powder and mixed with water and a little bit of sugar, makes a dark green paste that turns orange when applied to the skin.

Mehndi has anti-irritant, deodorant and antiseptic properties, and is used by Ayurvedic physicians for skin irritations such as heat rashes and skin allergies. The paste is also used as an antidote against heat and sunstroke and, in the past, the leaves were applied to bring down high fevers. Today, it may be applied to the body during the intense heat of the day, and people embarking on a long walk often apply it on the soles of feet. Because of its cooling properties, *mehndi* leaves and flowers are made into lotions and ointments that are used externally for boils, burns, bruises and skin inflammations. Antiseptic and nutritious to the head also, it is used as a hair conditioner and gives grey hair a red/orange tint.

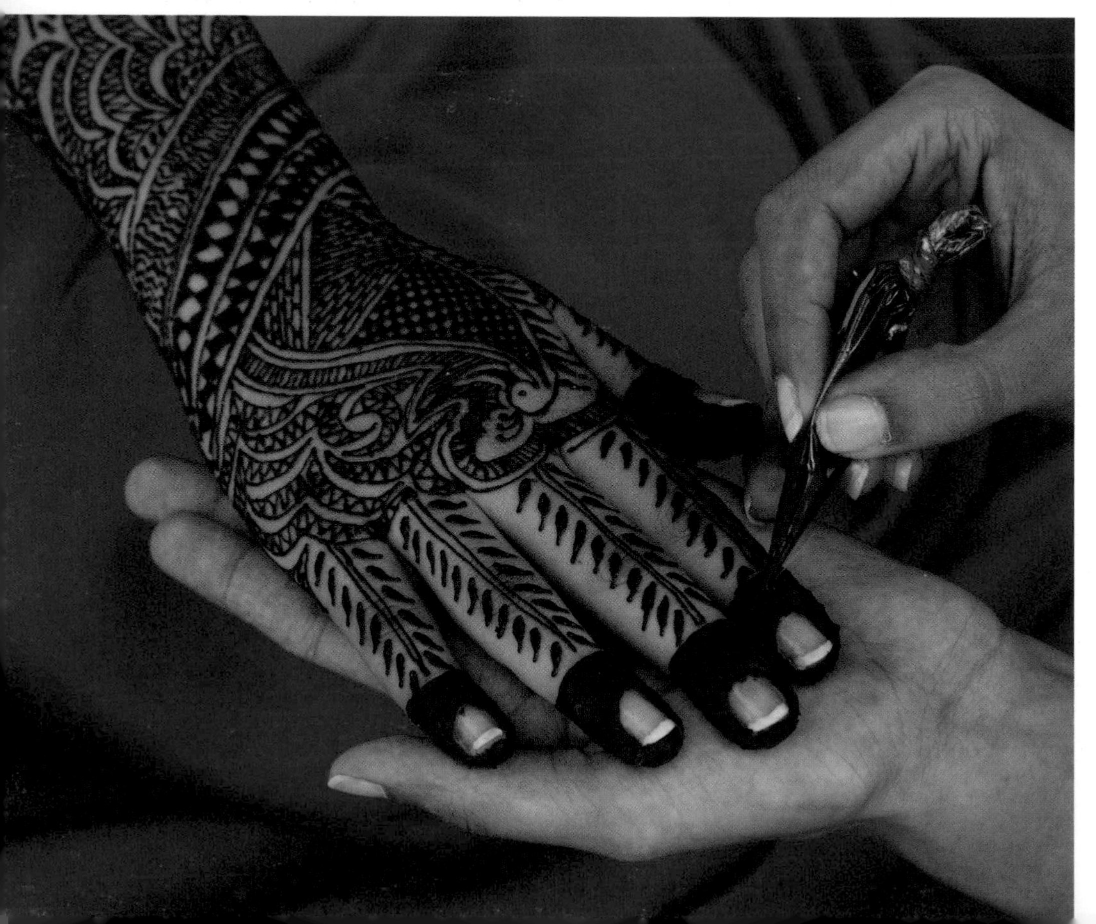

Historically, there are many references to this versatile plant. The Muslim prophet Mohammed used *mehndi* for healing and he also dyed his hair and beard with it. It is recorded in the *Qu'ran* that his wife and daughters used henna for decoration on occasions such as Eid celebrations and weddings. Some Muslim girls are named after the *mehndi* plant. Its small intensely fragrant white flowers make a wonderfully strong-smelling perfume that is favored by both men and women.

Over time, henna developed into a popular beauty aid, and the application of *mehndi* in intricate patterns on palms and feet is still an integral part of both Muslim and Hindu marriage ceremonies. It is considered a sign of love — the darker the coloration, the greater the love of the groom for the bride.

Sometimes, the *mehndi* is applied with the name of the husband-to-be hidden in the pattern; if he can't find it, he has to pay a forfeit! Often applied with the singing of songs, there are multiple patterns, most of which have cultural associations. In Rajasthan where these photos were taken, patterns typically have lines of v-shaped leaves, peacock feather patterning, a *bhandhej* (tie-dye) pattern, little acacia leaves and a *laheria* pattern (this literally

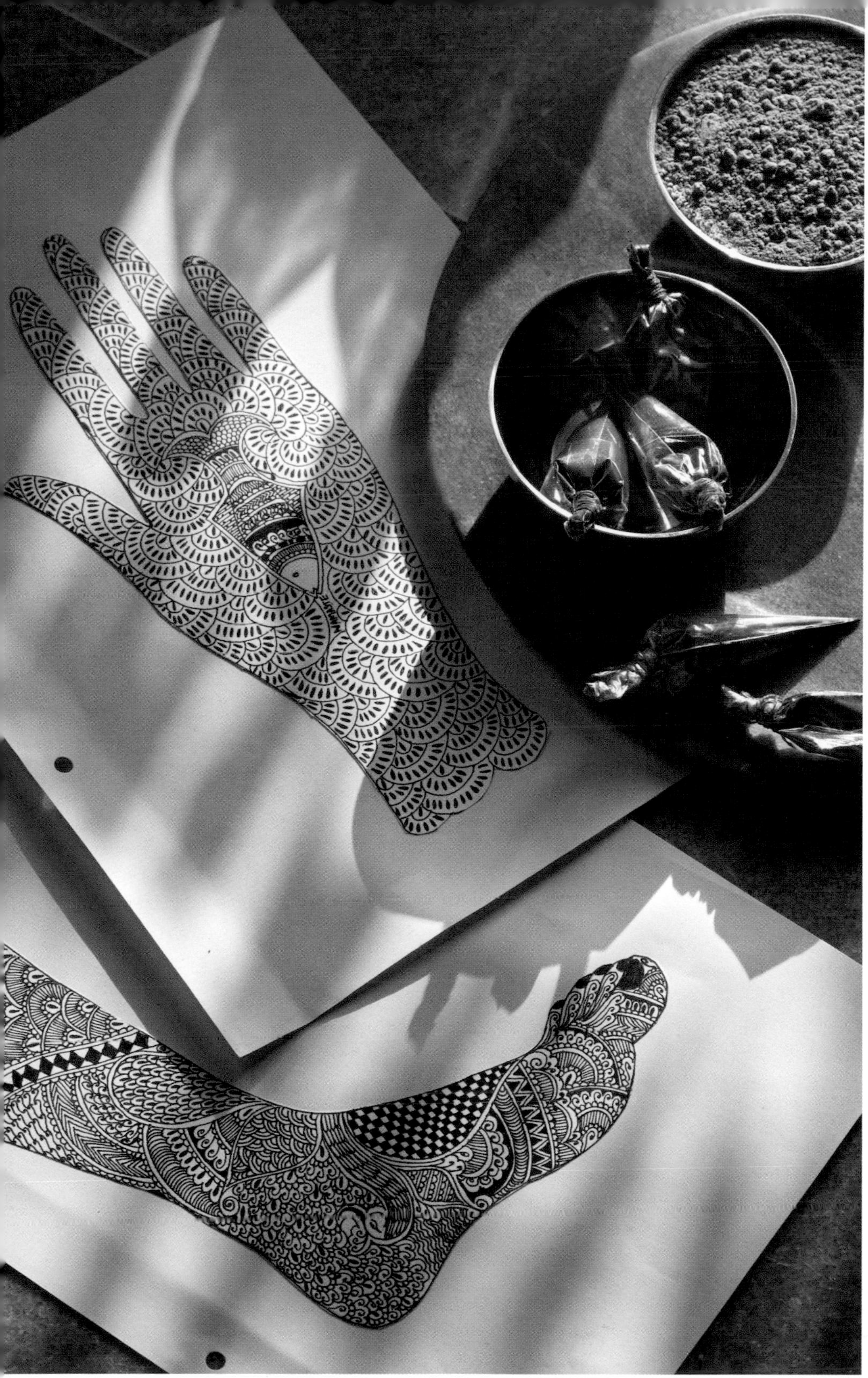

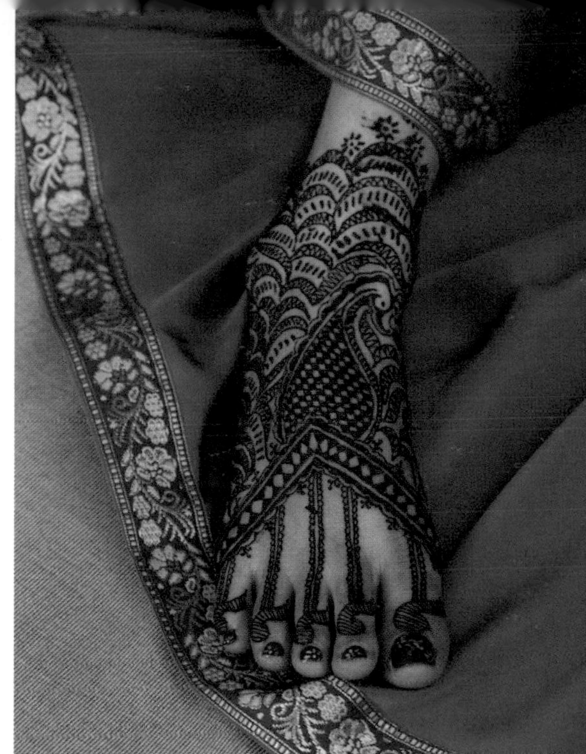

Drawings, powder, paste and examples of henna patterns on hands and feet photographed at the resort of Amanbagh in Rajasthan. The spa manager at the Aman spa there learned the art of *mehndi* application from her grandmother: Using a cone similar to the type of apparatus used for icing a cake, she painted hands and feet in intricate patterns. Different henna patterns indicate different geographical locations and cultural associations.

translates as "waves of the sea" and is found in geometric or floral patterns on brightly colored Rajasthani saris).

It isn't only at marriages that women decorate their hands and feet with *mehndi*. Many other festivals offer an excuse for girls to dress up and adorn themselves, and, increasingly, variations of traditional patterns may be applied as tattoo-type insignias on other parts of the body. Many visitors to India try a henna decoration at least once. As it is a safe, painless and non-permanent alternative form of body ornamentation that is gaining favor in the West, nowadays you'll find henna artists in popular tourist destinations such as beach resorts and bazaars all over India.

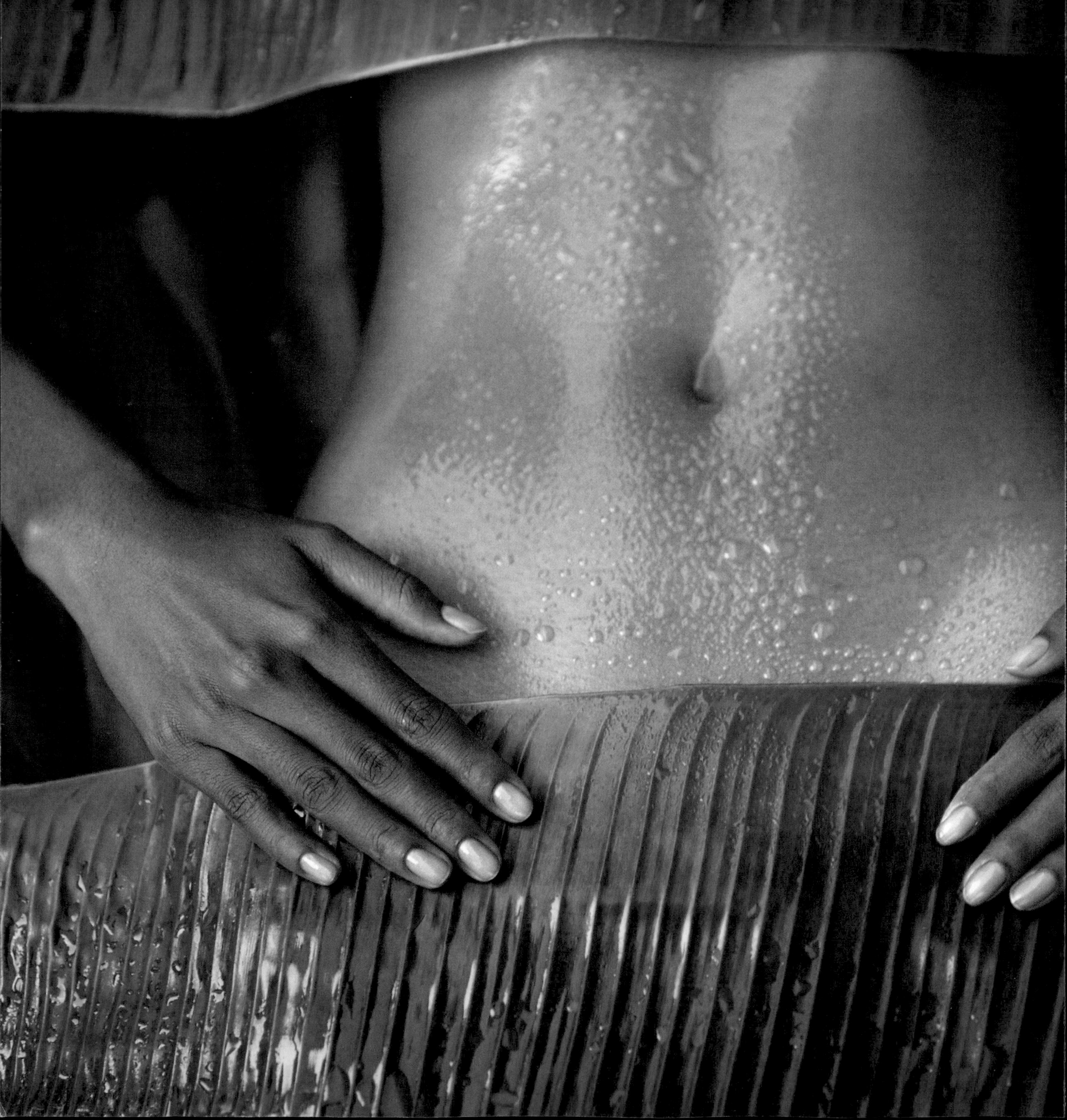

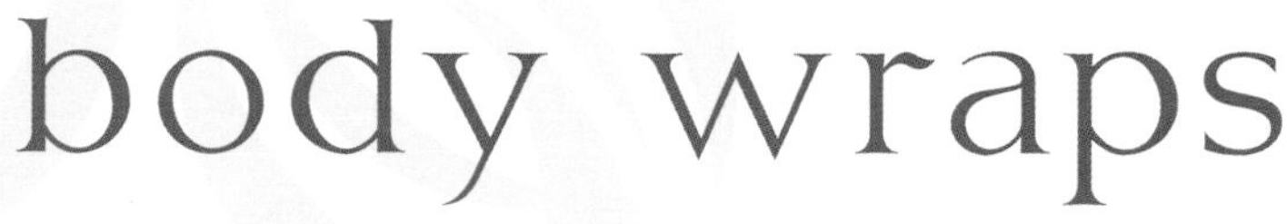

body wraps

There is something immensely comforting about lying swaddled in cloth, plastic or blankets while a warming, detoxifying paste is doing its work on your body. With its roots in Indian bridal tradition, as brides always have a wrap daily for a week prior to their wedding day, the body wrap in India employs a variety of ingredients. From fruits to flowers, herbs, spices and clays, a body wrap can be deeply nurturing.

Whatever the wrap components, the idea is that the warmth of the wrap allows ingredients to penetrate subcutaneously through the pores of skin. Some wraps are prescribed for their preventative and curative properties against cold and cough; others are used to alleviate muscle aches, headaches and fever. Others use minerals and ingredients from the ocean such as seaweed to encourage lymphatic drainage. All aim to increase blood circulation, encourage sweating to draw out unwanted toxins, cleanse internally and on the body's surface, and leave skin soft and glowing.

In a spa, a polish or scrub may precede a wrap: as skin has been freshly exfoliated, it is in an optimum condition to receive the properties of the wrap. We outline some innovate wrap solutions:

In the past, large leaves were used for wrapping, as they encouraged sweating, thereby removing toxins from beneath the skin's surface. Here, shiny banana leaves have been used effectively; in today's spas, these have largely been replaced by plastic, cloth, towels or cling wrap.

Ancient Indian Body Mask

Ananda spa, high in the mountains above the ashram town of Rishikesh, utilizes its natural pollutant-free environment with ingredients close to hand in this deeply cleansing ritual. First a combination of herbal roots with pure Himalayan spring water is applied to the body to slough off dead cells and prepare the body for the therapeutic clay application to come. This is followed by a *Multani mitti* total body mask; spiced with turmeric, sandal or other powders, it is applied evenly over the body which is then wrapped in a sheet. Whilst the mask works its magic, the client receives a facial pressure point massage. Pure bliss.

Anna Lepanam

Based on a clinical therapy from Kerala that was formulated for muscle strain and fractures, this skin-conditioning traditional treatment is called Navara *theppu* (*theppu* translates as "paste application"). The ingredients include Navara rice and a *bala* root decoction and, when the paste is applied to the affected area for 30–45 minutes daily for a period of 21 to 28 days, the healing ingredients penetrate deep into the skin and help to activate muscles after a serious bone fracture.

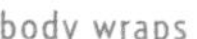

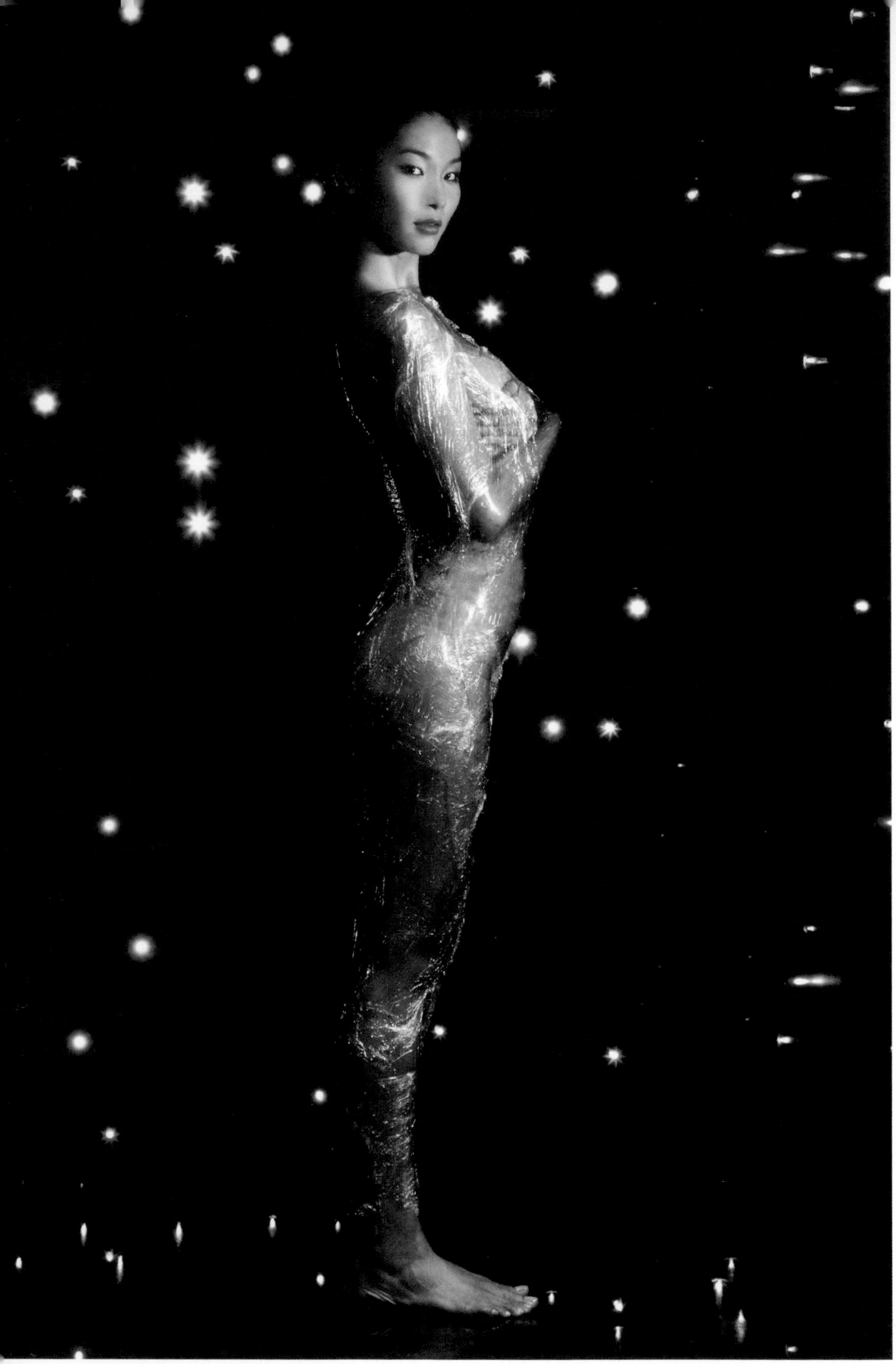

Left and below Wild mint and Nilgiri honey are used in a purifying mask at Aura spa, Park New Delhi. Spa director Megha Dinesh explains how it works: "The wrap is designed to minimize air supply to the skin so the body temperature rises, pores open, toxins are released through sweat and the wrap's contents are absorbed."

In an amended treatment at the spa at Rajvilas, Navara rice, milk and a *bala* root decoction are combined with turmeric powder, fenugreek seed powder and sandalwood powder into a gruel-like paste that is applied all over the body. The guest is then invited to lie wrapped in warm towels for about 20 minutes. Considered excellent for firming and contouring the body, it helps increase skin elasticity and flexibility of the joints.

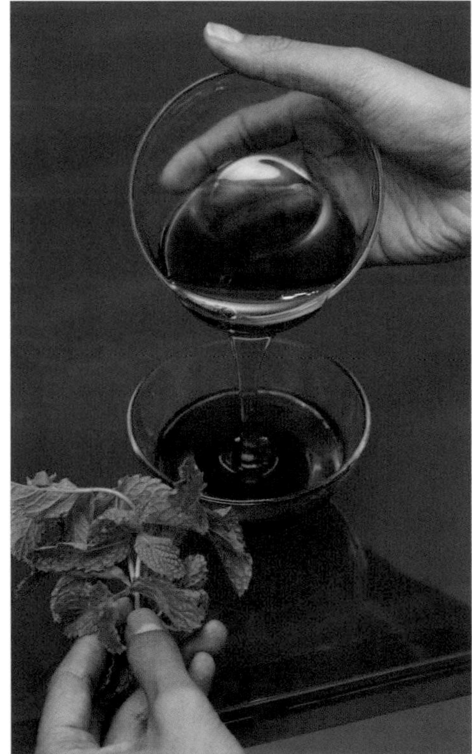

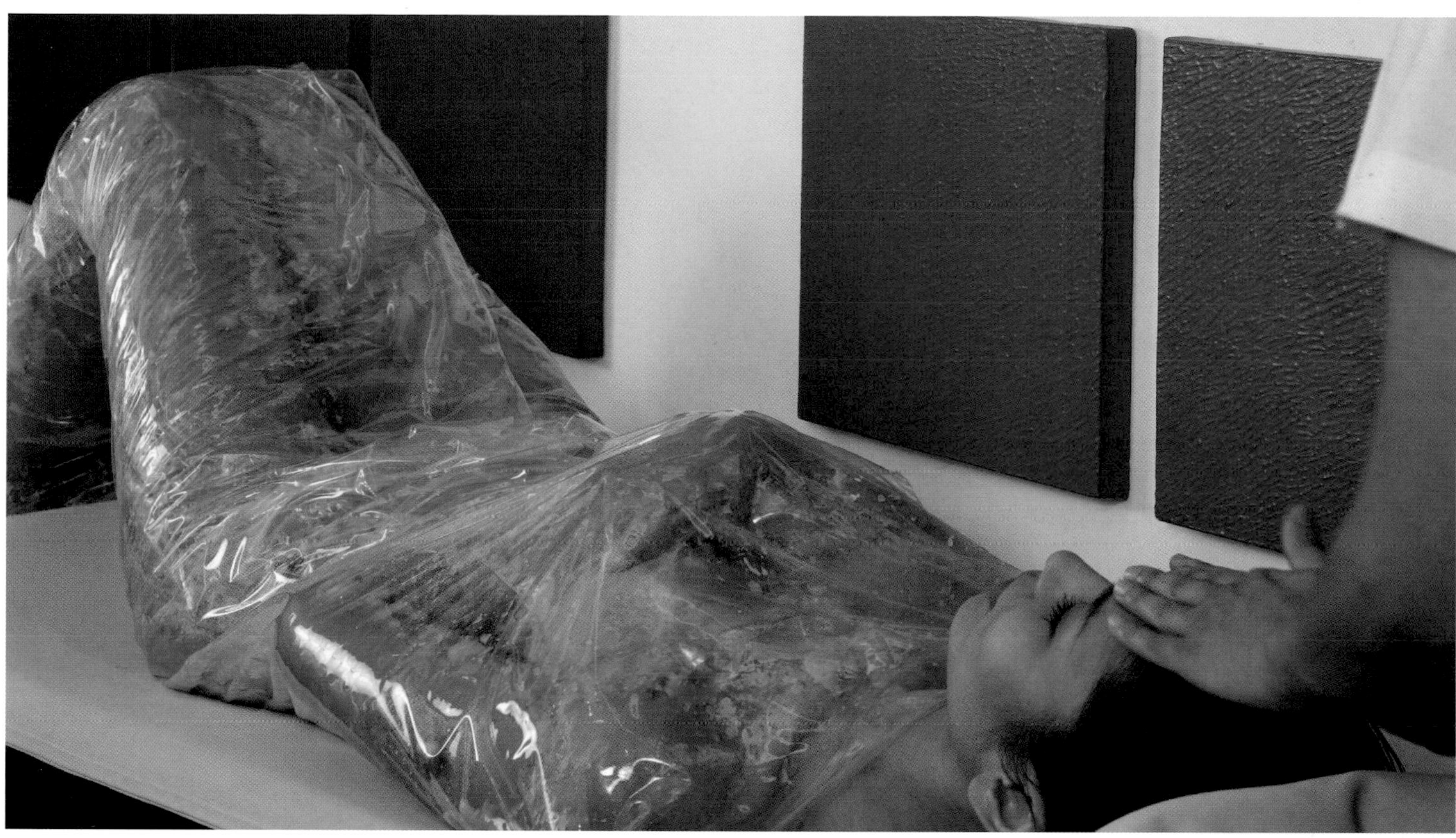

Enzyme-rich papaya is mildly exfoliating, so it removes flaking skin cells from the surface of the skin, making the body softer and smoother. When enclosed in cling wrap, the heat encourages the papaya to work in the subcutaneous layers too. You'll be amazed how skin texture is significantly improved afterwards.

Papaya Pamper

The beneficial effects of papain, the main enzyme contained in papaya, have been well documented. A popular meat tenderizer, it is also used as a home remedy for stings and bites as it has the ability to break down protein toxins. In beauty therapy, it is popular for its ability to fracture and remove cosmetic blemishes, skin secretions and dead skin cells. In keeping with their tradition of using fresh ingredients in treatments, Aura spas at Park Hotels offer a wonderful fruity papaya body wrap that is preceded by an oatmeal scrub. Ideal for sensitive skin, it leaves the body tingling and skin glowing after.

Saffron Secrets

Before Indian independence, when the princely states were at the height of their powers, certain ingredients were retained for the women of the Courts: rose petals were out of the range of mere mortals, and saffron — rare, expensive and golden — was drunk with milk by pregnant Maharanis in the belief that any progeny would be born with a golden, light complexion. Whether this worked or not is anyone's guess, but certainly its cost would have been prohibitive to ordinary people.

Nowadays, you'll find saffron in plenty of spa recipes and the Aman wrap at the spa at Amanbagh is a case in point. Consisting of a local clay and water mix with hibiscus, rose and saffron, it is applied all over the body directly after a 10-minute steam. As pores on the skin's surface will have opened up after the steam, the skin is super receptive to the healing and scenting properties of the ingredients. As the client lies, cocooned in clay and wrapped in a heavy towel, the therapist keeps contact with a gentle head massage for further relaxation.

body scrubs and polishes

Found not only in India, but in many countries worldwide, scrubs and polishes are wonderfully enlivening. In India, herbal or other natural ingredients (usually of an abrasive, but gently abrasive, nature) are combined with oil and massaged all over the body to increase circulation, open pores, boost metabolism and open the skin to receive the properties contained within the polish. A polish also exfoliates the skin's surface of dead cells that build up on the outer layer; these tend to give dull skin tone, so a polish literally does as it says. Skin is always smoother, brighter and more translucent after an exfoliating polish.

Scrubs and polishes can also be helpful for people with cellulite, although they do not constitute a miracle cure. Lumpy pockets of cellulite — unsightly deposits of water, fat and other wastes — build up on thighs, buttocks, hips and upper arms and not only look unattractive, but are difficult to dissipate. It is believed that these toxins and wastes become "trapped" within hardened connective tissue in cells — so releasing them is not easy. A healthy diet, a strong lymphatic system, regular exercise and vigorous skin "brushing" can all help.

Rich in minerals, clay polishes skin as it both draws impurities and toxins from deep within the body and smoothes surface texture. As it retains temperature, clay can be applied either cool or heated for different effects. This clay mix benefits from the addition of saffron, so the skin is nourished and revitalized too.

Traditionally, Indians used dry powder scrubs and polishes to reduce water retention and improve the elimination of waste products. Made from gram flour and oatmeal, found in most kitchens, it is called an *ubtan* scrub. Given to every Hindu bride to exfoliate, cleanse and symbolize the end of one life and the beginning of another, *ubtan* can be found all over the country. Clay is another popular product: Black clay is traditionally used in Rajasthan to both nourish and tighten skin and is applied externally on skin diseases. It is also used to wash the hair.

At Quan Spa at the JW Marriott Mumbai, the choice of body polishes and scrubs reads like a geographical tour of the Indian subcontinent. Usually offered in conjunction with another treatment — namely a wrap to infuse substances into the body system, a massage to improve circulation and also allow herbal oils to do their work in the deep tissues, a steam or a Vichy shower — they are deeply nourishing. Many have been composed with Indian ingredients and perfumes, and, whilst the

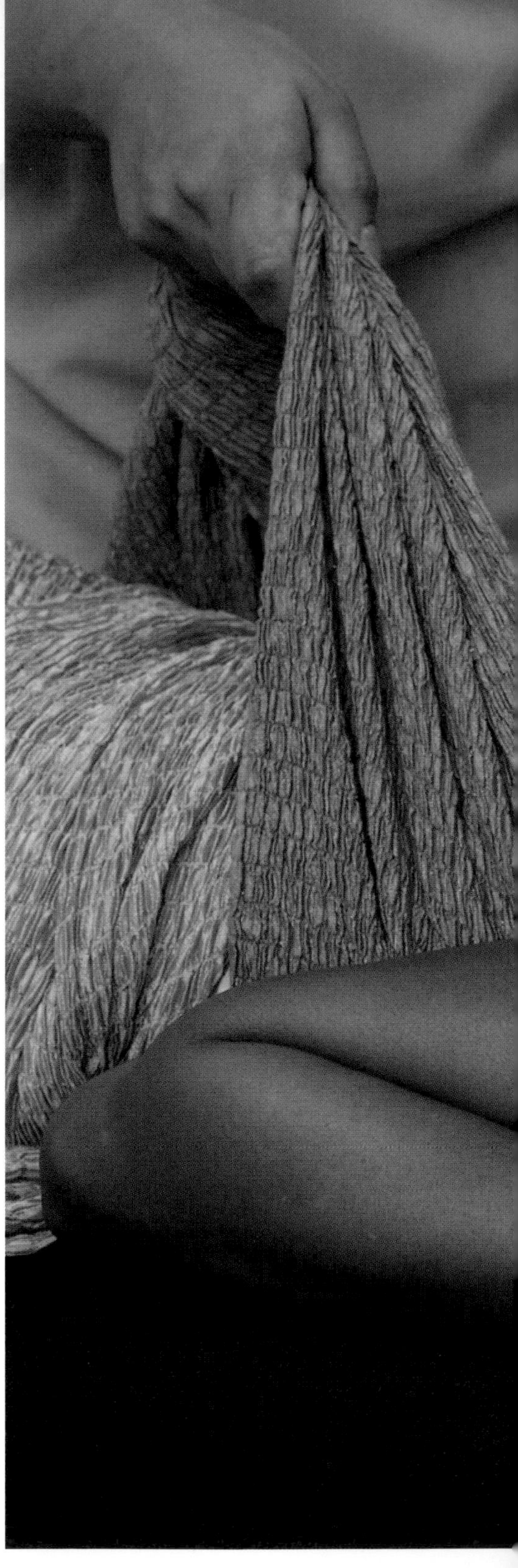

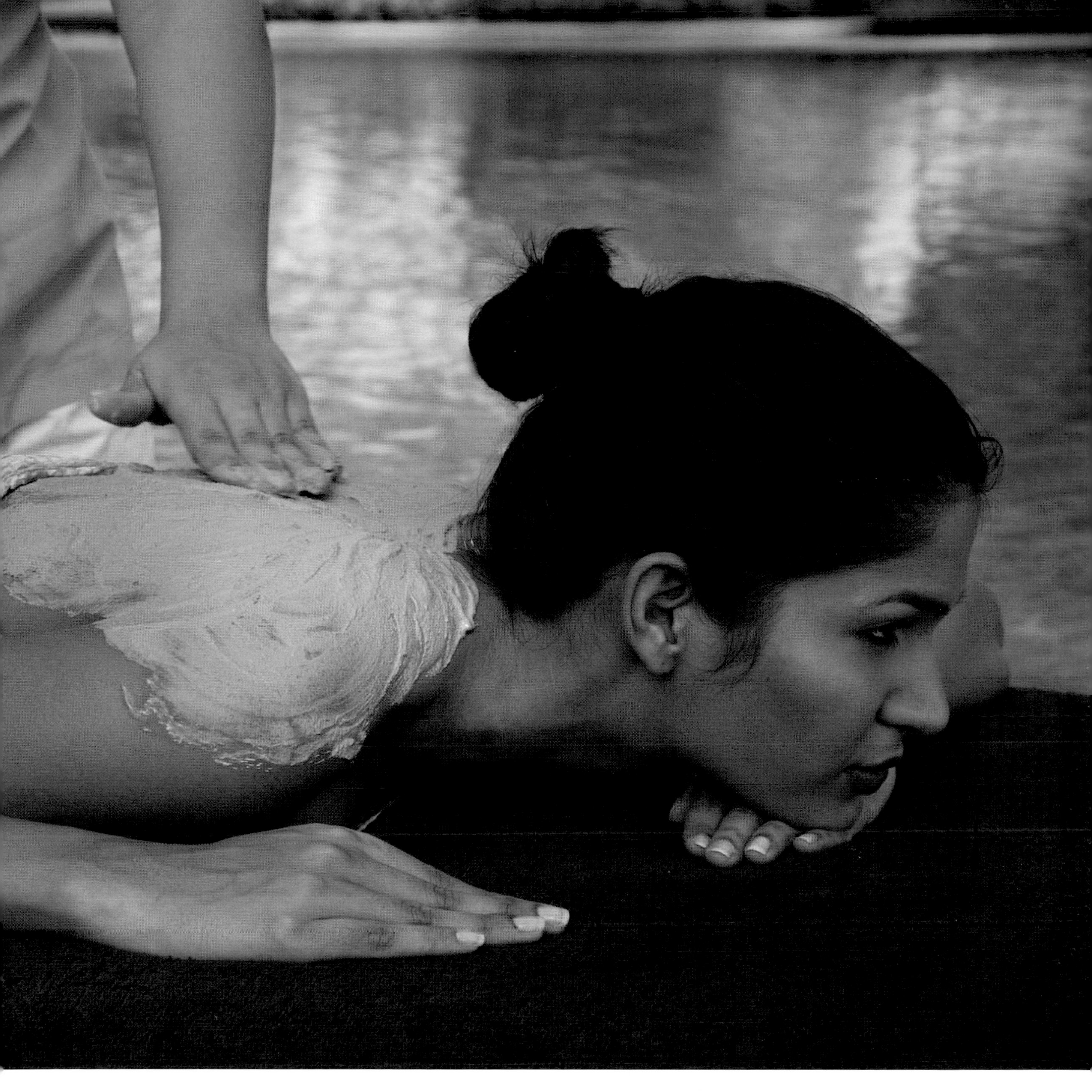

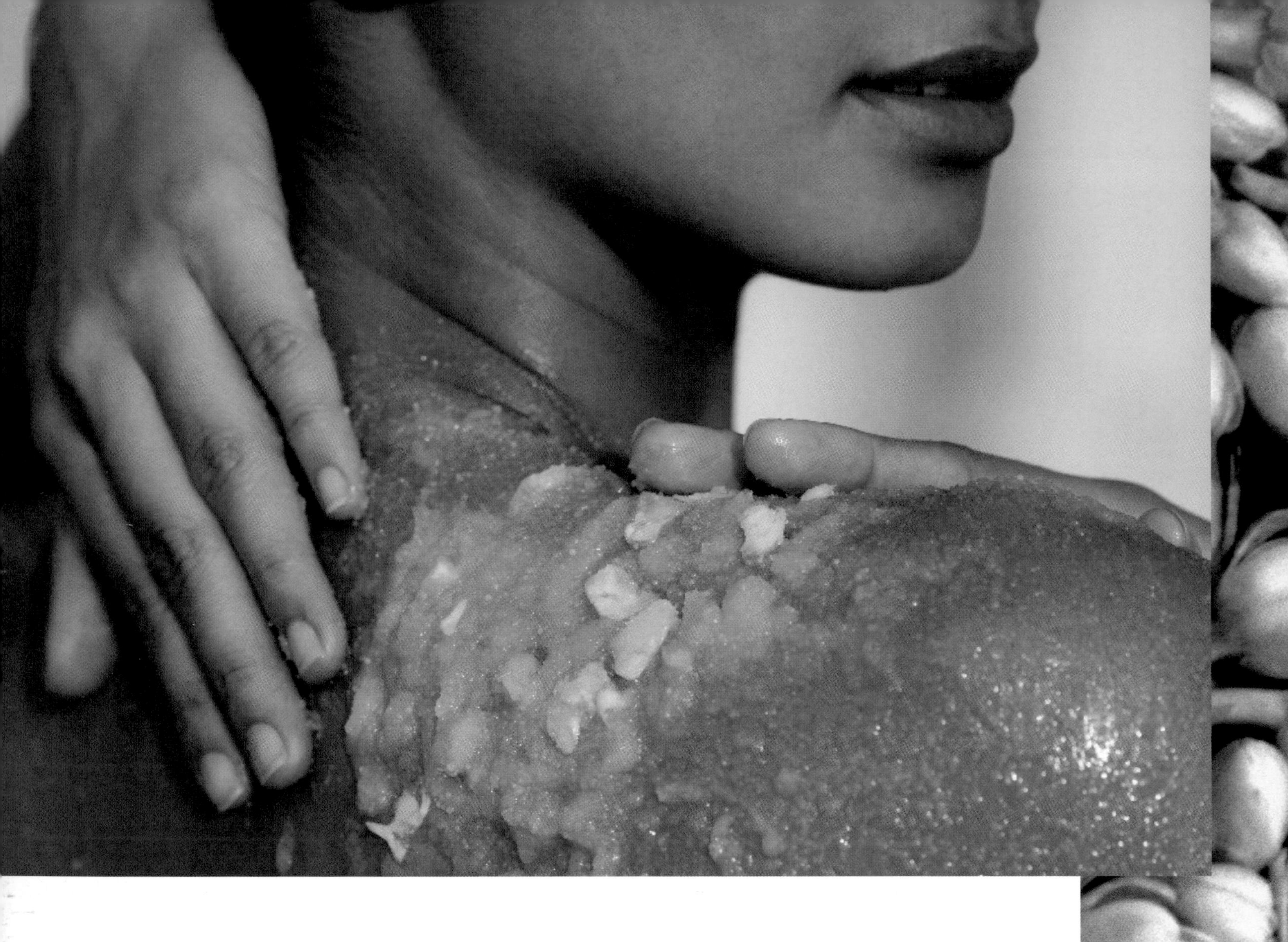

guest may choose which scent or ingredient he or she is drawn to, a high-quality herbal oil is chosen to suit individual *doshas*. Choose from the alluring menu below:

Allepey Body Polish: Drawing inspiration from the backwaters of Kerala, this is a coconut and cardamom combo that is antioxidant and full of nutrients.

Kollegal Body Polish: The Kollegal region has been India's source of sandalwood for centuries, so antiseptic, cooling sandalwood is combined here with high-mineral content mud, for an energizing, cleansing experience.

Madurai Body Polish: The temple town of Madurai in Tamil Nadu forms the backdrop for this polish; jasmine-scented oils, along with the lighting of oil lamps and ringing of bells, anoint the body for a balancing, aromatic journey.

Malabar Body Polish: India's Malabar coast was the port of call for Arab traders in their sturdy *dhows*, so this polish takes its name and ingredients from the Spice Trade; combined with a cooling lentil exfoliant to moderate the heat of the spices used, it is intense and warming.

Above Natural sea salt is used in many body polishes as it removes dry skin, increases circulation and leaves the body smooth and soft. It also re-mineralizes beneath the skin's surface, so is detoxifying and invigorating at the same time. This polish is mixed with jasmine petals and jasmine essential oil for an alluring Indian scent.

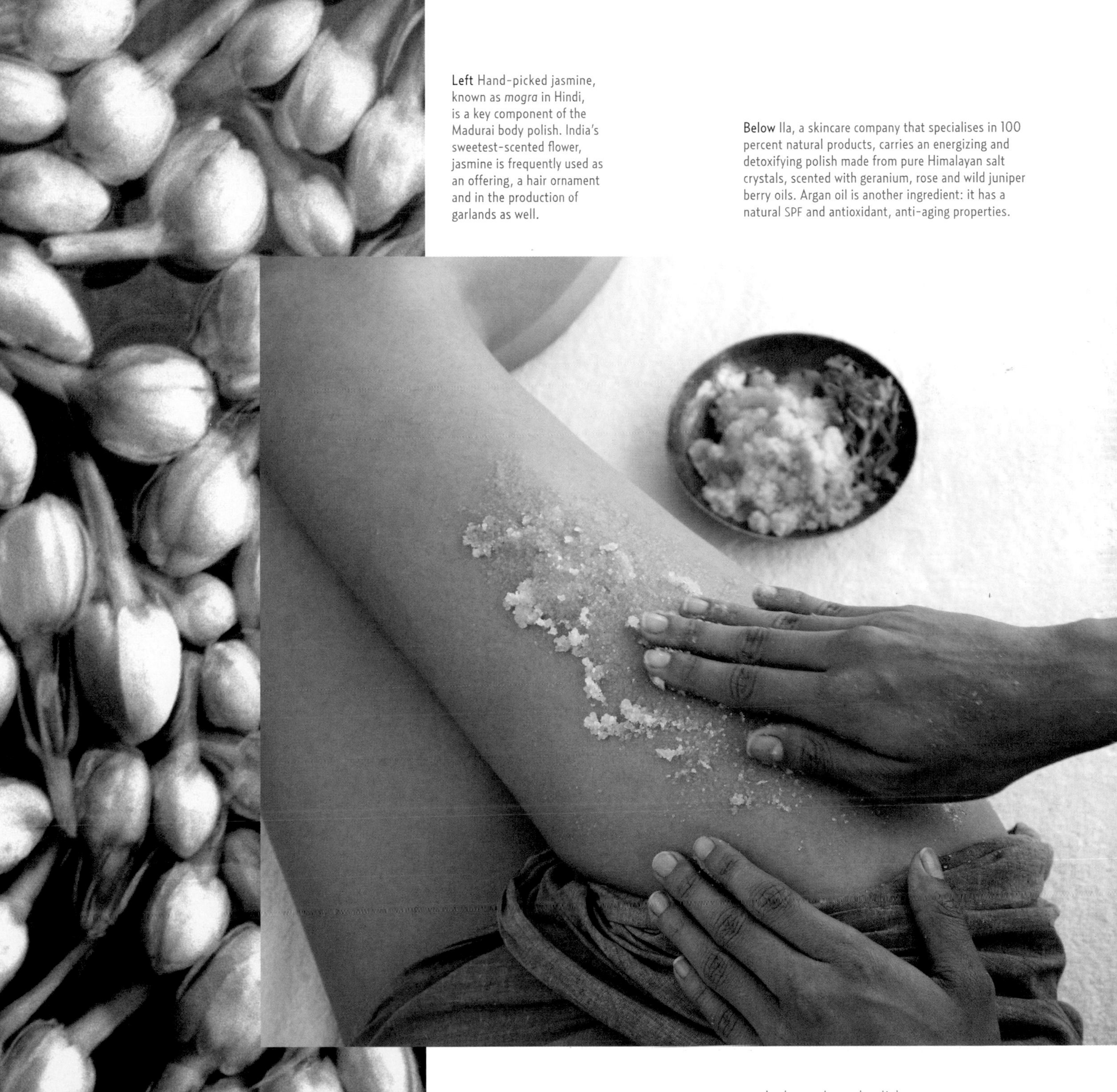

Left Hand-picked jasmine, known as *mogra* in Hindi, is a key component of the Madurai body polish. India's sweetest-scented flower, jasmine is frequently used as an offering, a hair ornament and in the production of garlands as well.

Below Ila, a skincare company that specialises in 100 percent natural products, carries an energizing and detoxifying polish made from pure Himalayan salt crystals, scented with geranium, rose and wild juniper berry oils. Argan oil is another ingredient: it has a natural SPF and antioxidant, anti-aging properties.

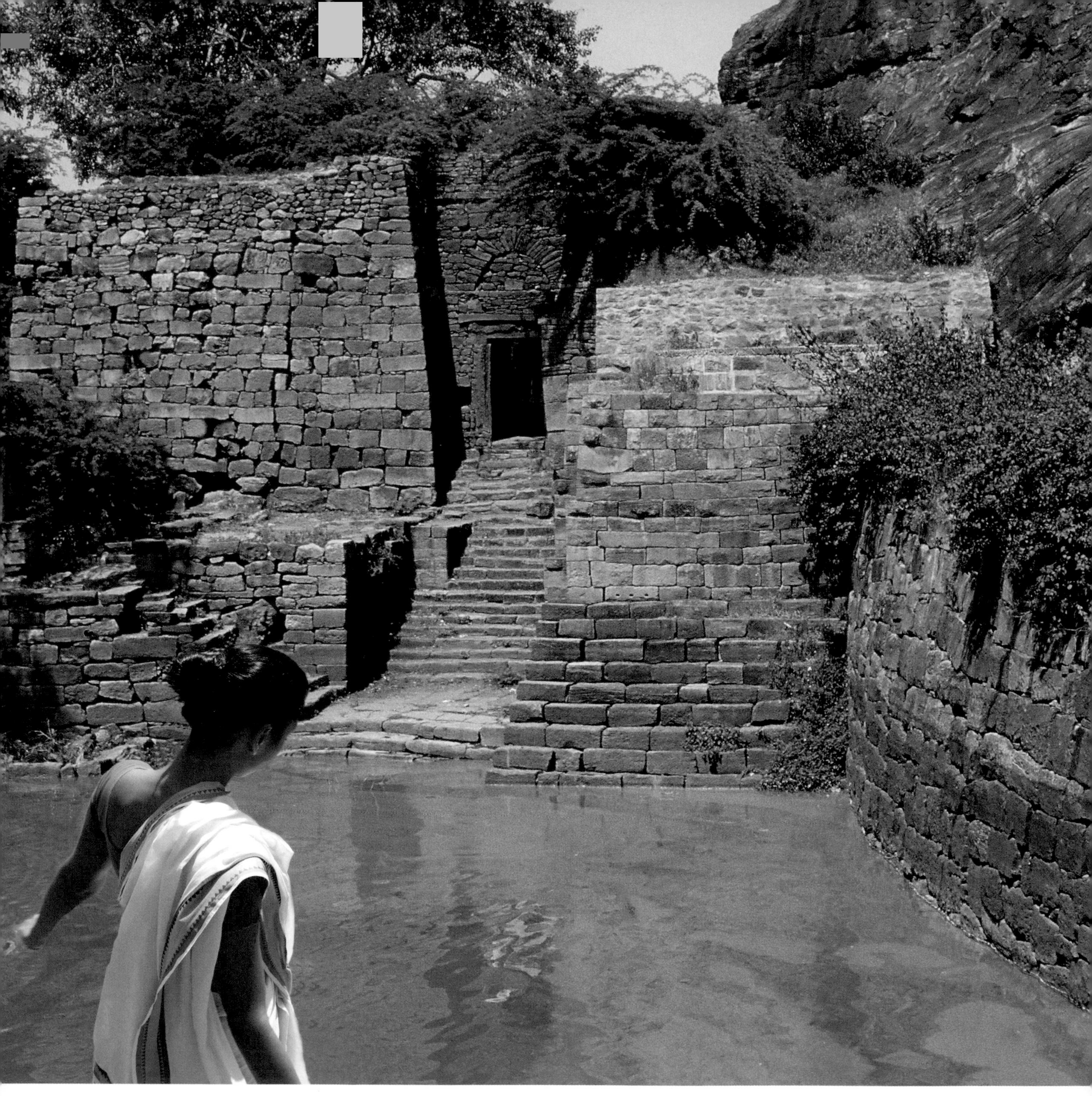

BEAUTY

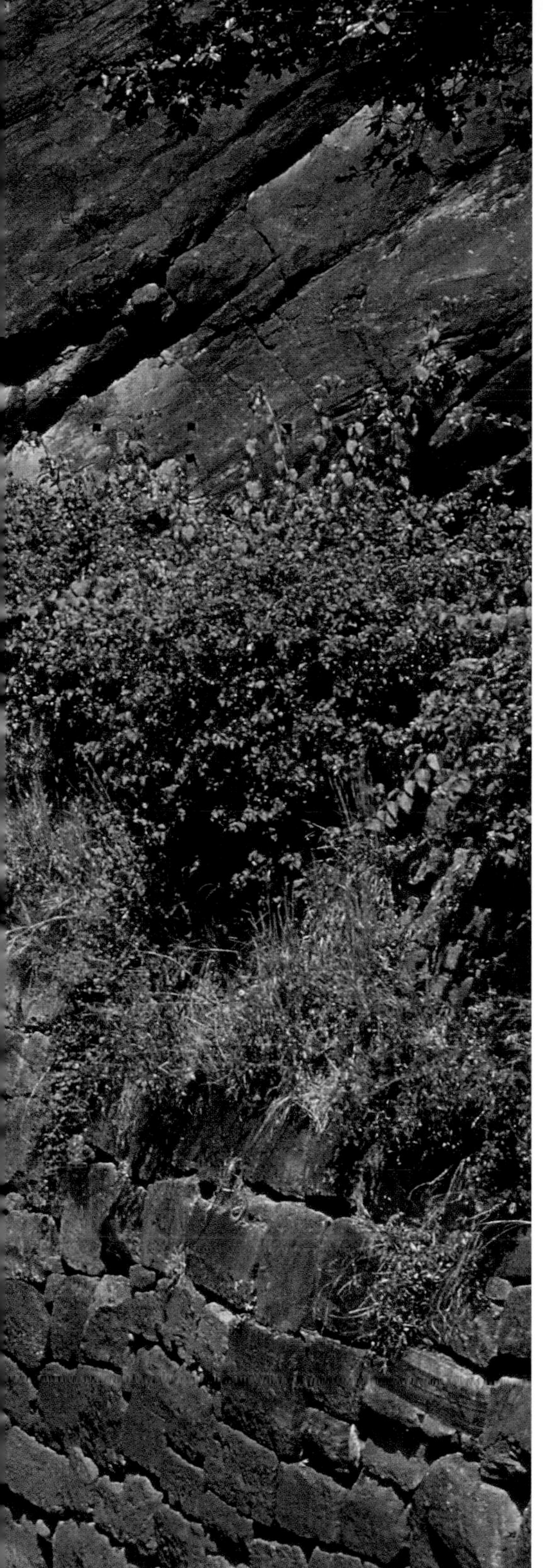

water therapies

Bathing traditions are widespread and deep-seated in Indian culture. For Hindus, ritual bathing is seen as a holy purification rite: Whether it is the washing of hands before a meal or a trip to a holy river, a dip in water is necessarily imbued with significance. Pilgrimages always involve absolution by water in one way or another as well. Muslims, too, use water rituals for both healing and purification, and are requested to perform ablutions before entering a mosque.

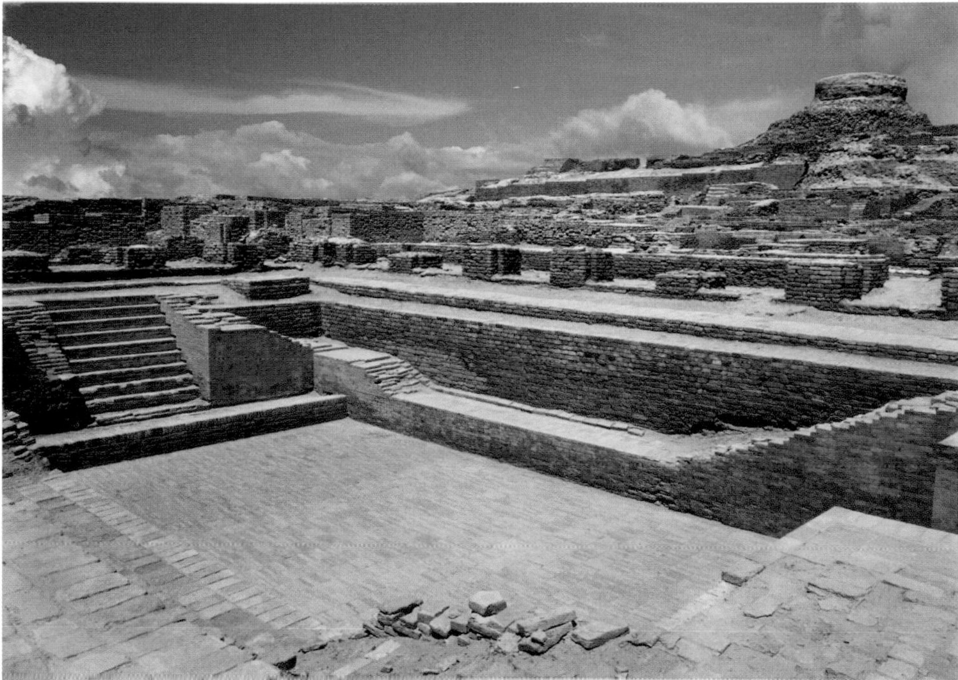

Left Dawn sees morning bathing on the ghats of holy lakes, rivers and tanks all over India. Traditionally, to cleanse in holy water is to wash away sin, greed, envy and evil in order to emerge physically and metaphorically pure. Devotees submerge themselves in the water, give offerings of water to their ancestors and pay homage to the new day. It's a ritual followed by everybody — rich and poor.

Above Situated on a north-south axis, Mohenjodaro's Great Bath has two large staircases leading down to the bath itself. In the ancient Indus River Valley civilization, it was almost certainly used for rituals as well as cleansing.

It is known that Indians prized both physical and mental cleanliness, and were bathing regularly far before most people in Western countries took up the practice. One of the most intriguing structures at the ruins of Mohenjodaro, one of the largest metropolises of the Indus Valley Civilization, is the 2-meter (6-foot) deep brick structure called the Great Bath. Waterproofed with tightly packed bricks and a layer of bitumen, it was surrounded by cloister-like rooms that are now believed to have served some religious purpose.

Whether bathing at Mohenjodaro was spiritual or physical or a combination of both is not known, but the elaborate water supply system and drainage network indicate that the Great Bath was a very important part of the city. This is backed up by reference to bathing in ancient Ayurvedic texts. These advocate that bathing be a daily ritual conducted to stimulate the body, remove fatigue, sweat and dirt and enhance *ojas* (subtle spiritual energy). The Vedic texts indicate that different *doshas* require different temperatures of water.

Elsewhere in India, there are numerous extant tracts on mental and physical hygiene. A 12th-century encyclopedic text from Karnataka called *Manasollasa* gives details of scientific approaches to bathing, whilst the 17th-century handbook written primarily for royalty *Sivatatvaratnakara*

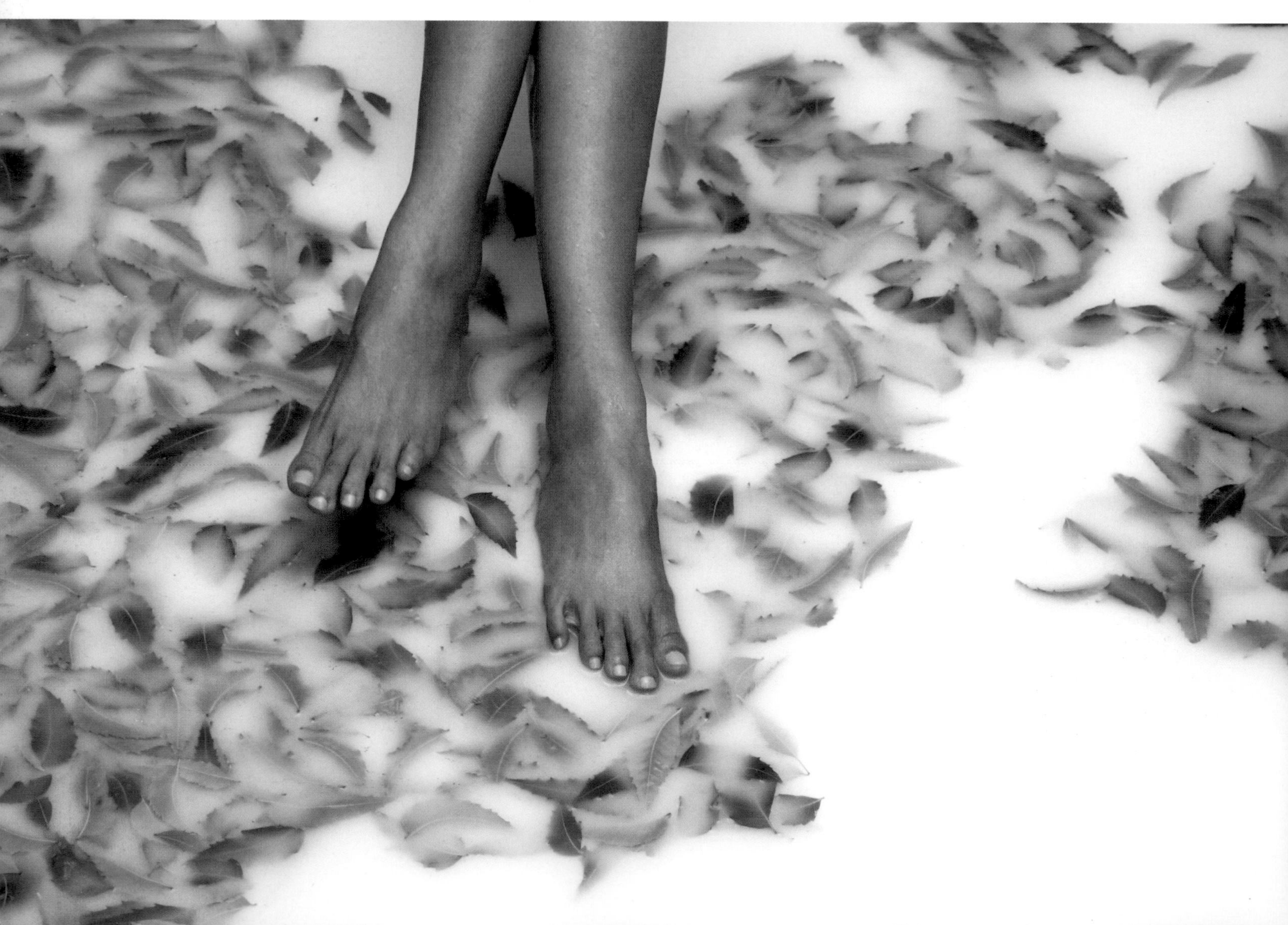

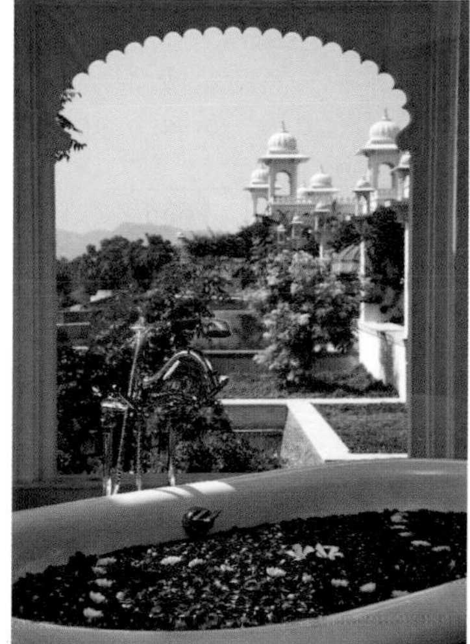

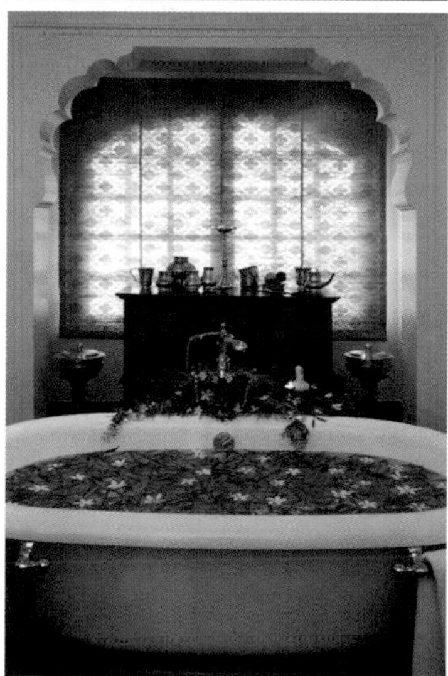

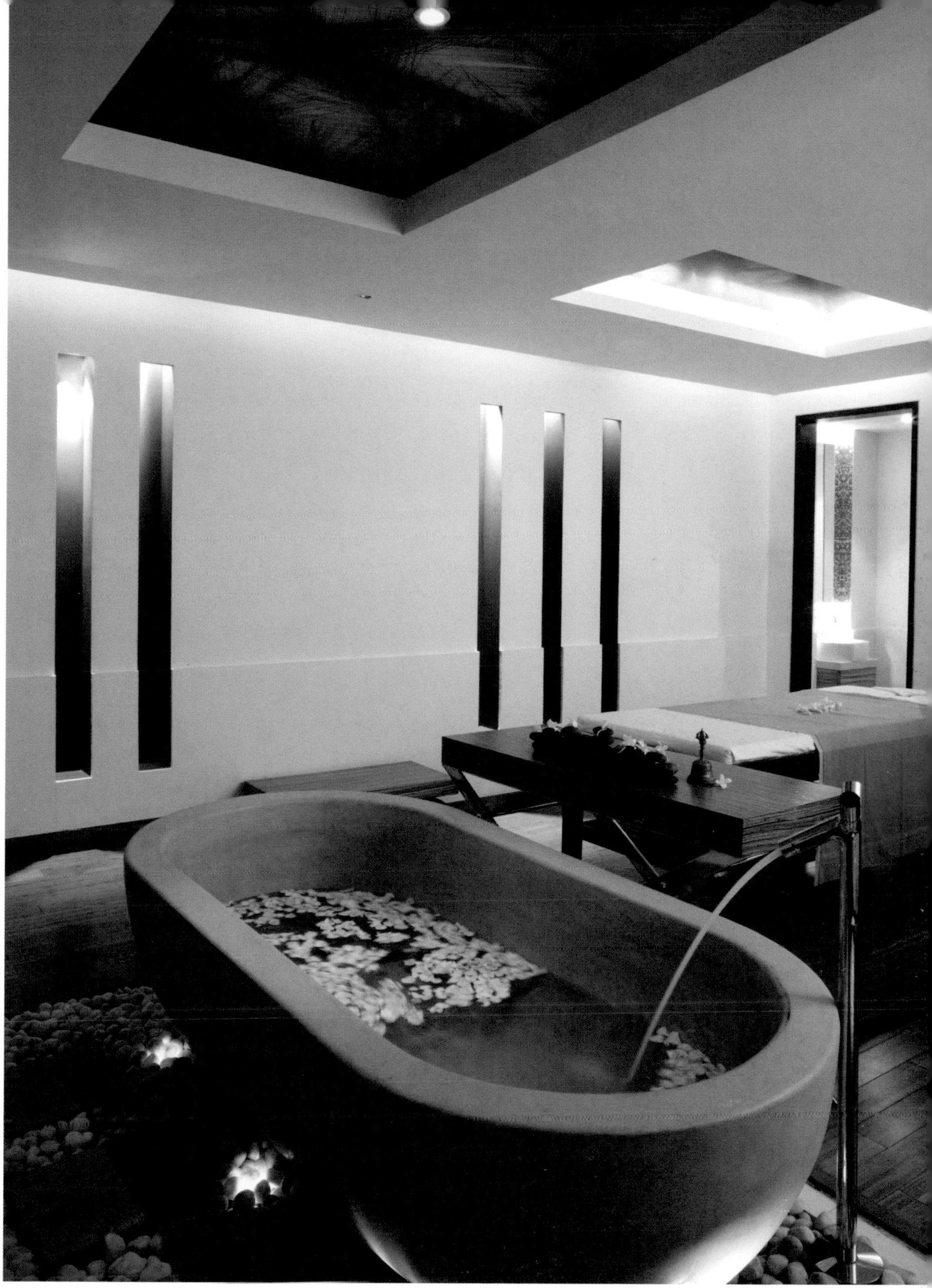

Left This milk and neem leaf bath is a purifying experience: even though the scent isn't particularly beautiful (think more vegetal than floral), it is deeply cleansing. **This page** Many of India's luxury spas offer cleansing, soothing rituals that involve a deep soak in a tub usually situated in a gorgeous spa suite. Clockwise from top left: A rose petal and milk bath immortalized by Rajput royalty offered at Udaivilas, a soft-scented floral bath at Quan spa and a deeply cleansing, leafy-scented neem leaf bath at Rajvilas.

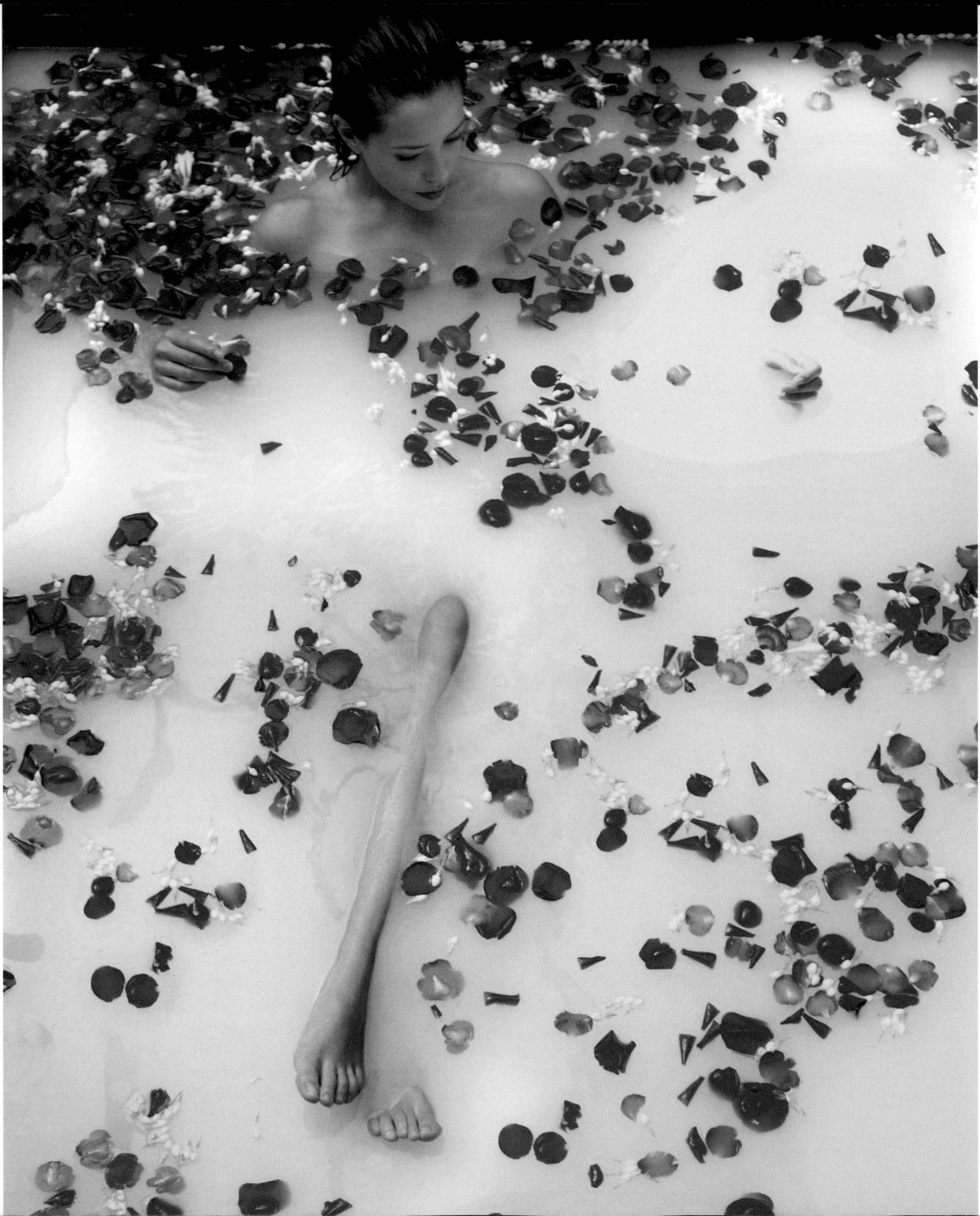

provides similar details about bathing. The tongue-twisting *Kanthiravanarasarajavijaya* written by Govinda Vaidya in 1648 gives a very picturesque description of a bathing *ghat* (public bath on a river-bank) and describes the importance of water supplies for bathing.

Soap was not traditionally used in Indian bathing. Paradoxically, the combination of soap and water — although cleansing — is de-moisturizing and accelerates aging. Indians preferred to use cleansing scrubs made from grains of gram flour, wheat husk or oatmeal to exfoliate and followed this with applications of oil after drying. Because many baths were public or semi-public, it was (and is) normal to keep the *sari* or *dhoti* on whilst bathing.

In 21st-century India, a variety of therapeutic, beautifying and cleansing baths are available at spas and clinics. Oil-infused or flower-filled baths often form the fitting finale to a relaxing, pampering sequence of treatments at a spa. They take their historical cue from royal bathing practices, and leave you scented, refreshed or invigorated depending on the bath's ingredients. Some bathing options are very simple, while others take longer to prepare: it's interesting to see how, in one way or another, they hearken back to ancient purification rites.

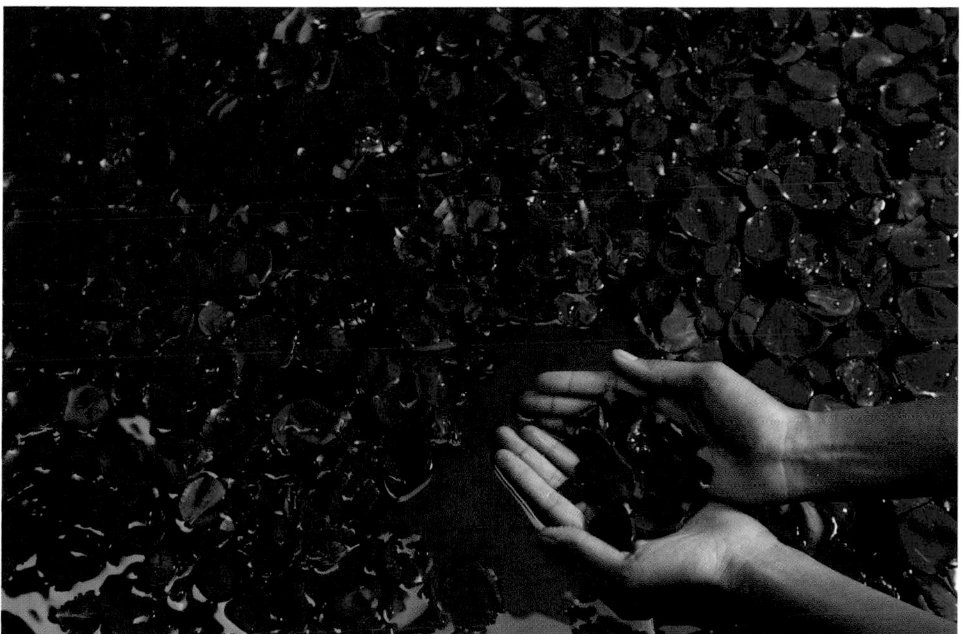

Left and above The rose petal and milk bath traces its roots to Rajput queens who would soak in stepwells after treating their bodies to a body scrub of turmeric, sandalwood, green gram flour and yogurt. Exfoliated skin would then be better prepared to absorb the moisturizing properties of the milk and the scent of royal roses.

Floral Baths

Oberoi Spas by Banyan Tree offer a number of specialty baths, including their visually arresting marigold bath. In everyday life, garlands of marigolds are often given to welcome visitors and the blossoms are used to adorn a home altar or are placed on little leaf boats with an oil lamp at evening *aartis* (prayer rituals). Even though they do not have any religious significance as such, their golden hues are extremely attractive, and when used in a bath the blooms have astringent qualities. After half an hour's relaxation in this gold-and-vermilion dream water, the skin feels firm and fresh.

Another floral bath with a difference is Quan Spa's interpretation of the milk bath based on an ancient Indian recipe. Milk has naturally occurring alpha-hydroxy acids that hydrate, exfoliate and improve skin elasticity, while *ahswagandha* root, also known as Indian ginseng, is used in a number of Ayurvedic remedies. It is one of the best herbs for the mind, clearing anxiety and inducing clarity. Rose petals, of course, provide a wonderful scent. Harnessing the power of water that flows around India's busiest city, their rose, milk and *ashwagandha* bath can be had as a single or couple's treatment or combined in a spa package based on the five elements of fire, water, air, earth and space.

Medicinal Baths

Hydrotherapy, of course, immediately comes to mind when one considers the bath in a spa setting. One of the famous Indian inventions is the hip bath: devised by naturopath Sri Lakshman Sharma in order to concentrate water between the ribs and thighs, it helps stimulate circulation in that region, so it's good for the urinary, digestive and excretory systems. The innovative arm and foot bath is a most important application in the case of bronchial asthma, as the reflex areas on the palms and soles are related to the lungs. It is also helpful for migraine sufferers.

In Ayurveda, medicinal baths are not overly used, though steam baths come under the category of some preparatory oleation and fomentation therapies. Described as a sudation process, medicinal steam is used to induce sweating and improve peripheral circulation to reduce high blood pressure and help in the absorption of medicinal particles present in herbal oils. The steam also augments the elimination of impurities in the excretory system and through other outlets such as sweat glands, kidneys and liver. Sometimes, a steam will also be prescribed for skin or muscle ailments, pain and swelling.

At Kalari Kovilakom, where Ayurvedic texts are followed to the book, steam boxes are part and parcel of the initial stages of the *panchakarma* regime. But the Palace to Ayurveda is also home to a pint-sized

Below Somewhat like the Japanese, Indians often cleanse themselves before entering a bath or shower. Brass vessels are favored. **Right** Made from rosewood, this bath at Kalari Kovilakom is purely medicinal. During a prolonged detox such as *panchakarma*, the skin often erupts with pustules as poisons are expelled from the body, so a soothing, medicated bath in this little tub helps surface healing.

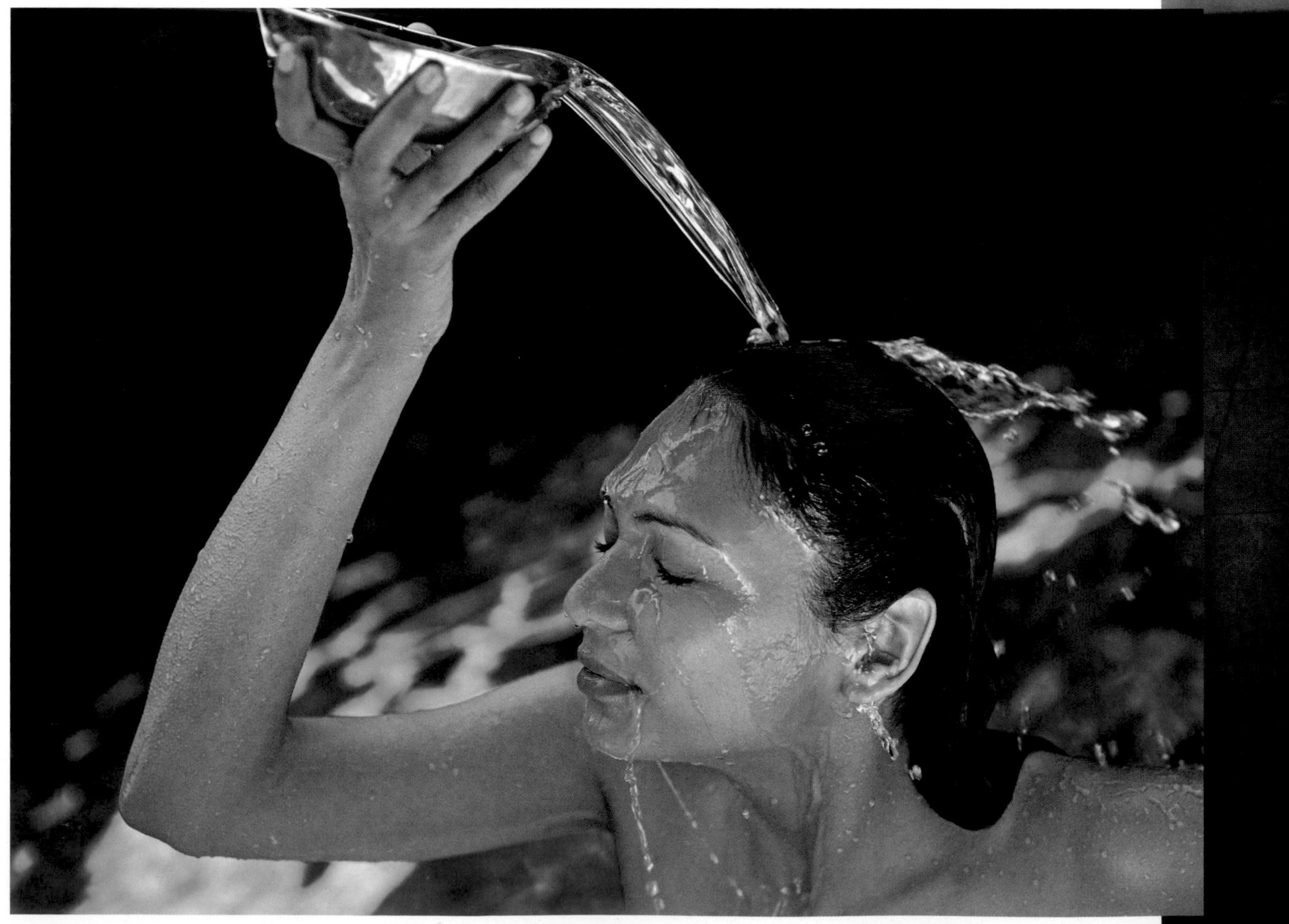

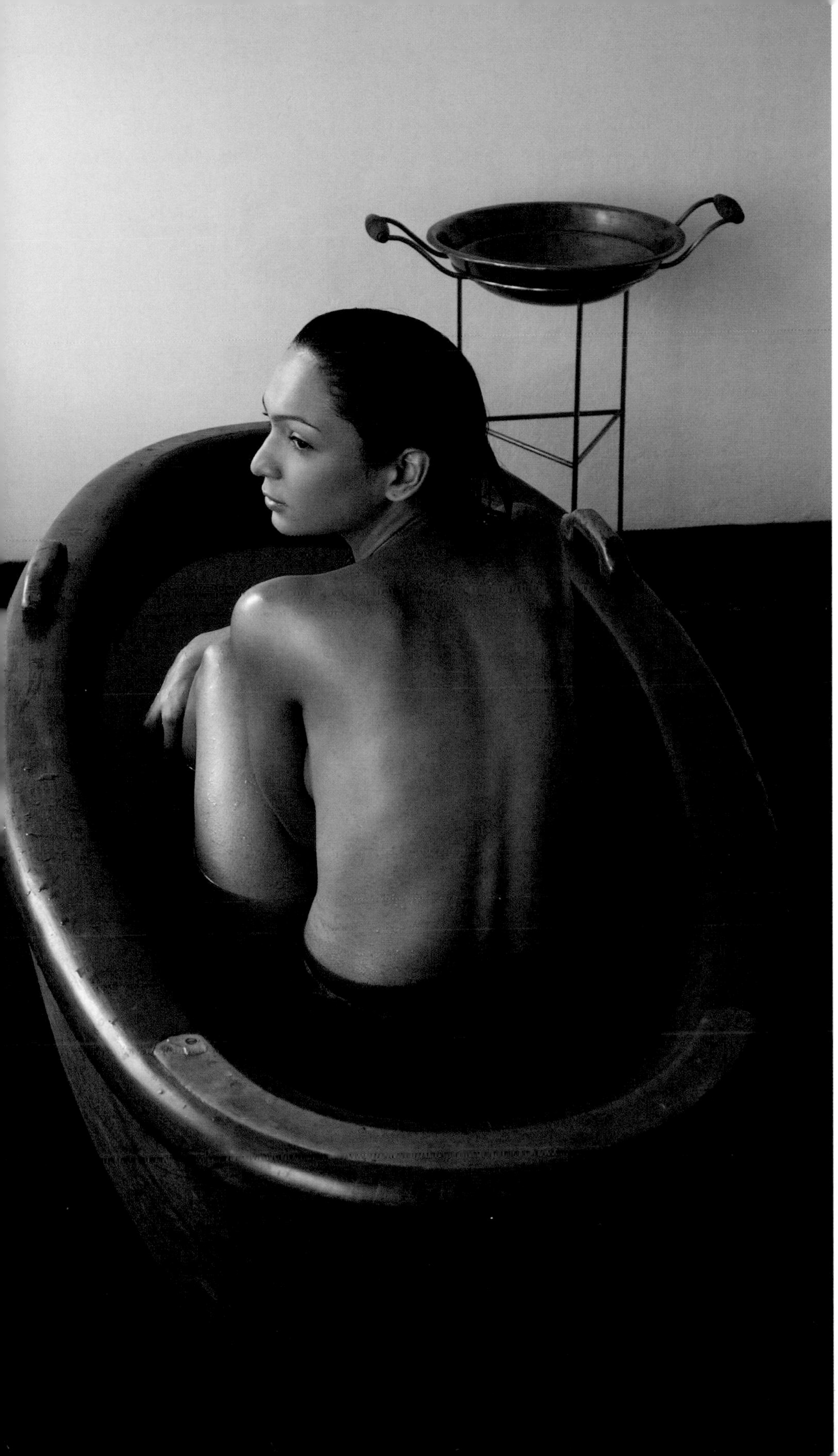

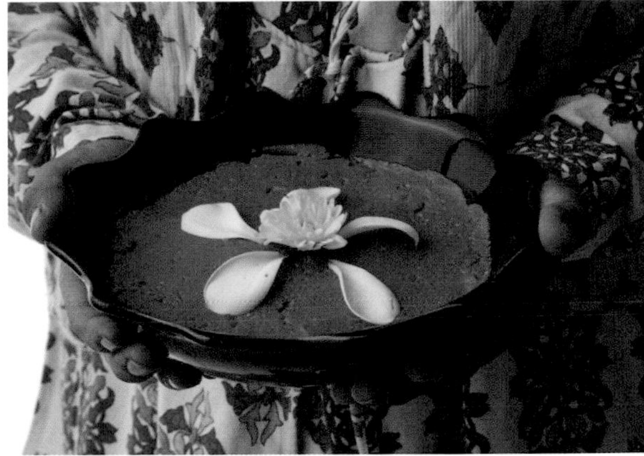

rosewood bath that often comes into its own at the end of a client's treatment. "After the *panchakarma* treatment, patients often break out in pimples as their toxins are released," explains Dr Jayan, "so this medicinal bath helps to restore skin conditions." Medicated warm water is also poured into this bath to soothe spinal problems, muscle ailments and skin conditions. Uterine or rectal prolapse are also helped by such baths, and people with hemorrhoids also find them healing.

One notable bath from the Himalayan region is the Bhutanese stone heated bath or *sman-chu*. Based on the Tibetan medical system known as *Soba Rig-pa*, it works on the same principle as hot stone massage. Using the healing power of heat from pristine mountain hot springs, the warmth from the water stimulates peripheral circulation and can also penetrate deeper, helping arthritic or rheumatic conditions. The Bhutanese often add herbs such as artemesia, sage and ephedra to the water, and often use a salt scrub prior to a dip.

Above Indians traditionally eschewed soap for an *ubtan* scrub for cleansing while bathing. This *ubtan* from Udaivilas consists of turmeric, sandalwood, green gram flour and yogurt. The turmeric leaves skin with a golden glow, while the sandalwood is soothing and antiseptic and the yogurt moisturizing and enzyme rich.

rasashastra

Healing With Gems, Crystals, Metals and Minerals

In Ayurveda, gems and precious metals are used to balance planetary influences, increase life force or *prana*, and cure certain diseases. Their preparation and prescription falls under the branch of Ayurvedic medicine known as *rasashastra* (literally "mercury medicine"). It developed relatively late in the Ayurvedic calendar, probably around the 8th century, but its practices were soon assimilated into mainstream Ayurveda. *Rasashastra* basically falls into two separate categories: *dehavaad* or the "treating of diseases" and *lohavaad* or the "chemical manufacture of medicines".

In Indian spas today, a prescription of gems, metals or minerals is rare: they are more commonly found in clinics and hospitals. However, the tradition of using such substances has found new life in a number of skincare formulations invented by entrepreneurial chemists and doctors. Tiny flecks of gold leaf or silver foil, or crushed diamonds and pearls, blended with botanical extracts, have found their way into innovative products. Facials using such ingredients are the latest in Indian skincare: Receive the elixir of life (gold) through the skin — and detoxify; use a crushed pearl exfoliator — and see the difference in your complexion. And, for the ultimate in anti-aging, dazzle with a diamond rehydrator; you can justify the extravagance, as it's doing you good.

Right Enriched with amino acids and minerals, this pearl mask from Shahnaz Husain is deeply rejuvenating.
Opposite Grounding stones used in therapy.

Metals and Minerals

Less exotic, but extremely powerful nonetheless, is the use of minerals and metals in Ayurveda. Because many metals and minerals contain certain impurities and/or toxins, they need to undergo a number of treatments before they are deemed safe to ingest. These processes are known as *shodhana* (purification) and *marana* (literally "kill"; heating and turning into ash), and may often be lengthy and complicated. For example, heavy metals such as mercury, gold, silver, copper, iron, lead and tin are heated and treated with such substances as cow's urine, milk, ghee and buttermilk before use. If they are to be taken in ash form, they are ground into a powder and incinerated; at other times they are added to water to create elixirs for drinking.

Dr Sreenarayanan of Ananda Spa points out that all Ayurvedic medicines are 100 percent natural, so it is unsurprising that minerals and metals are utilized. "Minerals and metals come from the earth," he points out, "and if they are purified properly, can be very powerful." He goes on to say that in 90 percent of cases they are ingested either as a *bhasma* (ash) or as pills, but such prescriptions must be accompanied by an extremely strict diet for the medication to work. He cites mercury for chronic conditions like cancer and arthritis; silver in rejuvenation treatments; gold for vigor and vitality as well as bone problems; iron for anemia and blood impurities; and lead for chronic skin conditions.

Gemstones

In India, jewels (often worn as uncut stones) are not only decorative, but are believed to hold certain powers. Some of these are emotional or superstitious on the part of the wearer, but others are distinctly therapeutic. Gem therapists say that the vibrational healing energies of a gem or metal may be transferred to a person if it is worn close to the body. Some people wear them for health reasons, others for luck, others for peace of mind.

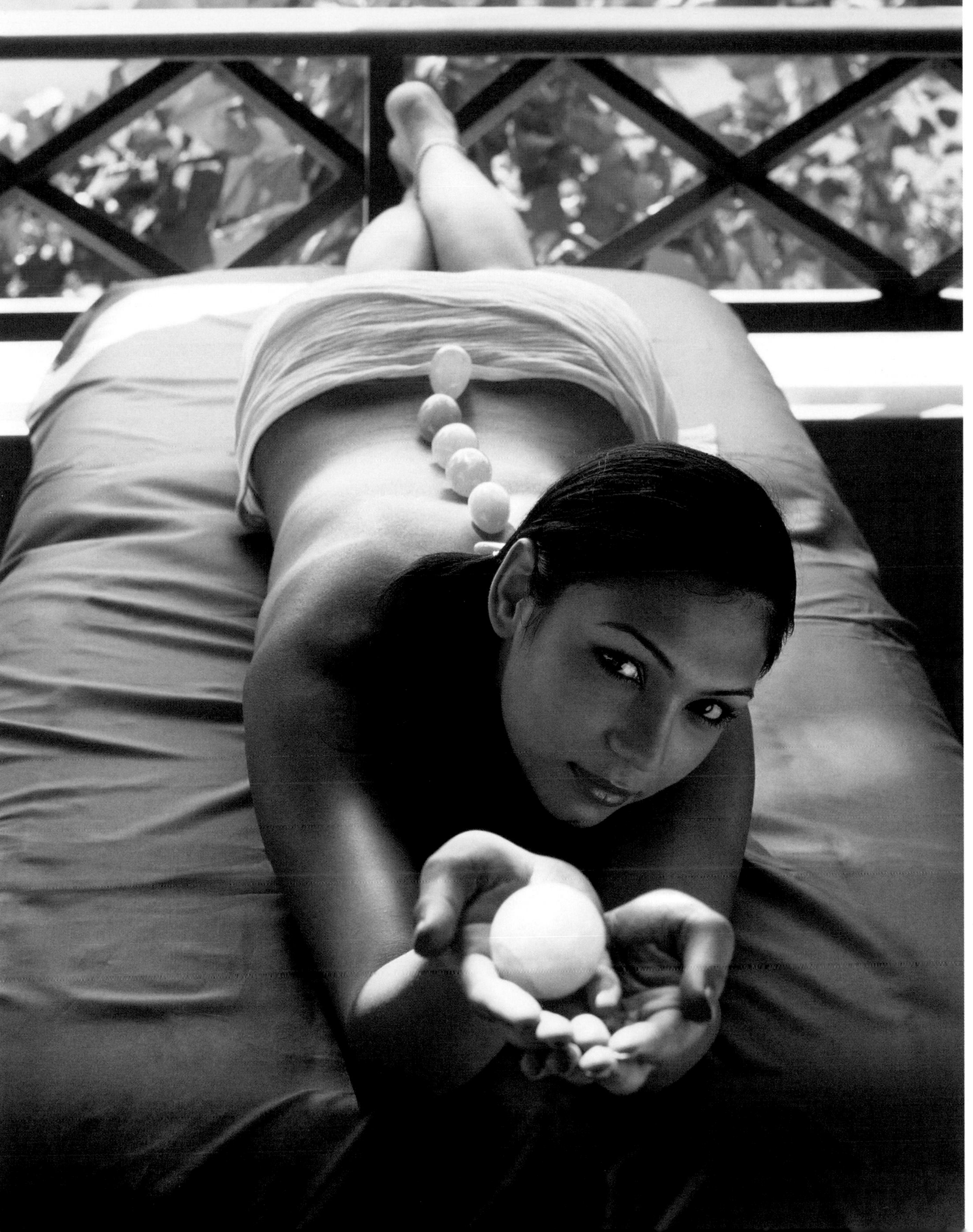

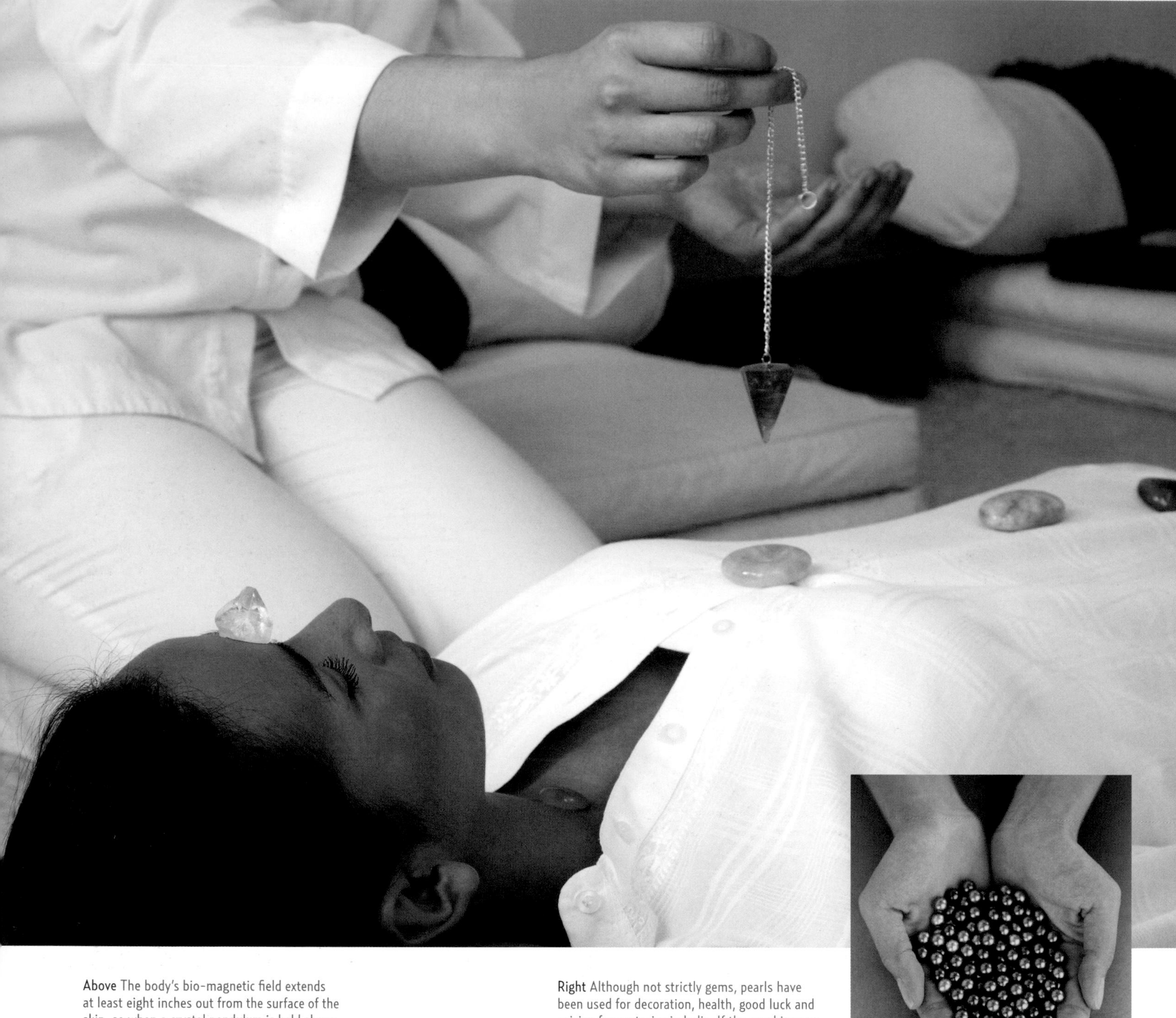

Above The body's bio-magnetic field extends at least eight inches out from the surface of the skin, so when a crystal pendulum is held above another crystal positioned on a *chakra* point, it is more than likely to move. This gives vital information to a crystal therapist, who is trying to free up energy flows and bring the body back to balance.

Right Although not strictly gems, pearls have been used for decoration, health, good luck and cuisine for centuries in India. If the pearl is your birth stone, it is said to be doubly powerful.

According to Dr Sreenarayanan, only certain stones have healing properties and they must always be purified before use. "Gems may be soaked in running water (preferably water from sacred places such as the Ganges) and the water is drunk for health benefits," he says, "Or they may be put in the husk of rice or left out in the sun. Another way of receiving the power of stones is to simply concentrate or meditate on 'special' stones; gazing on them in a quiet meditative manner dispels negativity and makes the mind calm and quiet."

He goes on to note that the use of gems and precious metals in this way is extremely ancient as it is rooted in Vedic astrological readings. The Vedas prescribed three methods to dispel negative planetary influences, namely the chanting of *mantras*, the wearing of gems and the taking of medicine. Today, many people choose to wear a *navaratna* or nine jewel bangle or a *rudraaksha* (string of medicinal beads) to keep harmful cosmic energies at bay. "If you wear your birth stone close to the body," asserts Dr Sreenarayanan, "your energy levels open up and your immune system is strengthened."

In this context, precious and semi-precious stones are easier to use than minerals and metals as they require minimal preparation. Their beauty, rareness and the effect of light rays passing through them are factors that make them useful in healing. If the stones are inlaid into jewelry items, they should be open-backed with gold as the preferred setting.

Crystals

Crystal therapy is another holistic therapy that utilizes the power of stones. Crystal healers believe that every living organism has an energy system based on meridian lines and *chakras*, so if appropriate crystals are placed on particular spots (ie *marma* points or *chakras*) sluggish or blocked energy is revitalized. Such therapy is also reported to be helpful with certain emotional issues. Some therapists use crystals in facials and massages too: warmed jade, turquoise and quartz used in a manner similar to hot stone massage encourages energy flow and carved, polished crystals placed on the facial *chakras* help cleanse and rebalance.

Crystal therapists hold that crystals are especially useful because they vibrate in the same energy fields as human beings, but for crystal therapy to be effective, a course of treatments is advised. "Depending on the person and their problems, this type of energetic work is most beneficial when received more than once," says one crystal healer, "a course of twice a week for a few weeks can be enormously helpful."

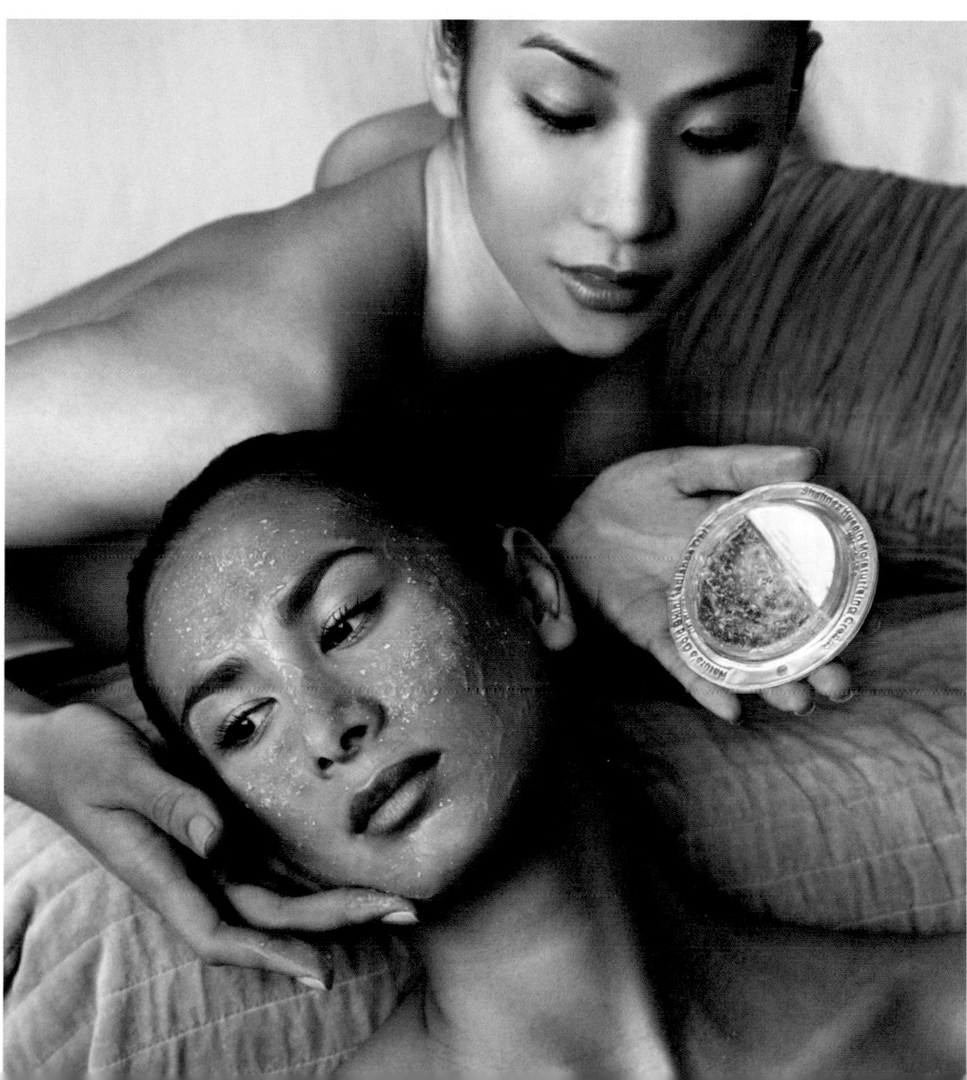

Go for gold: Eaten, injected or absorbed through the skin, gold is the ultimate elixir of life. Ingested in Ayurveda to boost the circulation and rejuvenate sluggish organs, it may also be injected to reduce inflammation in joints. Here, it is applied to the face as part of an absurdly luxurious four part facial treatment offered at Shahnaz Husain salons: aptly named the 24 carat gold collection, it is an extravagant treat.

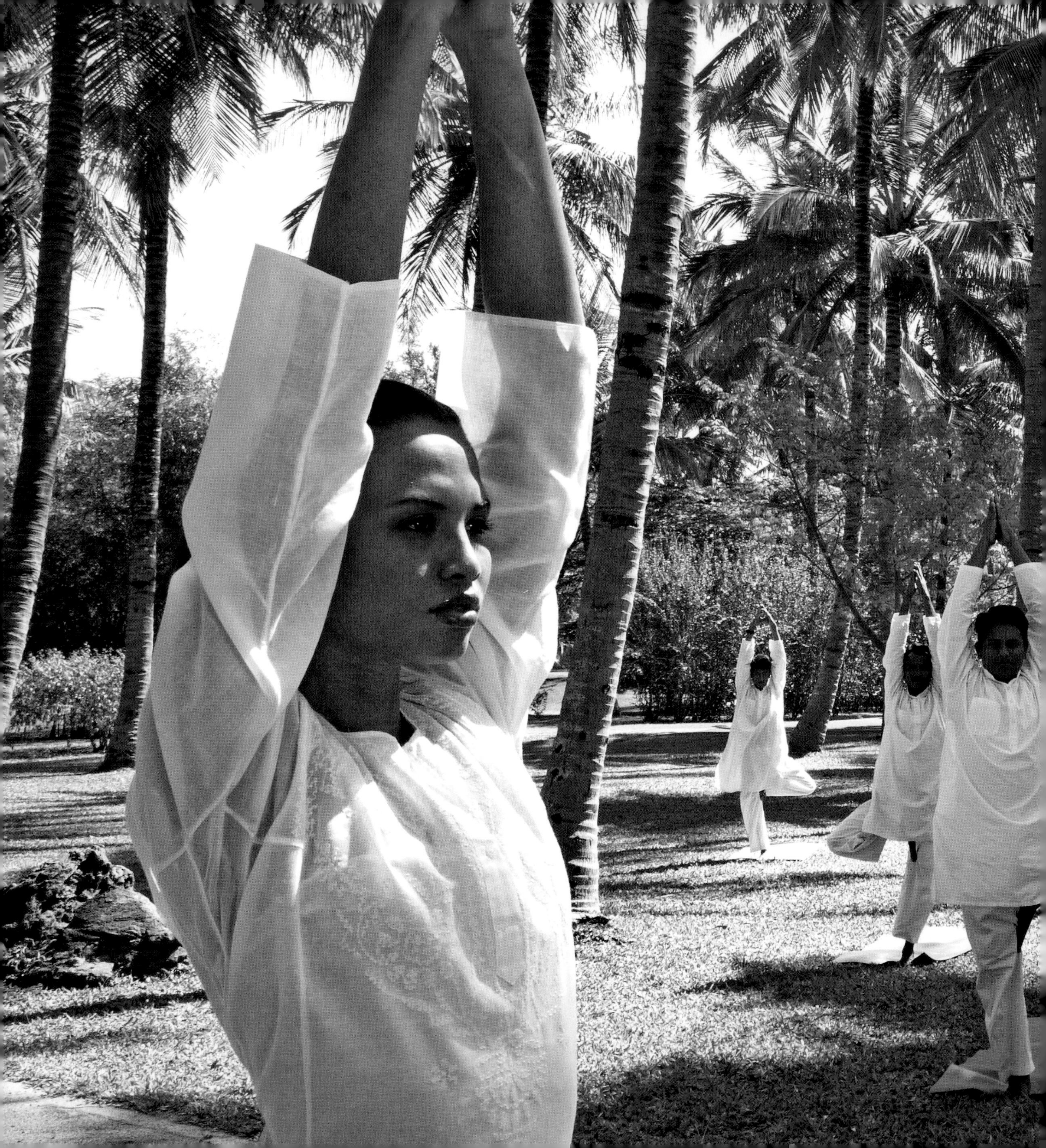

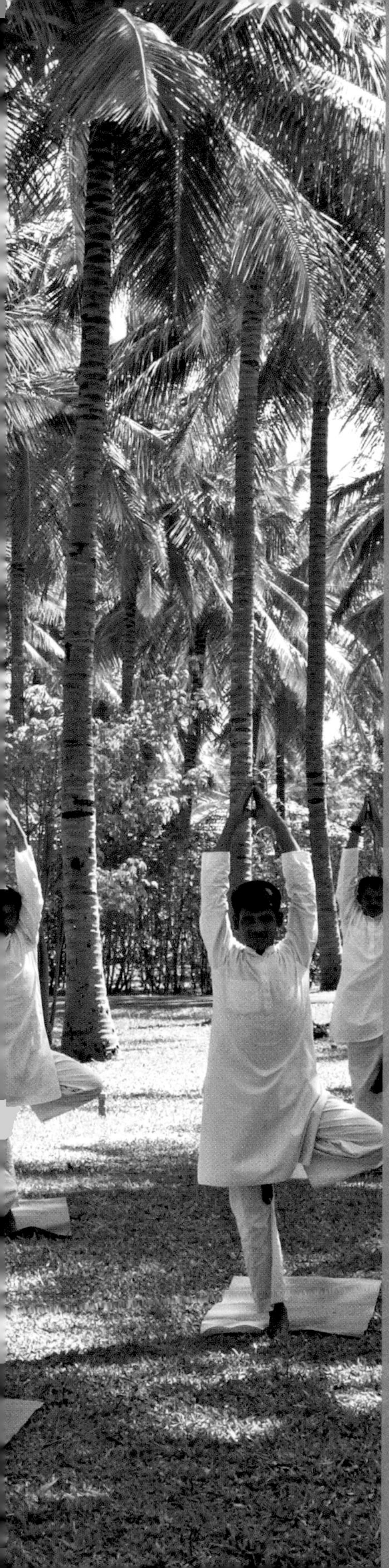

balance

A beautiful face and body cannot attain its greatest potential, if the mind and spirit aren't also nurtured, relaxed and fulfilled. In India, Ayurvedic physicians, yoga and martial arts instructors, gurus and teachers all stress the importance of a life lived in balance: one where mind, body and spirit work together in healthful harmony. This can be achieved with a number of practices that stress "mindfulness", such as meditation, yoga, *pranayama*, various physical/mental exercises and therapies that work to balance the *chakras*.

yoga

It isn't known exactly when the ancient art of yoga began, but there is archaeological evidence of various yogic postures dating back to around 3,000 BC. Many believe that it was Lord Shiva, the Hindu god, who created yoga, but the first written texts outlining its basic philosophy and practices probably date to the 2nd century BC. Called the *Yoga Sutras*, they were written by a certain Patanjali, and are believed to combine previous teachings into an organized system that continues to this day.

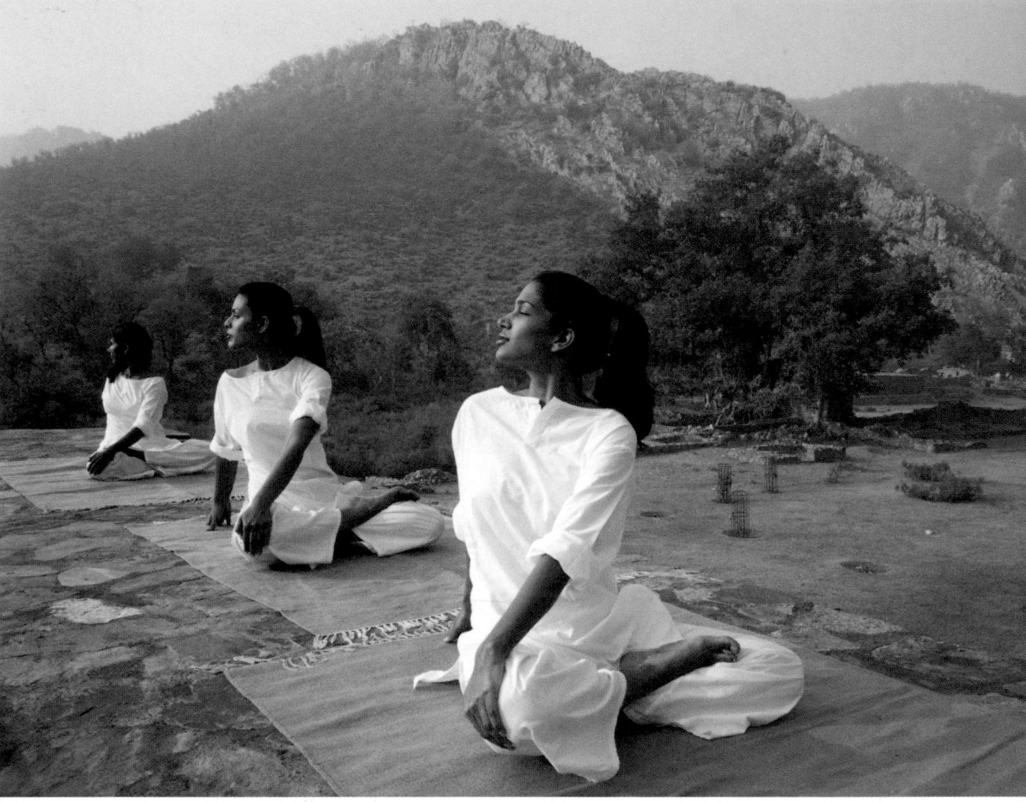

Above India offers some extraordinary places for yoga practice. Here, a teacher and two clients enjoy the early morning light atop a rampart of the deserted city of Bhangarh in the Aravalli hills not too far from Jaipur. It is one of the mind-expanding trips organized by the Amanbagh resort.
Right An inspirational illustration depicting some of the different yoga *asanas* on the perimeter, and a lotus-posed devotee showing the positioning of the seven *chakras*.

Patanjali states that yoga is a methodical practice, the ultimate aim of which is the attainment of perfection. Through the control of both physical and psychical elements, disciplined activity, spiritual exercises and the conquest of desire, one can attain salvation. He outlined an eight-limbed path (*ashtanga*) to reach this ultimate stage: *yama* or abstention, not doing bad things to other people; *niyama* or observance, things you should do to yourself; *asana* or postures; *pranayama* or breath-control and breathing exercises; *pratyahara* or withdrawal of the senses, controlling them and being aware of them; *dharana* or fixed attention (concentration); *dhyana* or contemplation (meditation); and *samadhi*, the final stage of super-consciousness (equivalent to the Buddhist concept of Nirvana).

Today, there are many different styles of yoga, but in general, yoga involves repetition of postures (*asanas*), followed by resting poses, breathing exercises (*pranayama*) and meditation. Hatha yoga, a term often heard, is not actually a style of yoga but a path that ultimately leads to the path of self-control (*raja*). In addition to the main styles of yoga listed overleaf, there are many other forms that are more recent additions to the practice such as Bikram Yoga and Power Yoga.

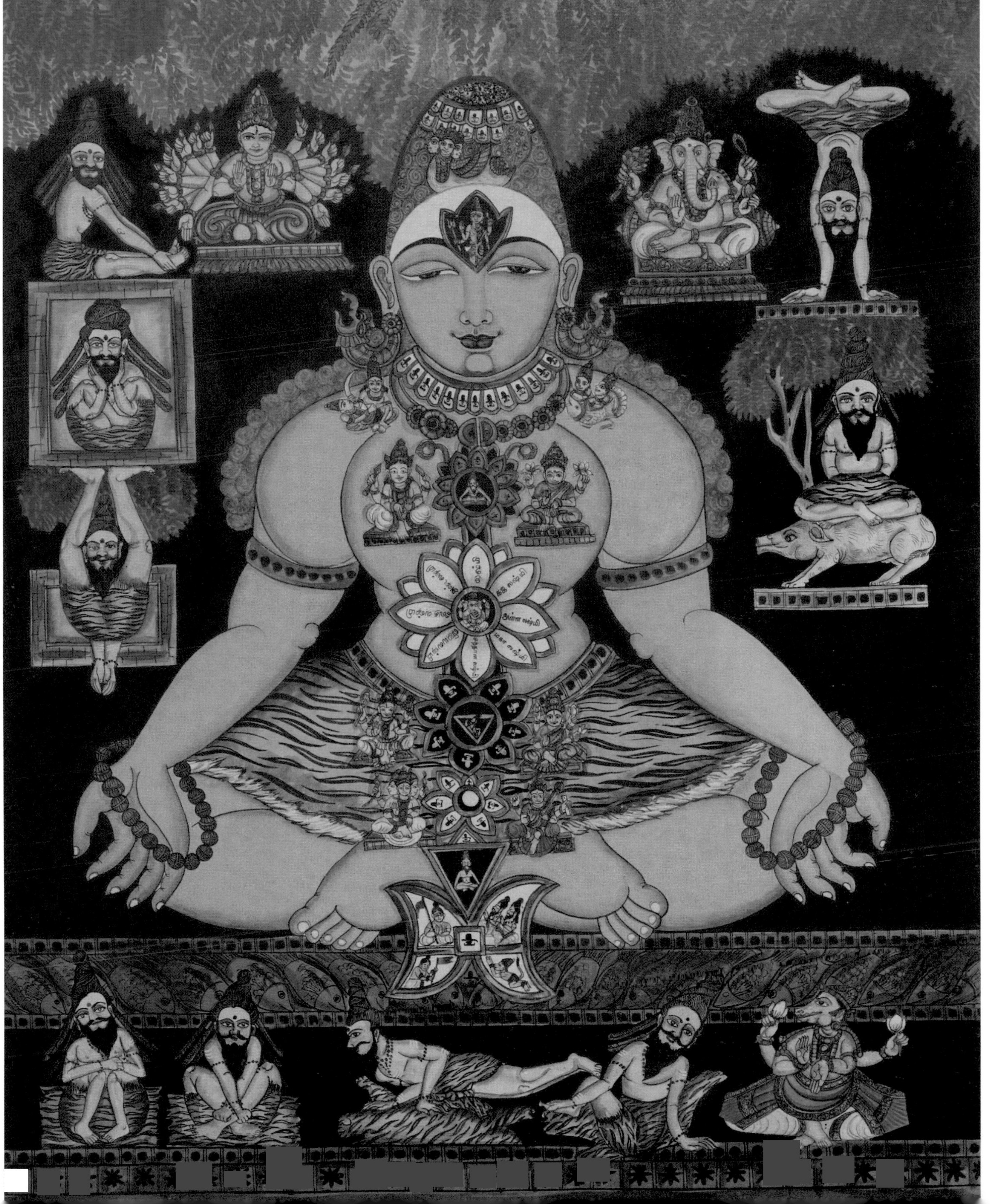
அன்ன லக்ஷ்மி
மகா லக்ஷ்மி

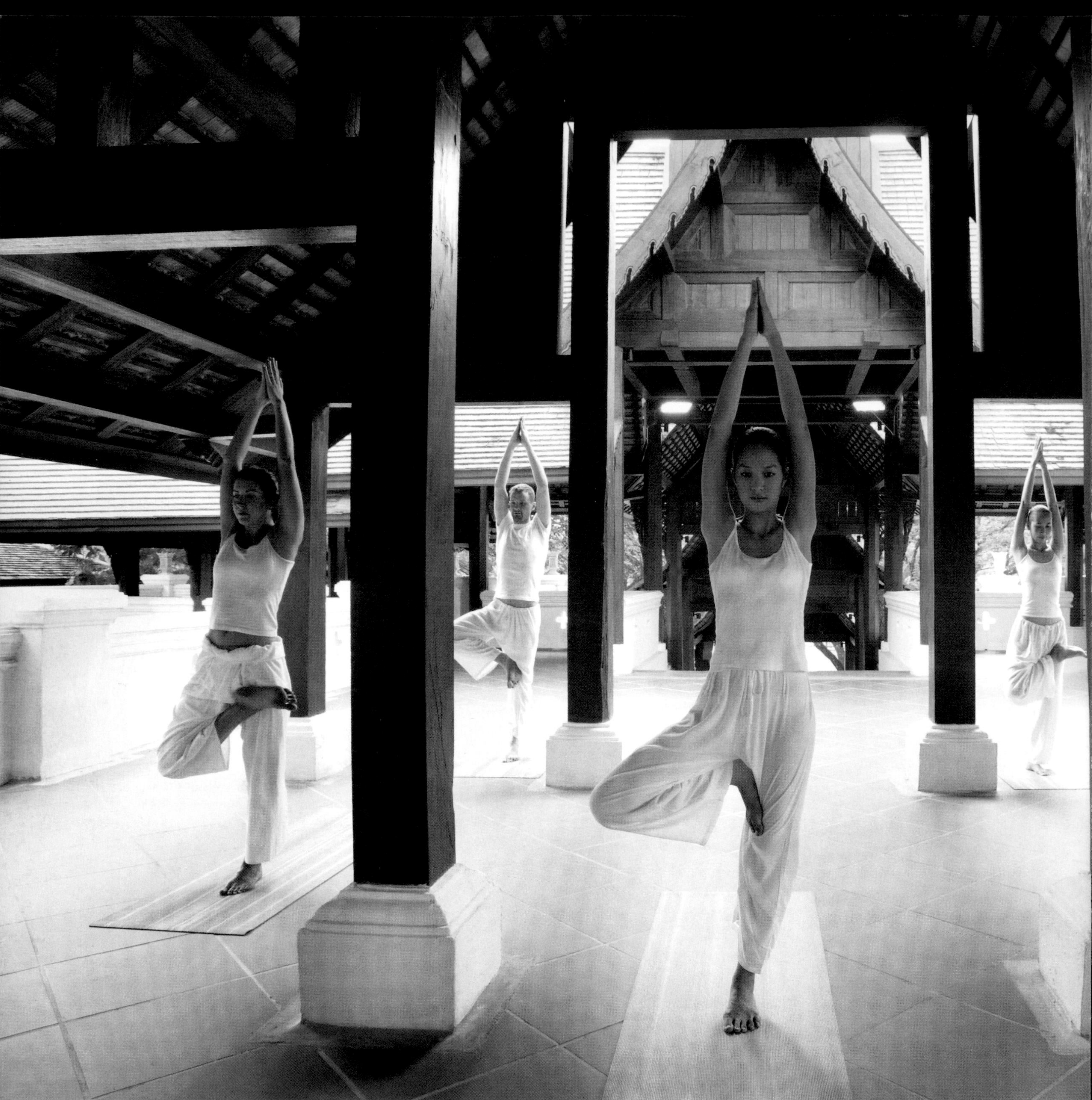

BALANCE

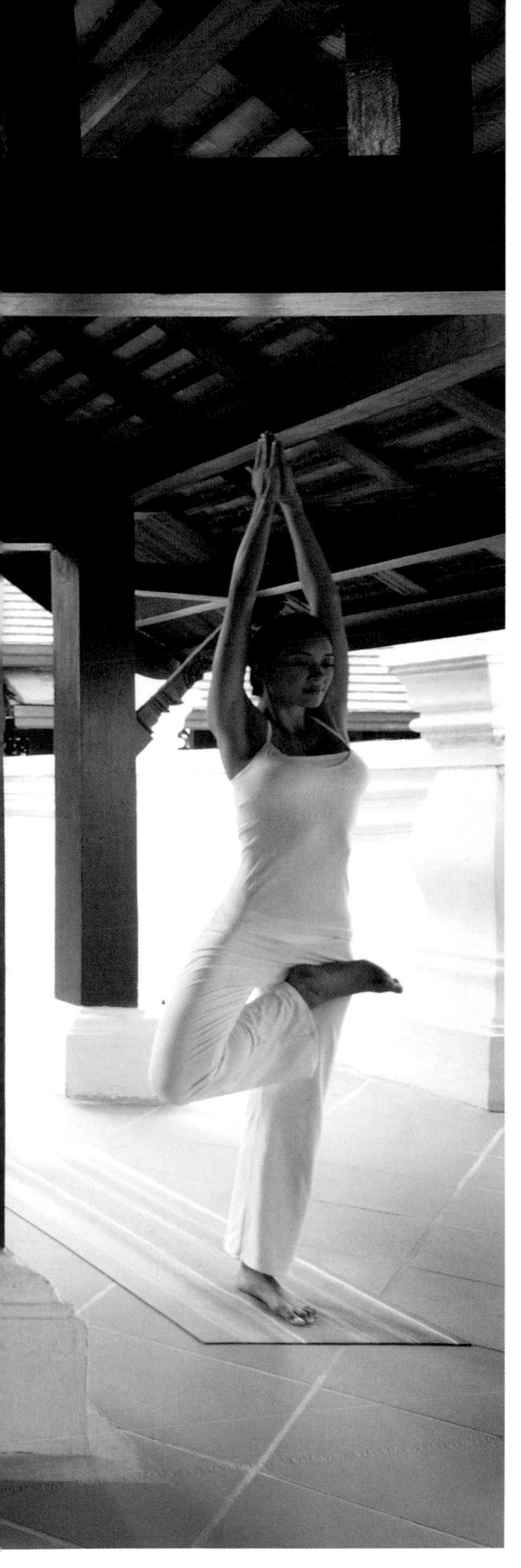

Iyengar Yoga:
The yoga teacher BKS Iyengar, born in 1918, started this style of yoga in Pune. The Iyengar concept includes work to achieve correct and accurate alignment and practicing with an astute consciousness of how to build a stronger *asana*. The aim is to make sure every pose is completely in line. Props such as straps, blocks of wood or blankets may be used.

Ananda Yoga:
This classical style focuses on gentle postures designed to move the energy up to the brain and prepare the body for meditation. It is not at all aerobic: it looks inwards, but nonetheless places emphasis on proper body alignment and controlled breathing practice.

Ashtanga Yoga:
Formulated by Sri K Pattabhi Jois, a yoga master based in Mysore, this system involves synchronizing the breath with a progressive series of postures. It concentrates on the flow from one pose to the next, on the breath (*ujjaipranayam*) and on strong, physical poses. During an *ashtanga* session, an intense internal heat and a powerful, purifying sweat is produced, so that both body and mind are exercised to their full potential.

Sivananda Yoga:
This is a traditional type of yoga that focuses on connecting the body to the solar plexus where it is believed an enormous amount of energy is stored. Comprising repetition of *asanas* followed by resting poses, it also focuses on breath, dietary restrictions, chanting and meditation.

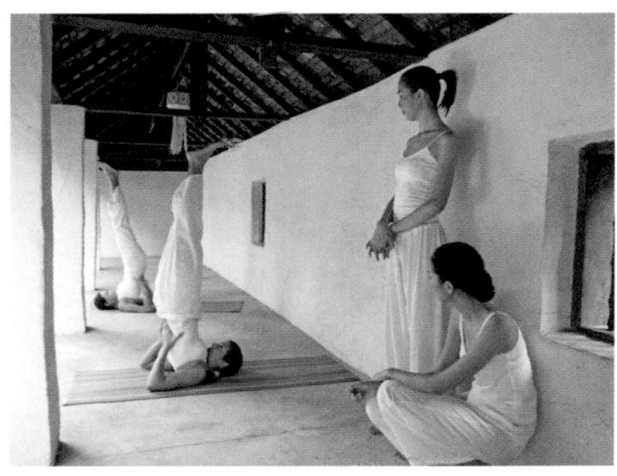

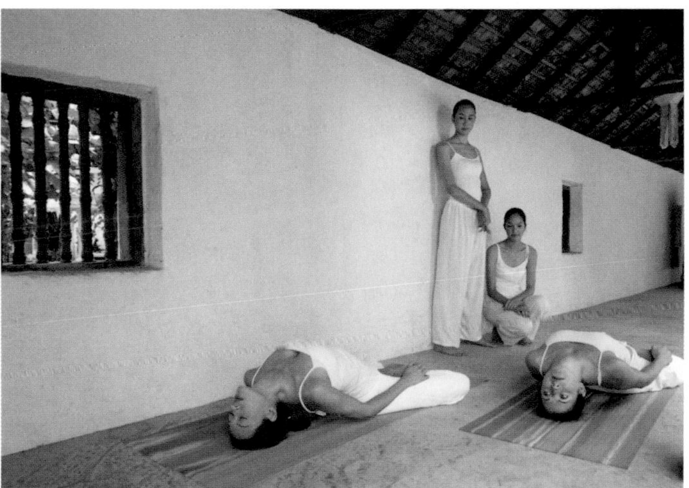

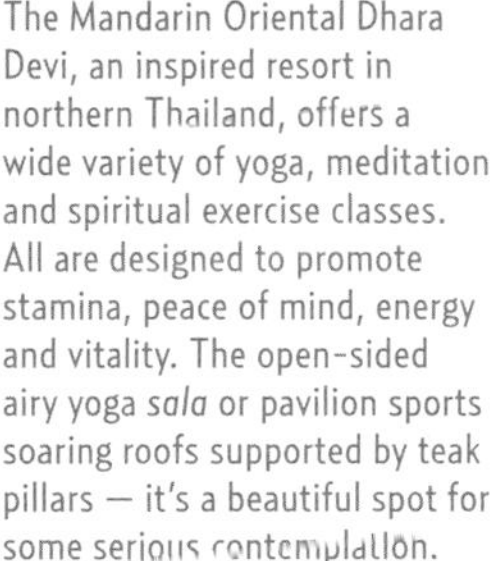

The Mandarin Oriental Dhara Devi, an inspired resort in northern Thailand, offers a wide variety of yoga, meditation and spiritual exercise classes. All are designed to promote stamina, peace of mind, energy and vitality. The open-sided airy yoga *sala* or pavilion sports soaring roofs supported by teak pillars — it's a beautiful spot for some serious contemplation.

Shiva, the lord of yoga, is depicted in three stylized Thai paintings in different meditative positions. Thailand has embraced yoga in many of its spas and healing centers.

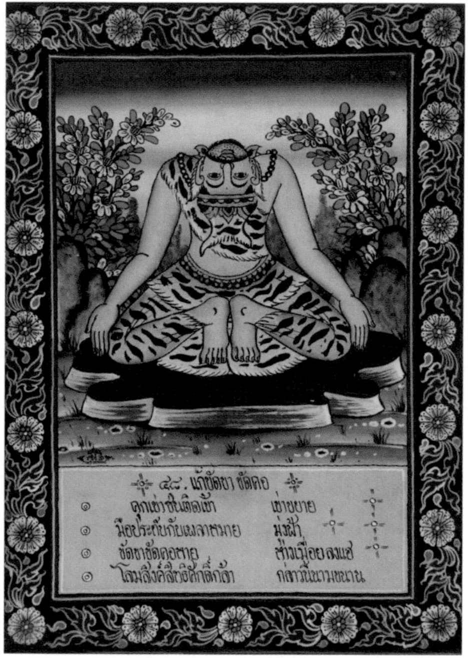

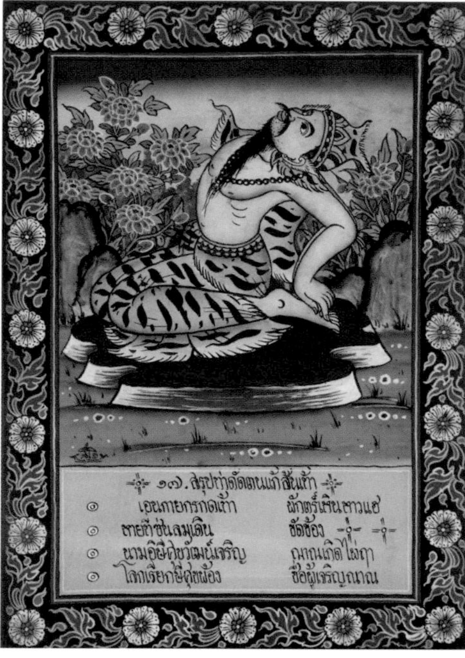

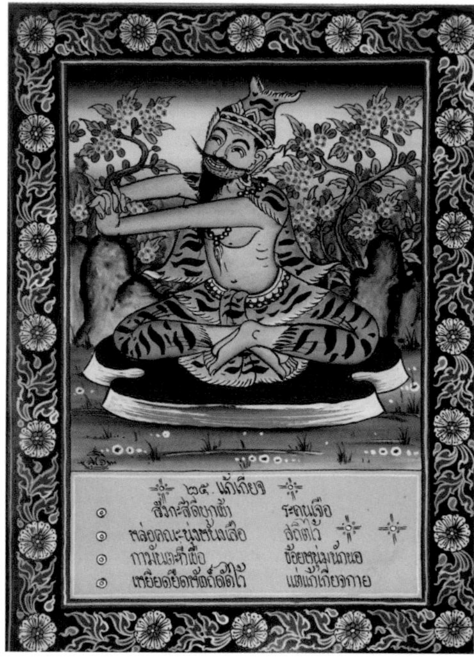

Kundalini Yoga:

The aim of this form of yoga is to awaken and reach one's spiritual potential. Using the metaphor of a serpent coiled at the body's bottom *chakra,* practice unwinds the serpent and helps it to rise upwards in an attempt to reach the top *chakra,* which is the highest possible. It concentrates on postures, chanting, meditation and breathing exercises.

Viniyoga:

Viniyoga is a term used to describe the yoga taught by Sri T Krishnamacharya, a descendant of the 9th-century *yogi* Nathamuni. His son is the current *viniyoga* lineage holder. *Viniyoga* aims to make yoga relevant to every situation and every individual person, and concentrates on postures, breath, meditation and prayer.

The benefits of yoga are many: Taken from the Sanskrit, *yoga* means "union" or "joining", so the ultimate aim of yoga is to join with the Almighty. This may not be within the reach of many, so, on a more prosaic level, yoga confers many less ambitious benefits. Physically, practitioners report increased flexibility, better lubrication of joints, massaging of internal organs, toned muscles and detoxification of the entire body. These are joined by mental, spiritual and emotional benefits as well. Devotees often report transformations in their lives once yoga is practiced regularly. Stress, anxiety, ill health, unhappiness and anger are replaced by peacefulness, vibrant health, service, and love towards all creation.

Many Indian spas, hotels, resorts, retreats ashrams and healing centers offer yoga. People also often attend yoga schools or *sala*, and there are literally hundreds of inspired settings in India (and outside India) in which to practice this ancient art (see photo on page 100).

Right A painting depicts the Hindu *sapta rishis* or seven sages who are extolled in the Vedas and other Hindu literature. They are regarded as the patriarchs of the Vedic religion, so have perfected many of the teachings in the Vedas. The sage at center bottom is in *urdhva-padmasana* or elevated lotus position.

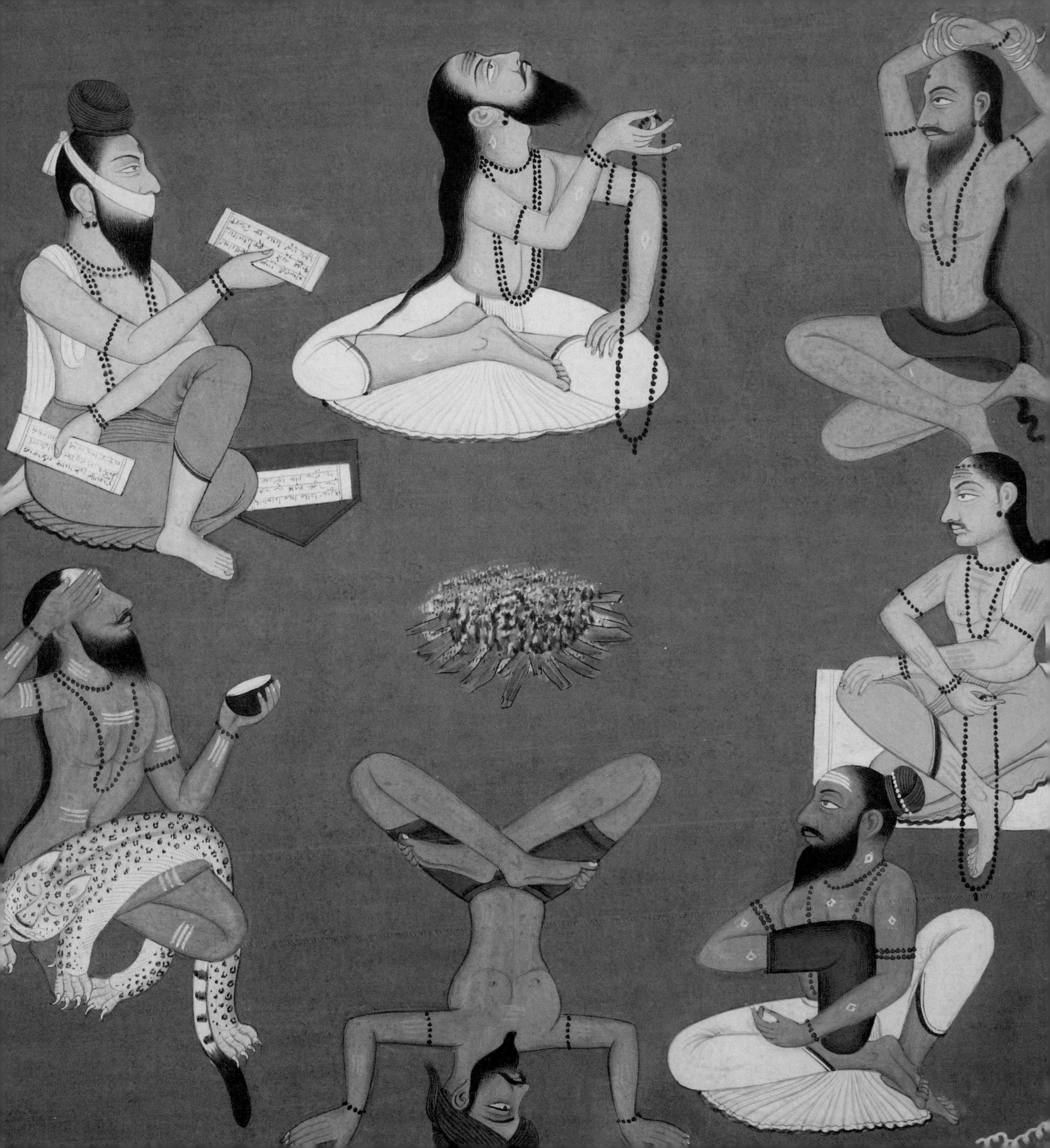

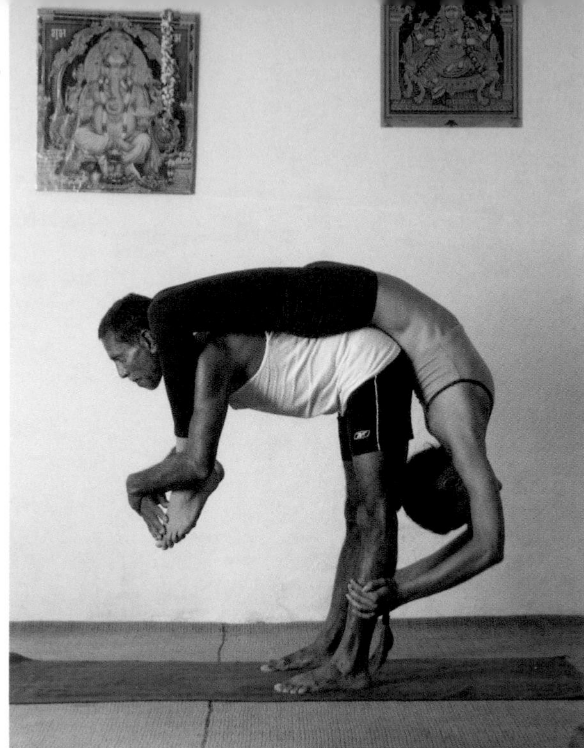

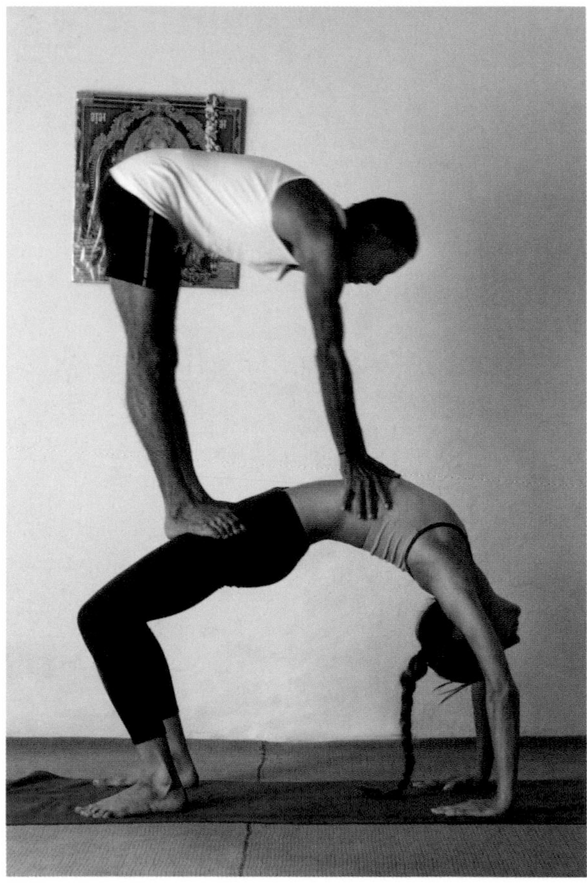

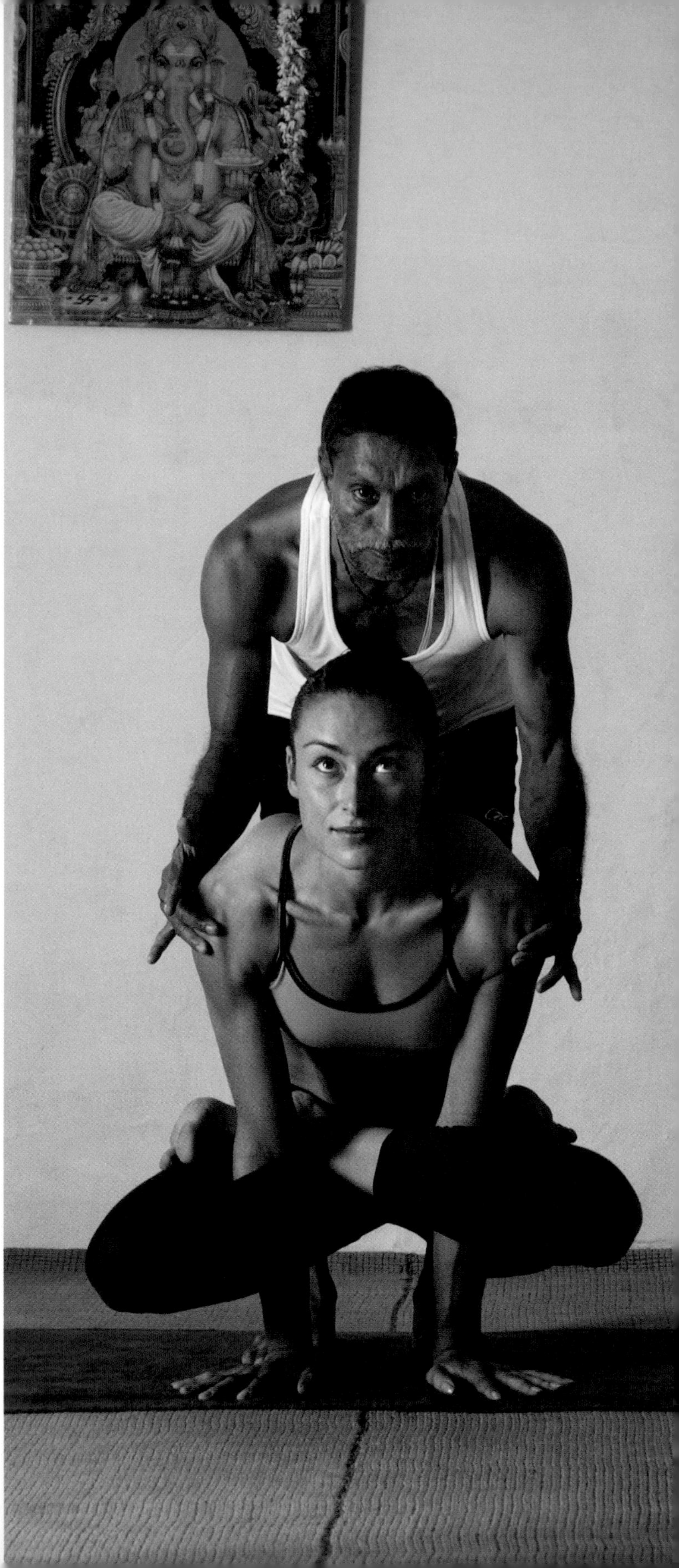

BALANCE

A relatively low-key, but top-notch, yoga school in Mysore is the Mandala Yoga Sala housed in a 100-year old house on Dewan street in the Laxmipuram area. Set up by Harish Bheemaiah, the school is renowned for its excellent tuition by *acharya* (teacher) Mr V Sheshadri and his son. Sheshadri was a student of Yogaratna Sri B N S Iyengar (not to be confused with B K S Iyengar) and has achieved recognition at both international and national levels. He helps students push beyond their limits with a unique style of adjustment (he often sits or stands on them!).

Opposite, top left *Urdva danurasana* or "intense back bend".
Opposite, bottom left *Uttanasana* or "forward bend".
Left *Kukkutasana* or "rooster pose".
Below An adjustment to *uthita trikonasana*.
Right, top *Virabhadrasana 1* or "warrior 1".
Right, middle *Urdva mukha shvanasana* or "upward facing dog".
Right, bottom *Adho mukha shvanasana* or "downward facing dog".

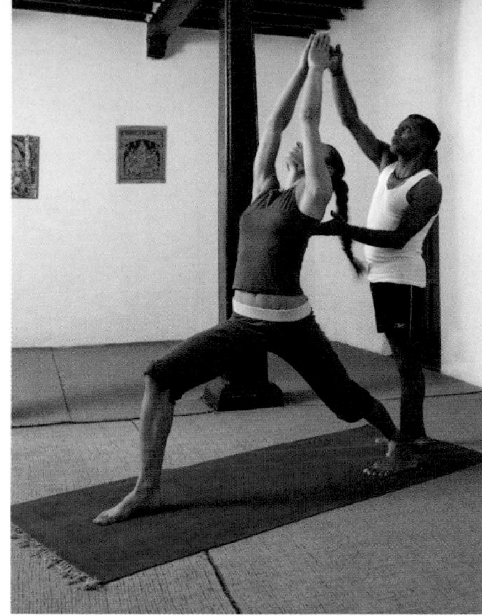

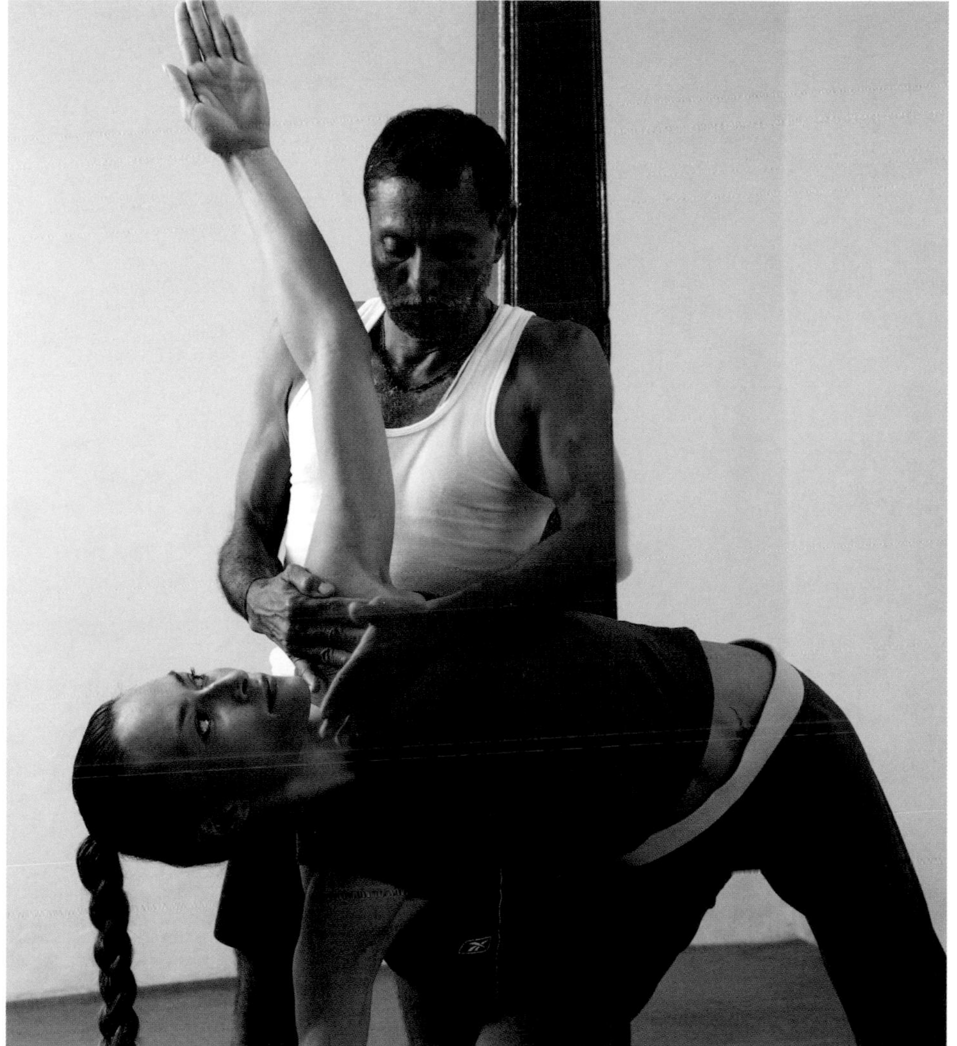

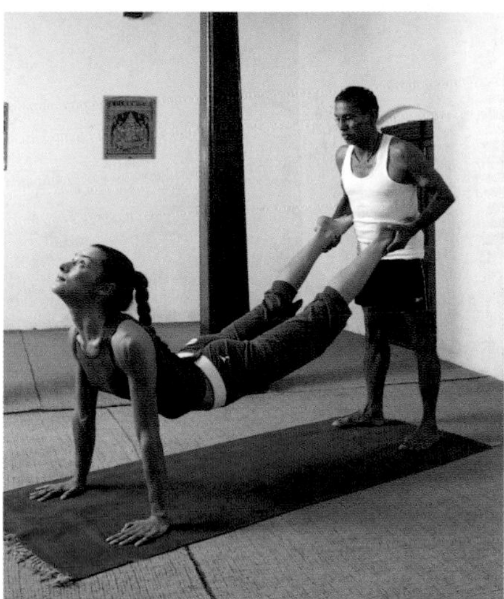

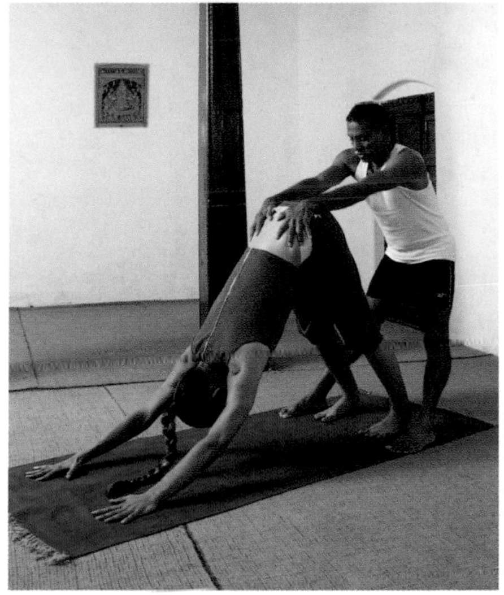

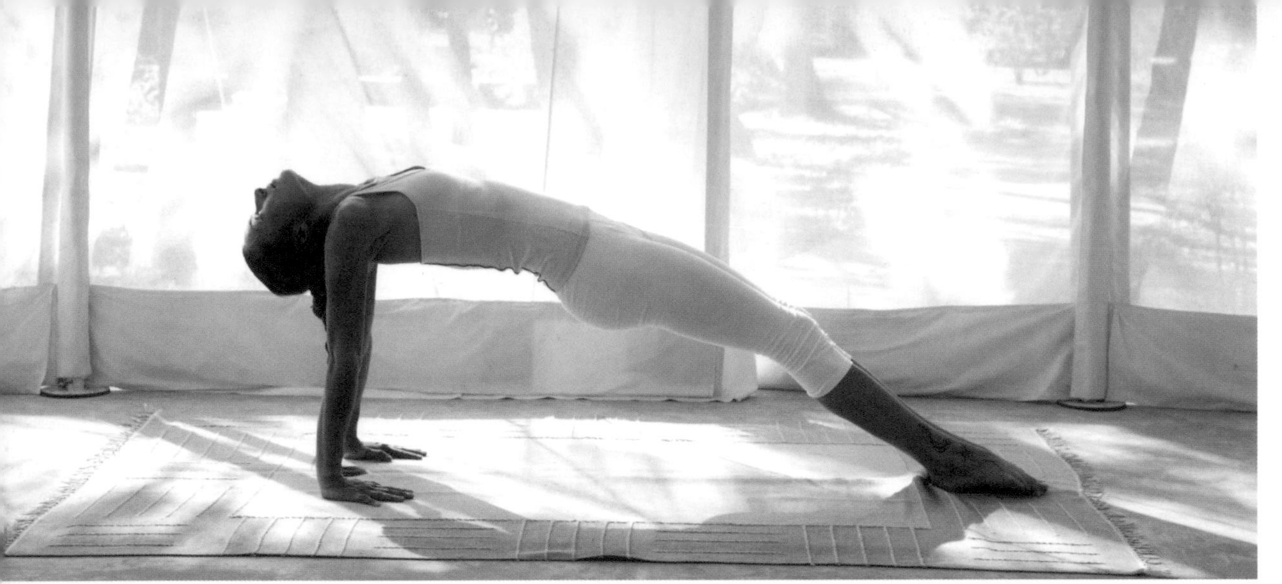

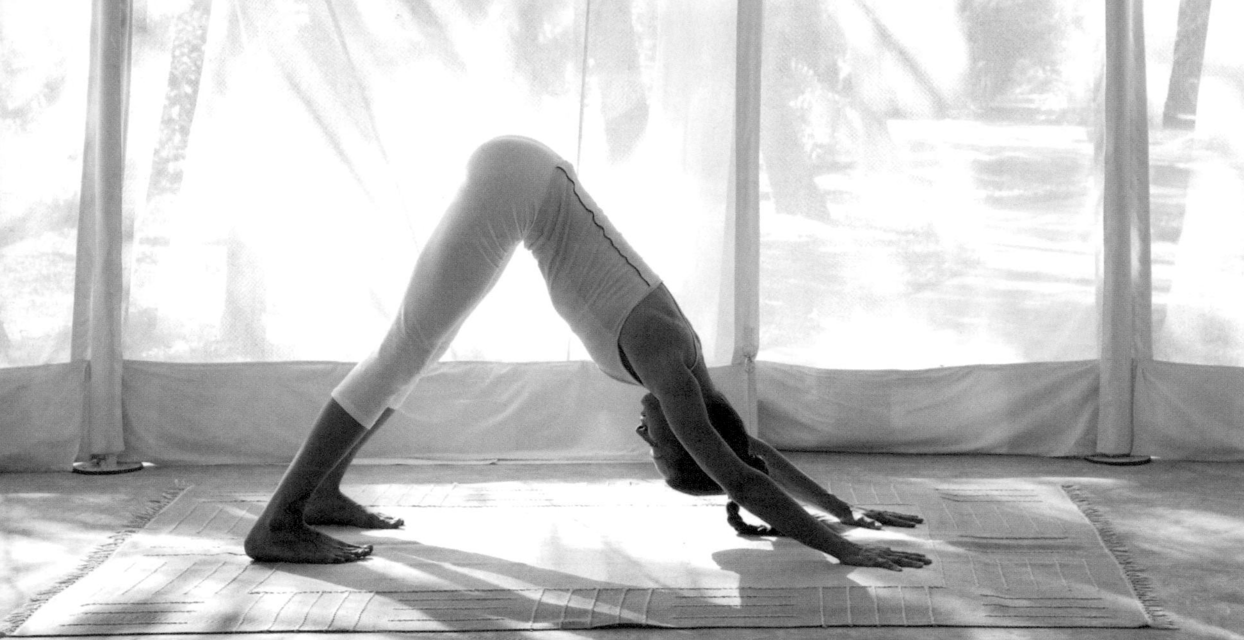

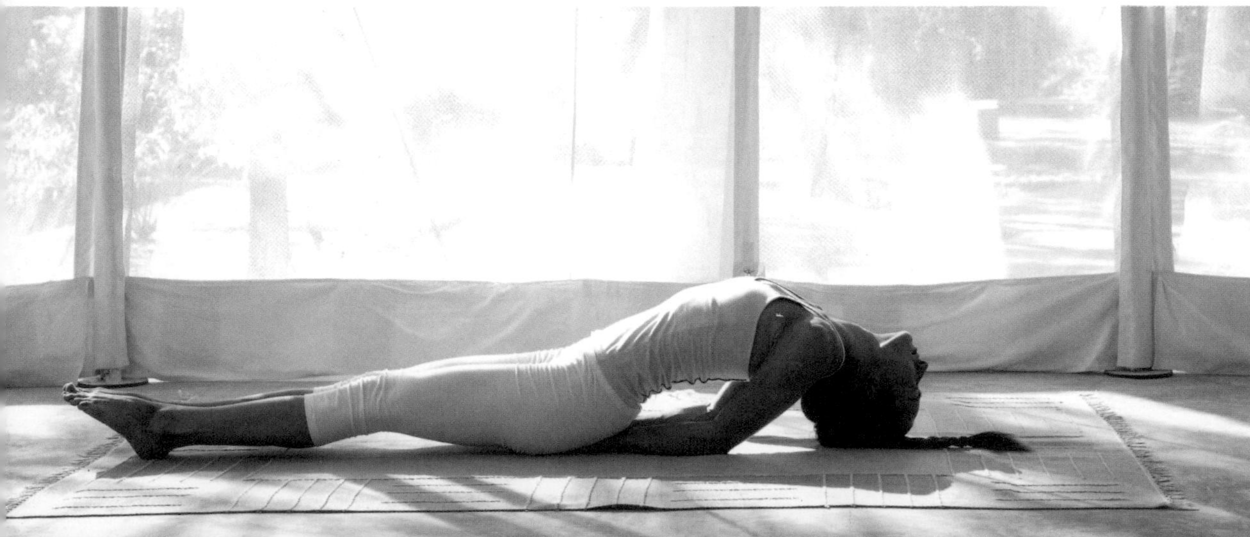

Shreyas Retreat, just outside Bangalore, combines five-star facilities with an ethos that can best be described as boarding school basic. As the owner explains, it is about "living an ashram-style life with daily yoga, meditation sessions, organic vegetarian food, no alcohol, community service and farming". For those who want to immerse themselves in India's ancient wellness traditions, it offers innovative tuition and plenty of peace and quiet, but does not skimp on creature comforts. It markets itself as a place that helps guests to find their "inner core."

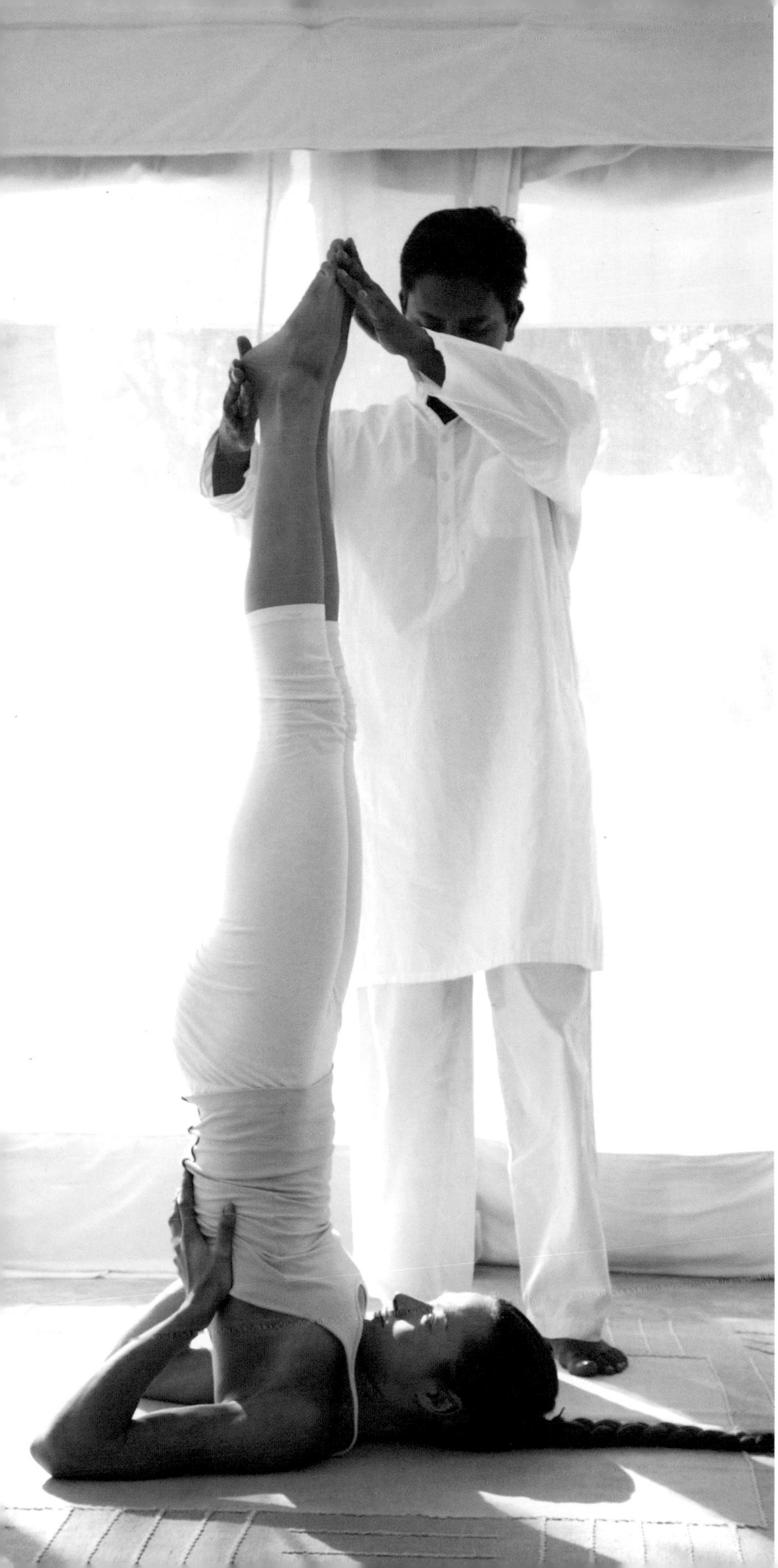

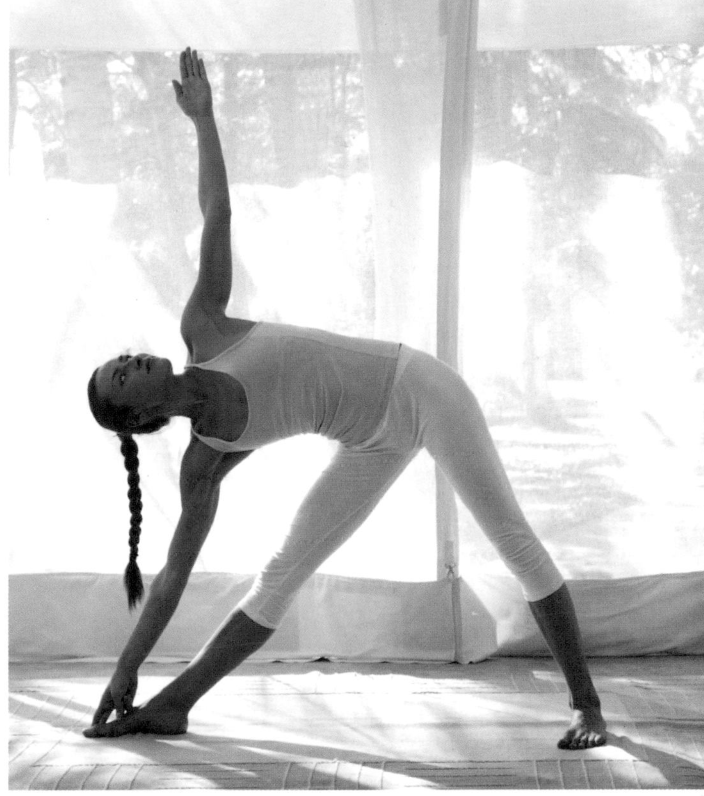

Aided by Shreyas instructor Bharat Kumar Patra, our model and yoga teacher Yana Odnopozov demonstrates some of the different *asanas* in the yoga repertoire. *Asanas* should be "steady and comfortable" according to Patanjali and Yana looks nothing if not poised in these photographs.

Opposite, top *Punatanasana* or "east extension posture", an *asana* that helps strengthen shoulders and wrist joints.
Opposite, middle *Adho mukha svanasana* or "downward facing dog", one of the postures in the Sun Salutation series.
Opposite, bottom *Matsyasana* or "fish posture", helpful for neck and spine.
Left *Sarvangasana* or "supported shoulder stand", a posture that helps with thyroid disorders.
Above *Trikonasana* or "triangle pose": Maintained to strengthen knees and calf and thigh muscles, this posture is good for the spine.

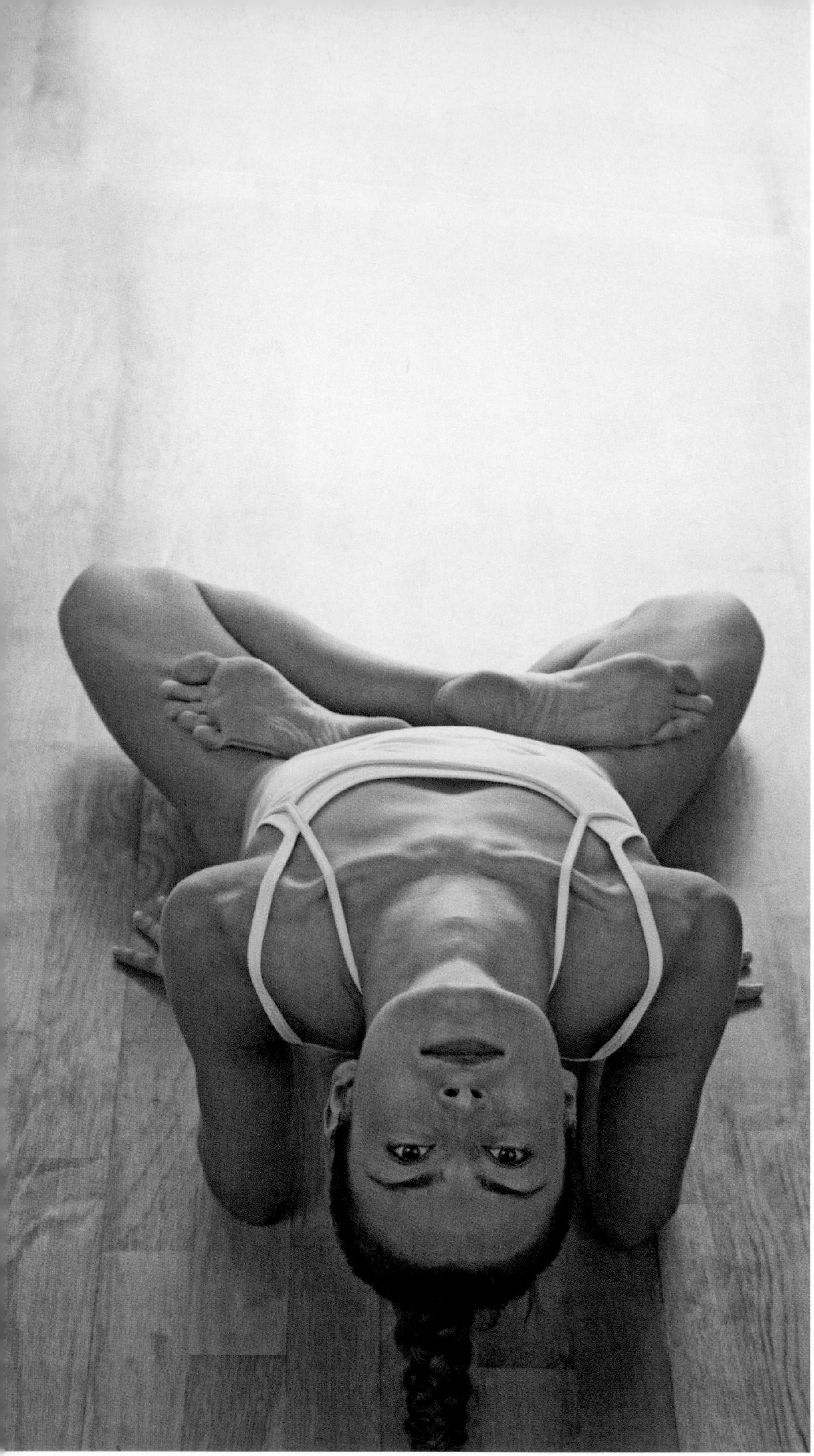

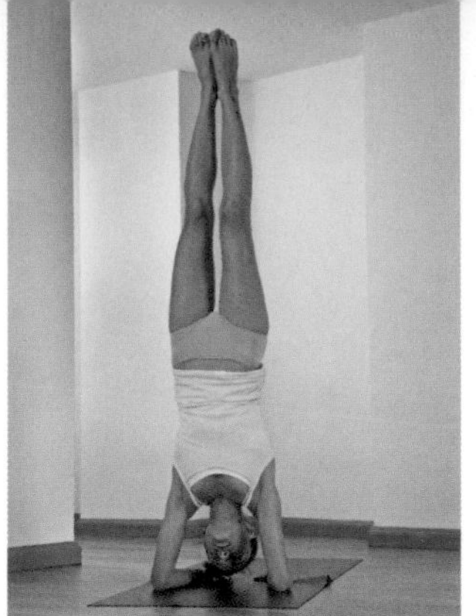

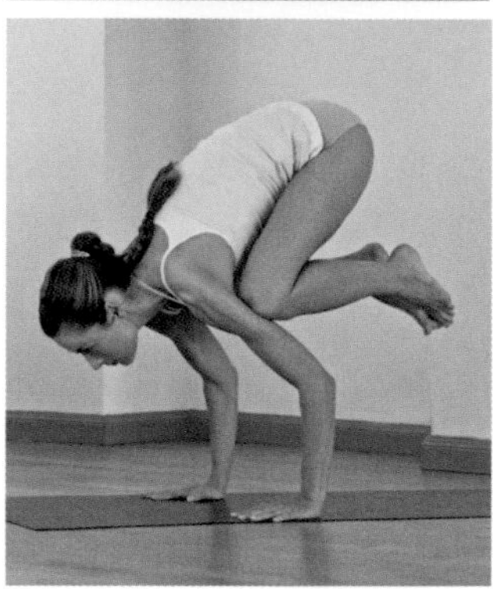

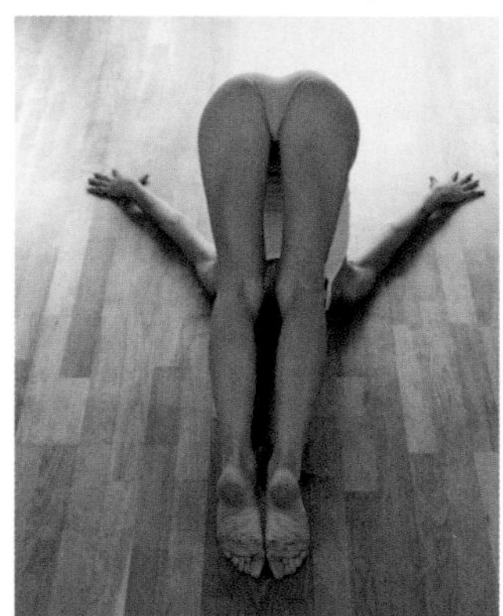

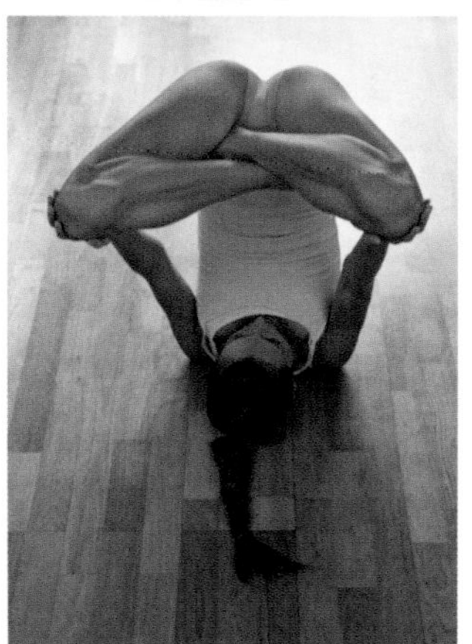

Far left This is a variation of *padmasana* or "lotus pose"; usually performed sitting upright, here the practitioner leans back.

Left, top to bottom
The headstand, known as *sirsasana*, is a major pose in yoga. Hands and arms can be used in a number of different ways to support this pose which stretches the spine and builds neck muscle.
The crane pose or *bakasana* is a yoga posture that stretches the knees, hamstrings and lower back. It is one of the easiest balance arm postures in the yoga repertoire.
This posture is known as *halasana* or "plough pose" (*hala* in Sanskrit translates as plough). As the plough makes the hard ground soft, the veins are stretched here to reduce stiffness in the body. Another variation of *padmasana*.

Right *Parsva bakasana* or "side crane pose" gives an intense stretch in the lower back and requires good upper body strength. The lower arms bones (ulna and radius) act as supporting beams and the legs are bent at the knee. This is a variation of the side crane posture, as the participant has stretched out both her legs to one side.

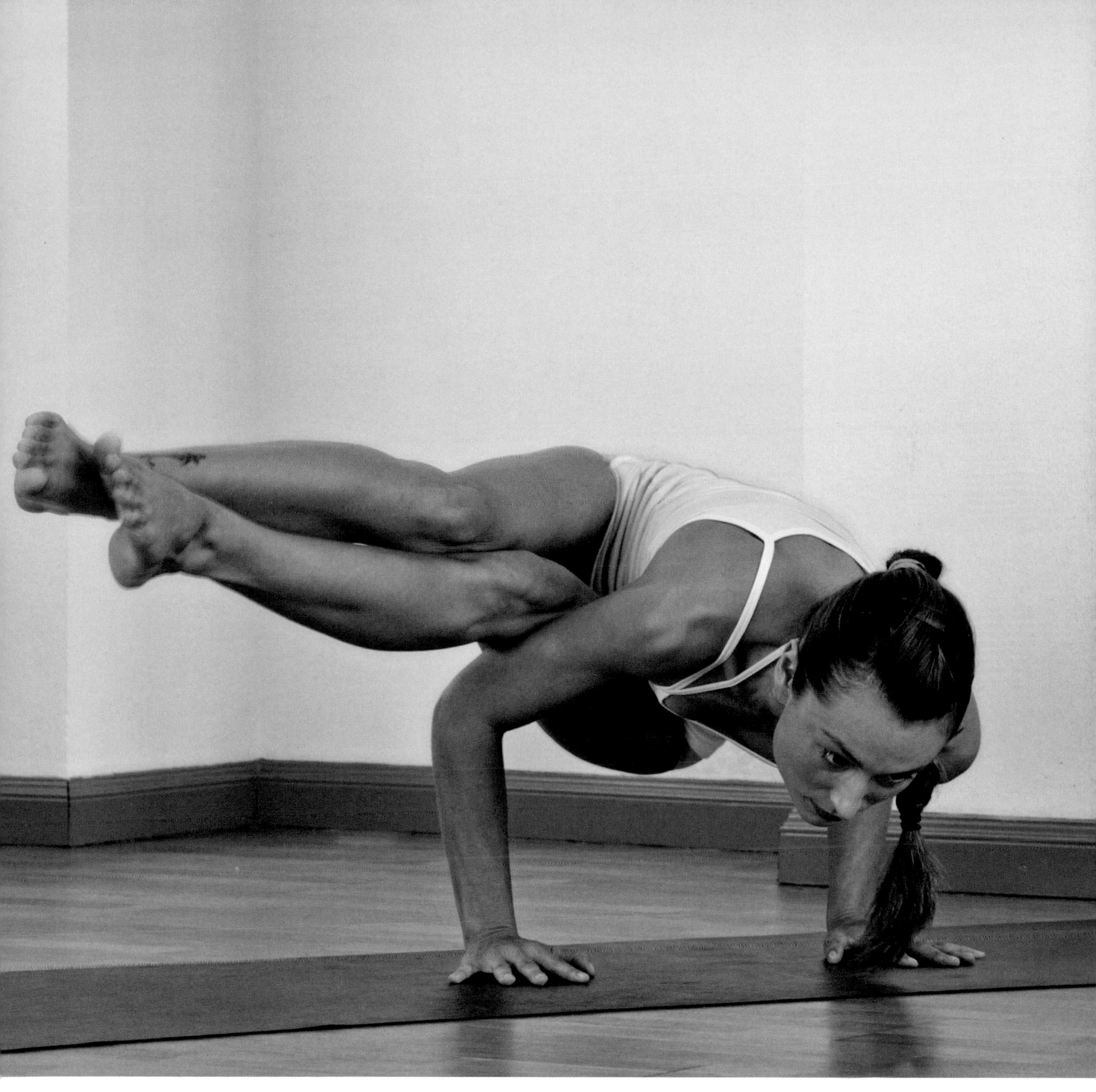

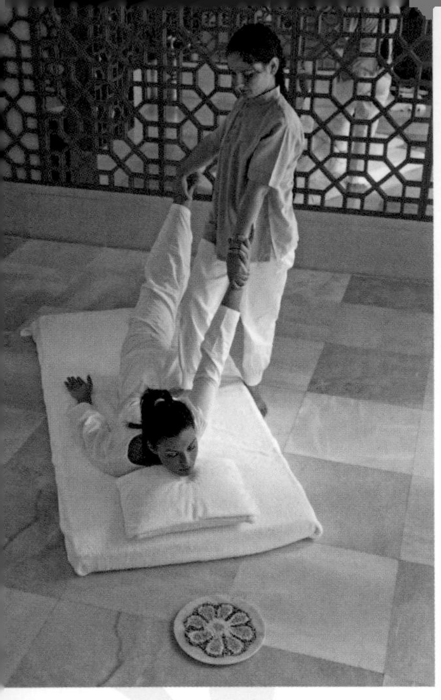

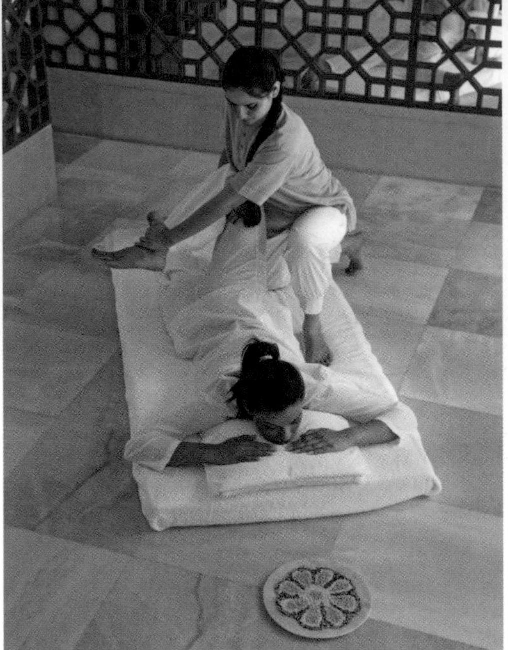

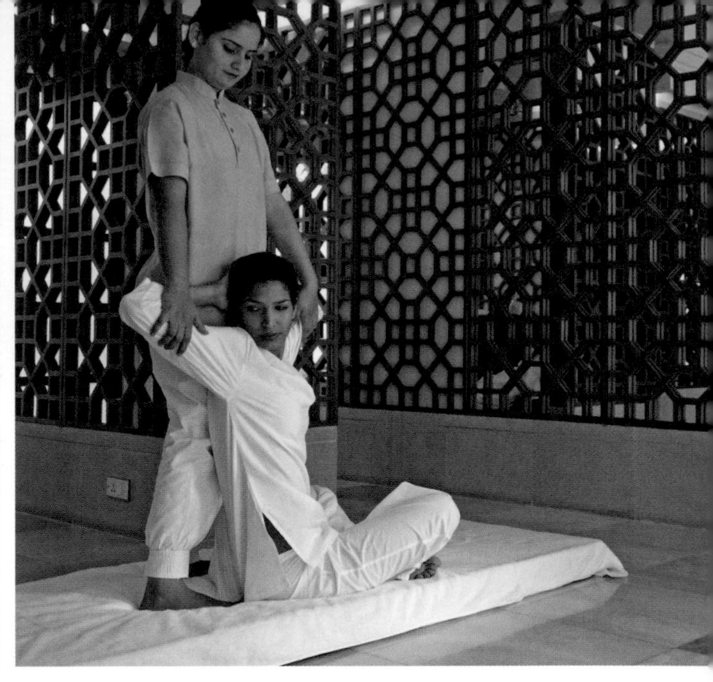

amulya uphar Lazy Man's Yoga

Similar to Thai massage, but based on the stretching facilitated by yoga postures, Amulya Uphar is a unique technique offered at Rajasthan's Amanbagh. Translating as "Priceless Gift" from the Hindi, it is an oil-free treatment that takes place on a mattress on the floor, with the client wearing a loose *kurta* pyjama suit. The therapist works on the client's meridian lines and acupressure points, manipulating the body into different positions to open up energy channels that in turn stimulate sluggish blood circulation, movement of lymph and the flow of *chi*.

First of all, clients are prepared for the body work with a foot wash with a hot towel to remove negative energy and a gentle touch on the solar plexus and crown *chakra* to let them know they are in safe hands. Lying on their back on a mattress on the floor, they are requested to breathe normally before the massage begins. This always starts with the feet as it is here that the body weight rests: Using thumbs and the palms on the meridian lines, reflex points are awakened on the soles, then the masseuse moves up the legs to stomach and hands, shoulders and head. After this, the client turns over and the therapist works on the legs, back, neck and head.

Amulya Uphar is quite a physically demanding experience, with the therapist sometimes sitting on the client, and often pulling him or her into somewhat contorted positions. The cobra pose, for example, has the therapist kneeling on the pressure points of the client's thighs while holding both hands and pulling them backwards. At certain points the client may be requested to breathe in or out in order to facilitate the opening up of the body, but the therapist — by listening to the body — knows how far it can be coaxed, stretched or twisted.

Amulya Uphar can be an amazingly de-stressing experience, with many clients reporting deep relaxation, relief of tension and increased suppleness afterwards. As with Watsu, a similar practice offered in water, it works best if clients give themselves up entirely to the therapist by relaxing completely.

Such yogic stretching is offered at other venues in India and overseas: Essentially, the body is being assisted into yoga *asanas* and stretches without having to make any effort itself. It has all the benefits of yoga, but much less of the hard work!

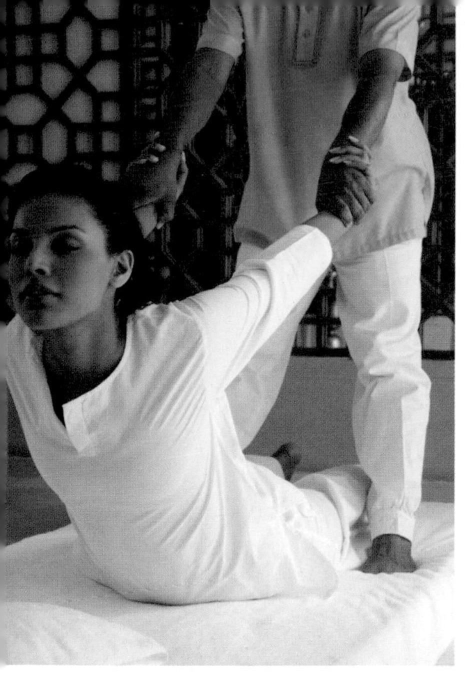

The skilled Amanbagh therapist pulls, turns, manipulates and stretches the client's body to simulate certain yoga postures and stretches. All the while, she works along the energy lines, using acupressure, reflexology and internal organ massage. The aim is to clear blockages of *prana* and give the client a full body workover to improve overall health and create a feeling of wellbeing.

From far left Pulling arms and legs stretches the abdomen; hamstring stretch; twisting from the waist to free up muscles in the upper arms; pulling the client towards *dhanurasana* or the "bow pose" to stretch shoulders and elongate the spine.
Right Another "bow pose" angle.
Below Stretching arms to work on the triceps.

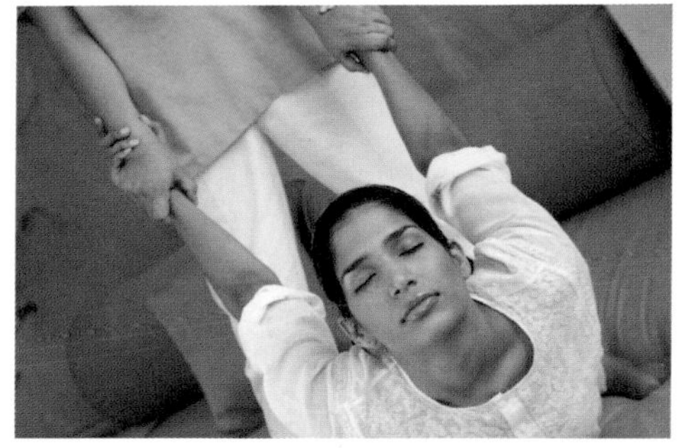

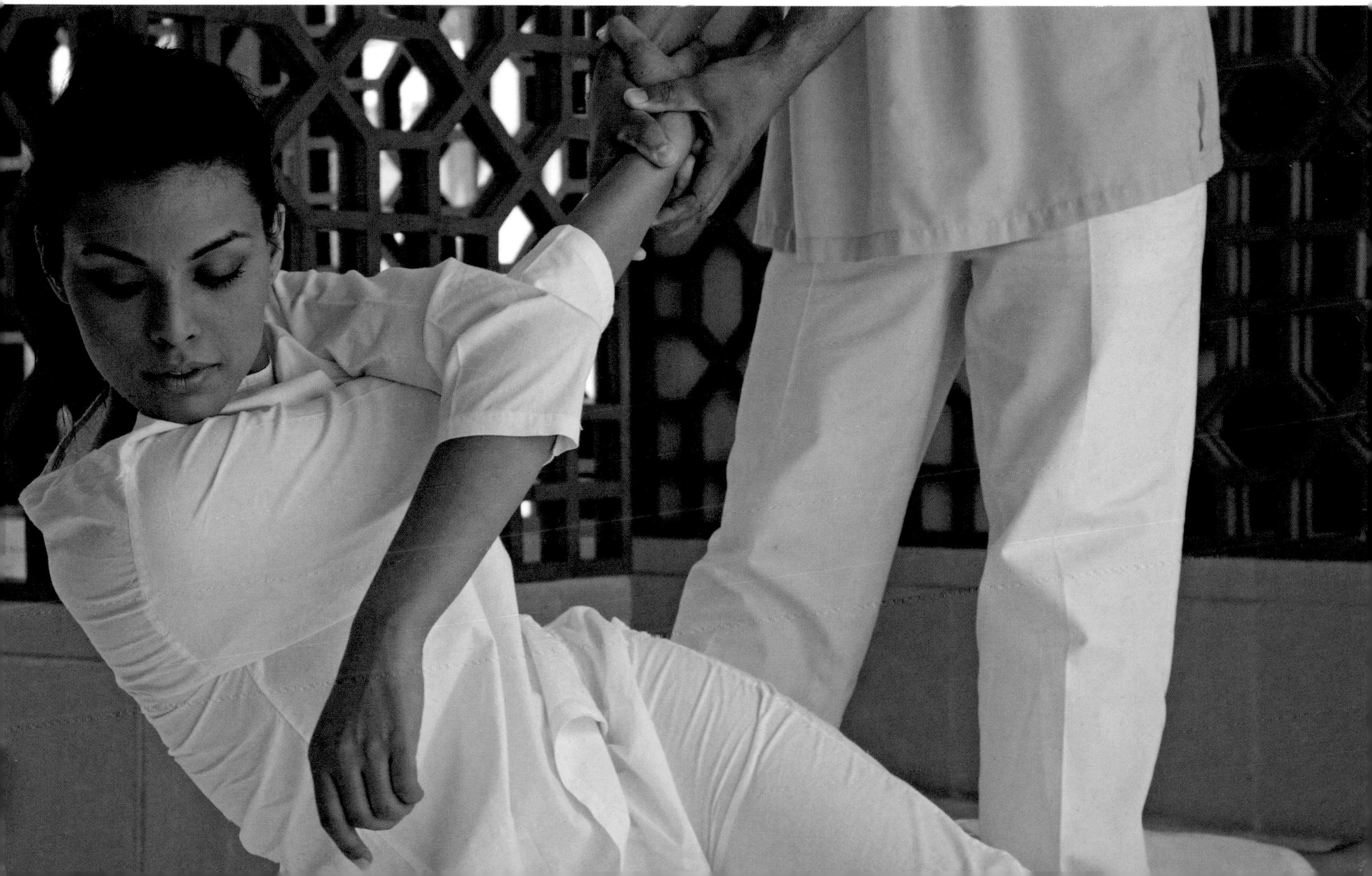

pranayama Therapeutic Breathing Exercises

Taken from the word *prana* meaning "vital energy" or "life force" and *ayama* that means "control" or "extension/expansion", *pranayama* comprises a series of breathing exercises that calm the mind, improve the condition of the abdominal and chest area, and eliminate toxins from the body. Originally expounded by Patanjali (see page 100), it is all about the expansion of the vital force through regulated breathing processes.

Regular *pranayama* practitioners report that they are calm and balanced, their minds are focused and they have increased vitality and longevity. According to Patanjali, *pranayama* awakens the brain and the cerebrospinal nerve centers enabling them to reach their highest potential. Be this true or not, research suggests that it is beneficial in treating a range of stress-related disorders and it relieves symptoms of asthma.

All the exercises follow a sequence of inhalation (*puraka*), holding (*kumbhaka*) and exhalation (*rechaka*). The main focus is on correcting bad breathing habits and concentrating on the here and now. Inhalations should be deep, complete and focused, filling the lungs completely, while exhalations are slow, deep and uniform. Ideally, the latter should take twice as long as the former, and at the end of a *rechaka* the lungs should be emptied to the maximum extent, their tissues contracting as much as possible. In the case of *kumbhaka*, there is no question of speed or movement: it is simply stopping all breath by holding all the respiratory apparatus tight and still.

There are a number of *pranayama* exercises and all should be practiced in a sitting posture. Choose from the half a dozen sitting postures laid down by Patanjali: the simplest, least strenuous one is *swastikasana*, but more advanced yoga practitioners may prefer the lotus position or *padmasana*, the traditional recommendation for *pranayama*.

Sessions usually start with a prayer or a simple *om*. Practitioners are encouraged to sit in a relaxed posture, with spine straight and shoulders relaxed. After a couple of such introductory exhalations, the hands are rubbed together to stimulate the circulation, and a gentle self-massage is given to the face and back of the neck.

Before the breathing session begins in earnest, it is recommended that the process known as *kapala bhati* takes place. *Kapal* is a Sanskrit word for "forehead", while *bhati* means "lighting" or "glowing". It is a *kirya* or cleansing process that is practiced in a meditative posture with spine and neck erect, and eyes closed. A session of rapid breathing, with active and forceful exhalation followed by passive inhalation, it has no *kumbhaka* or holding of breath stage. All the nerves reverberate during this exercise, you may even sweat profusely and, on the exhalation, most people experience a flapping movement in the abdomen.

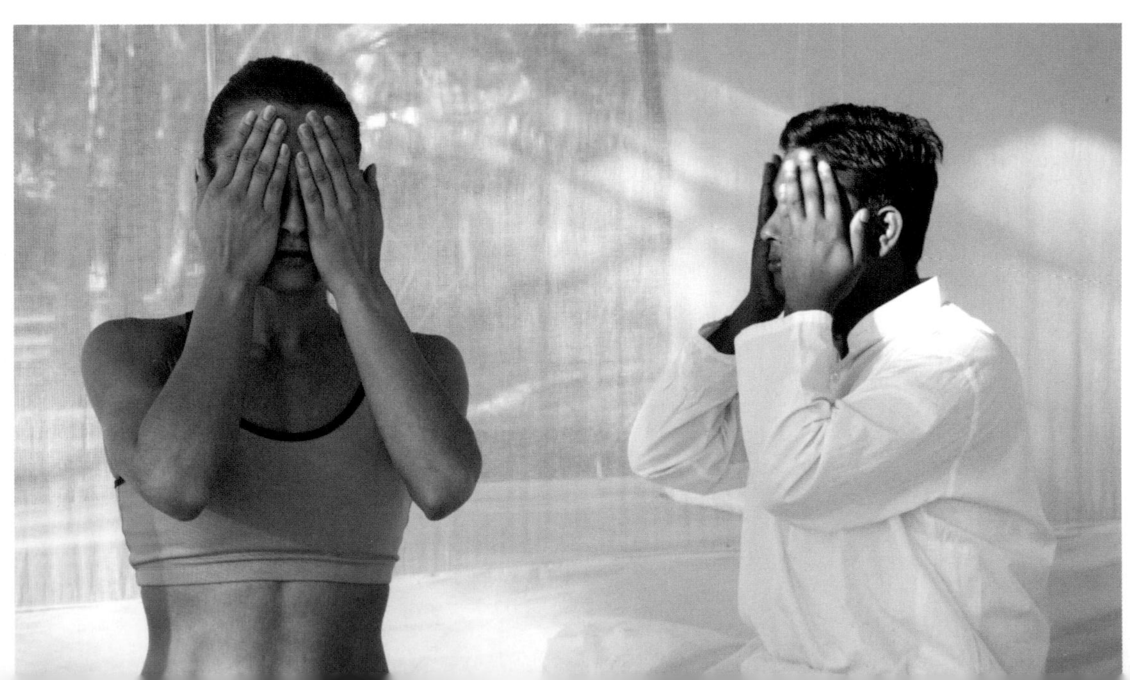

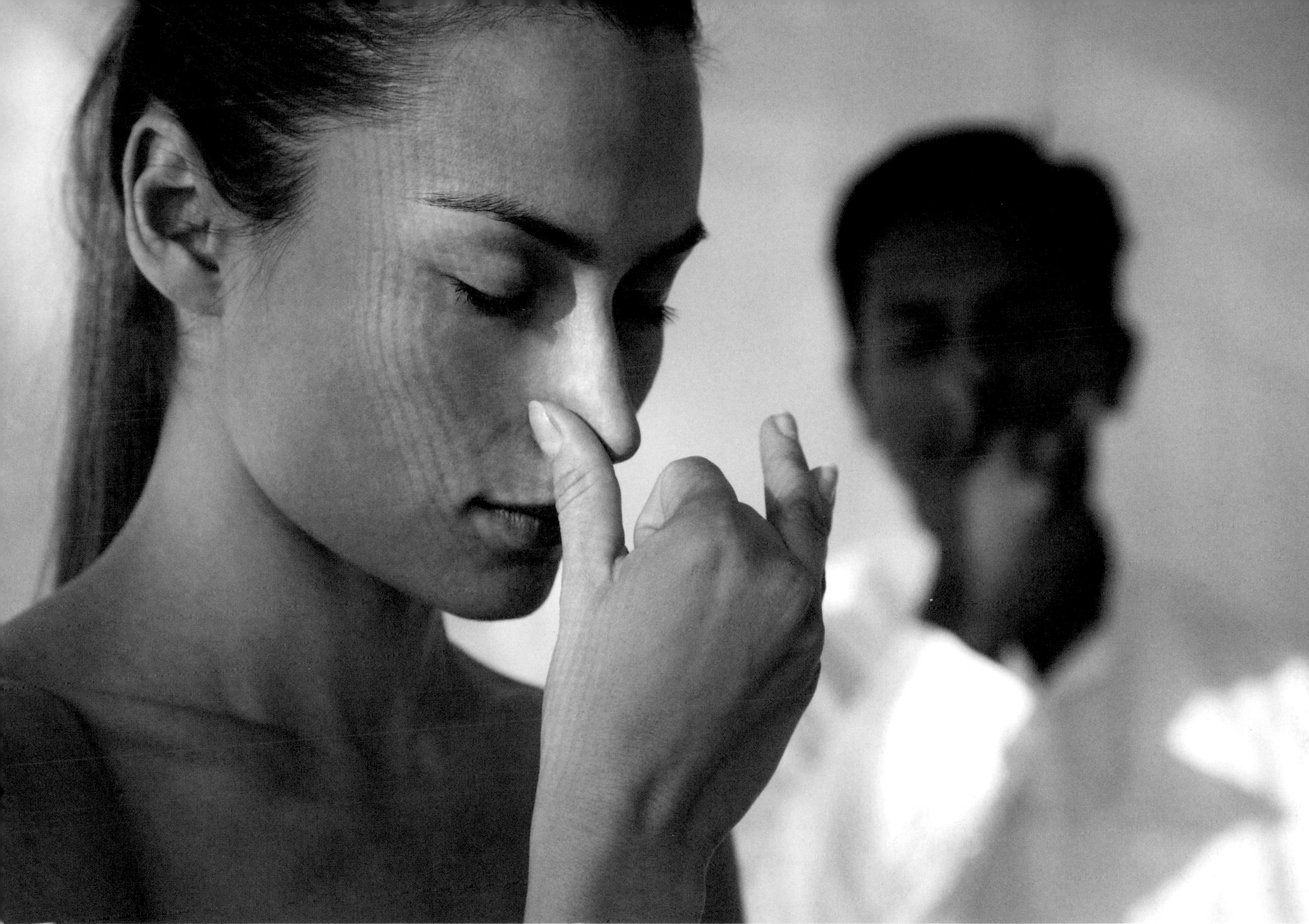

Left Shreyas Retreat runs regular *pranayama* sessions in conjunction with yoga. They always start with the practice of palming. During this, hands are rubbed together to stimulate circulation and a gentle self-massage is given to the face and back of the neck.
Above *Nadhi sodhana* or "alternate nostril breating", a very particular *pranayama* practice, calms the mind, balances the mental state and stimulates both sides of the brain as both nostrils flow freely.

As *kapala bhati* is an extremely dynamic experience, it should only be done for about a minute, as this is enough time to give a massaging effect to the inner organs as well as balance and strengthen the nervous system. It also helps set up the lungs and entire respiratory tract for the breathing exercises to follow.

Vhustrika is often the first exercise: Translating as "bellows breath", it is a breathing technique used by yogis to build energy, tone the respiratory muscles and induce a feeling of alertness and mental clarity. As suggested by the name, the breath imitates the action of a bellows. Essentially a method of controlled hyper-ventilation, it comprises a series of inhalation/holding/exhalation sequences that focus on the thoracic and chest region. Active inhalation with chest out and shoulders rising slightly is followed by holding, then active exhalation to bring the chest back in. These sequences help promote proper diaphragmatic breathing, oxygenate the blood and purge the lungs of residual carbon dioxide.

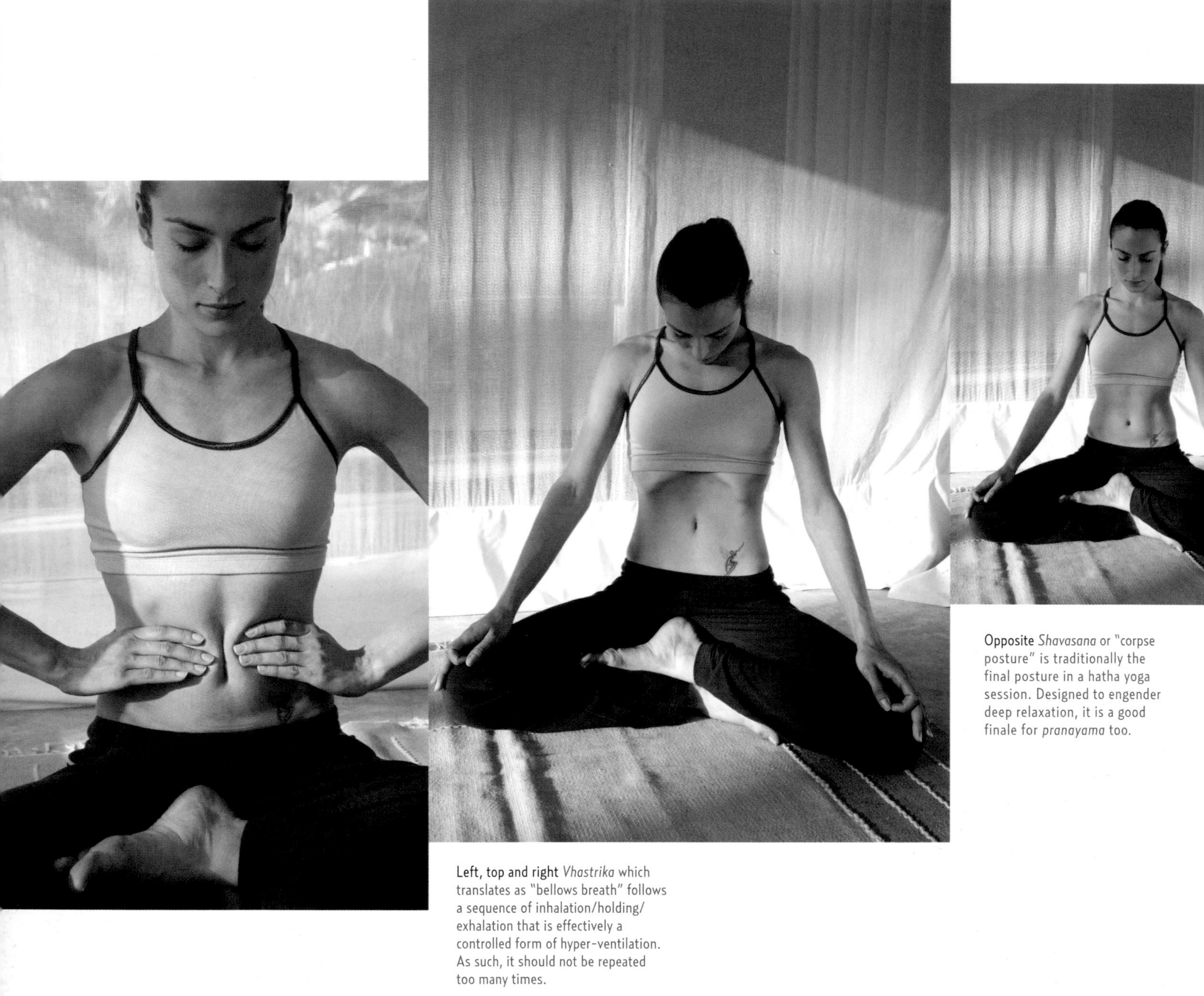

Opposite *Shavasana* or "corpse posture" is traditionally the final posture in a hatha yoga session. Designed to engender deep relaxation, it is a good finale for *pranayama* too.

Left, top and right *Vhastrika* which translates as "bellows breath" follows a sequence of inhalation/holding/exhalation that is effectively a controlled form of hyper-ventilation. As such, it should not be repeated too many times.

Alternate nostril breathing or *nadhi sodhana* is another technique. *Nadhi* is the word for "psychic passage", a specific pathway through which *prana* flows, and *sodhana* is "purification", so this sequence is designed to facilitate smooth flow of *prana*. It should not be practiced if the nasal passages are blocked; in fact, in any *pranayama* series, if the breath feels forced, stop immediately.

In *nadhi sodhana*, the flow of breath is controlled by either the thumb or the ring finger of the right hand in what is known as the *nasika mudra* (see photo of hand position on page 115). First of all, the right nostril is blocked with the thumb, and air is slowly exhaled through the left nostril. When the lungs are completely empty, the practitioner inhales slowly through the left nostril, then closes the nostril with the ring finger. He or she then exhales completely out of the right nostril, inhales through the right nostril, and blocks again with the thumb. It is a good idea to mentally count five seconds for each inhalation and six seconds for every exhalation. The whole process should be repeated a few times for maximum benefit.

Another technique is *uddiyana bandha* (*uddiyana* means a "jump upward", *bandha* is a "lock"). Basically, it means the contraction of particular muscles in the body that are locked or held tightly in a certain position. There are four main *bandhas* associated with *pranayama*; the other three are *jalandhara bandha* (bending the neck forward and setting the chin below the throat), *mula bandha* (contraction of the anal sphincters and the pelvic floor) and *jilva bandha* (holding the tongue on the roof of the mouth).

In *uddiyana bandha*, the thoracic diaphragm is moved to an extreme upward position, held, then released. Practitioners sit in the lotus position with hands in the *chin* mudra (index finger touching the thumb and other three fingers relaxed), and focus on the lower abdominal section of the body. The sequence is as follows: Breathe out completely, contract the lowest *chakra* at the bottom of the spine, suck in the abdomen, lock in the chin with the chest, and hold the breath. Keep steady for as long as is comfortable, then release from the chin and abdomen, and exhale. *Uddiyana bandha* can take quite a time to master and novices should never exceed their individual capacity.

In general, *pranayama* modifies normal breathing processes considerably, thereby creating substantial internal pressures and stretches. Added to this, is the need to keep the whole body focused from top to bottom, thereby releasing any held tension and stress. *Pranayama* classes are offered at many venues throughout India and elsewhere and many find it a wonderful exercise before a meditation session.

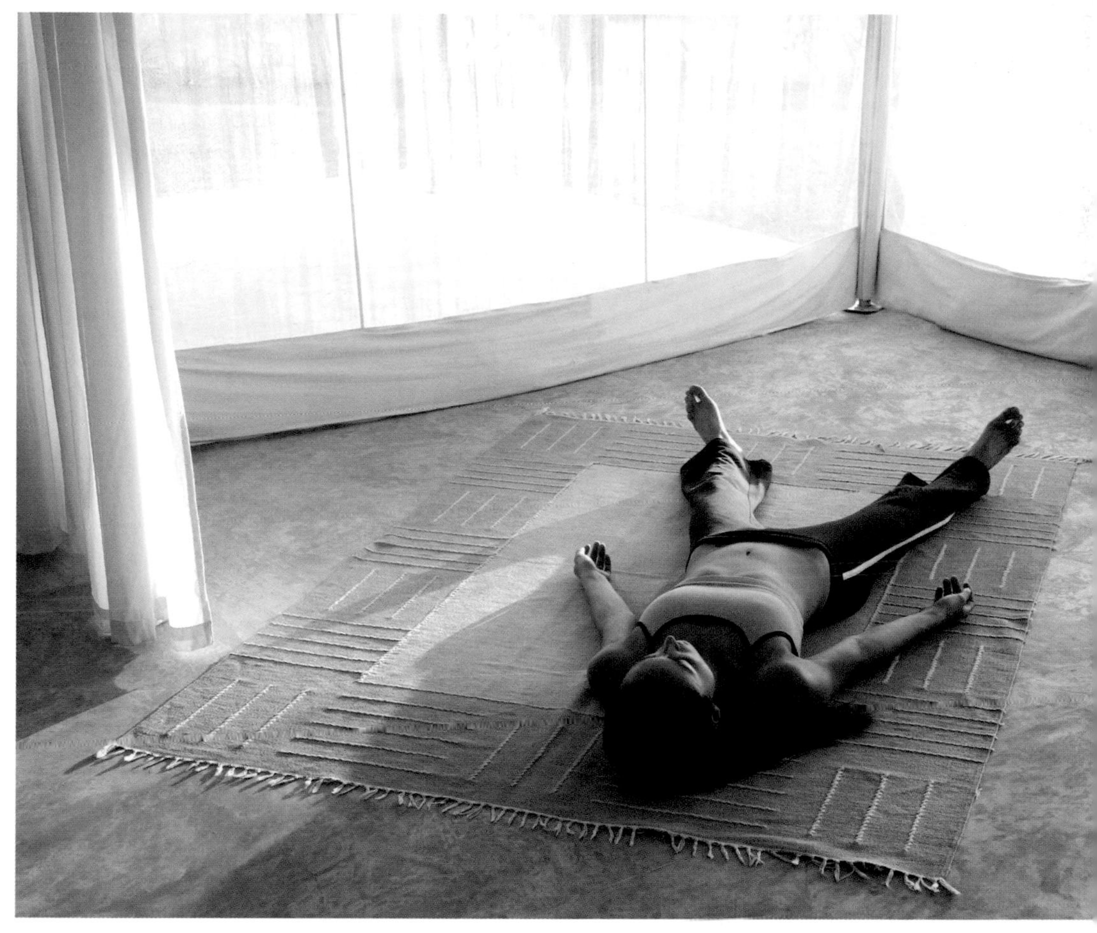

meditation

Rooted in many of the world's great religions, meditation has been used as a healing therapy for centuries. Today, it is experiencing a renaissance in popularity with many doctors prescribing meditation as a way to lower blood pressure, improve performance, relieve insomnia and promote relaxation. It is safe and simple; it needs no complicated machinery or drugs; and it can balance on a physical, emotional, mental and spiritual level at the same time.

Above Meditation has long been practiced both in a secular fashion and as a Buddhist or Hindu practice. Here we see a detail of the hands and feet of the Buddha; 14th century, Sukothai Period, housed in the Prasat Museum, Bangkok. **Right** An evening meditation session atop one of the roofs at Amanbagh. Using fire, it comprises ritual and chanting, to give thanks for the day.

Meditation and Hinduism

Meditation originated in India with yoga, one of the six schools of Hindu philosophy. First mentioned in the *Puranas*, the *Vedas* and the *Upanishads* (Hindu holy scriptures), it was later outlined by Patanjali (see page 100). Its aim is to still the mind, body and soul, alleviate suffering and promote healing. How this is done varies: *Japa* yoga advocates the repetition of a mantra, hatha yoga is aimed at raising spiritual energy, raja yoga works with breath, *surat shabd* yoga uses sound and light to meditate, and *bhakti* yoga or the "yoga of love and devotion" aims to concentrate practitioners' focus on a particular devotional subject.

Viewed as a method of attaining physiological and spiritual mastery, meditation is central to Hinduism. The seven *rishis* or great sages were master meditators and today's *sadhus* or wandering mystics employ meditation, along with asceticism, renunciation, celibacy and yoga with the ultimate aim of attaining enlightenment. However, one does not need to be a Hindu to practice Hindu meditation. Many Hindu meditative techniques are secular in nature — and everyone is welcome to try them.

A popular choice for those serious to learn more about Hinduism and meditation is a visit to an Indian ashram. Neither a temple nor a monastery, an ashram is a more like a retreat. The idea is to lead a simple life, develop a positive attitude and come away with an understanding

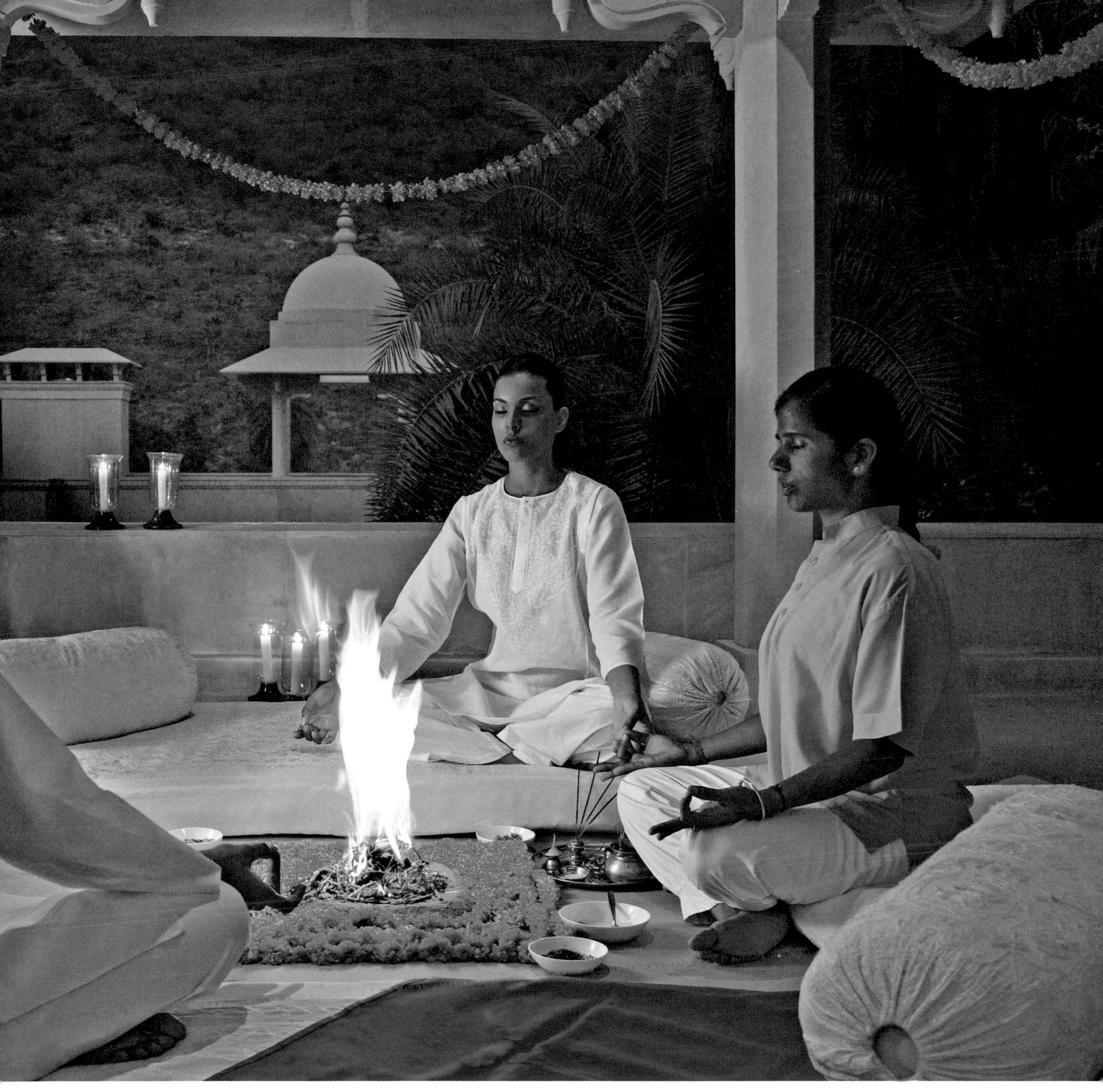

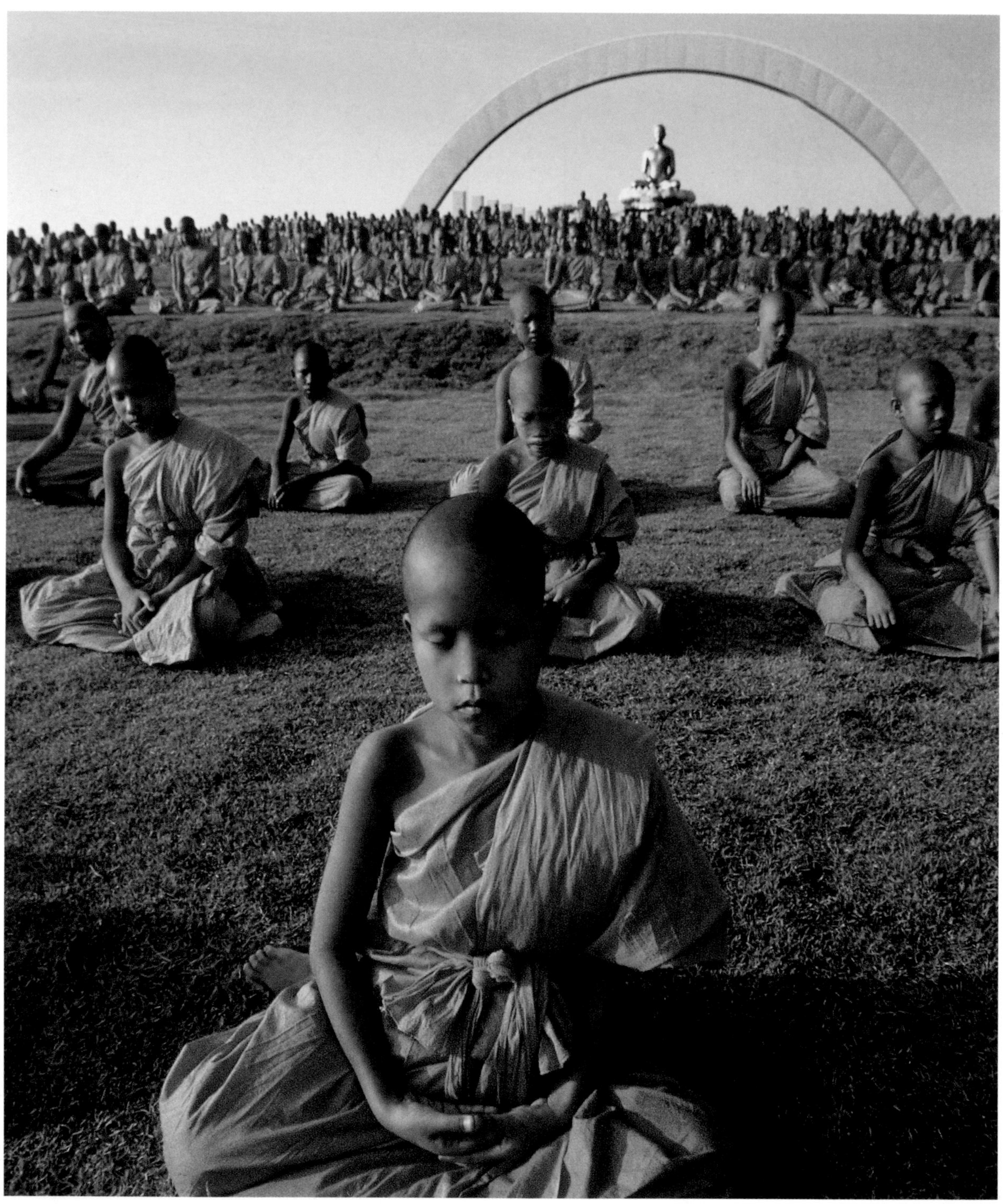

Right Novice monks in "resting pose" during meditation. **Opposite** Many spas and retreats offer meditation sessions these days. Here a client focuses on the inner mind during a session at Prana Spa, Bali.

of selfless service. A 15-day visit usually includes a *sadhana* course where yoga (see pages 100–111), meditation, *pranayama* (see page 114–117), relaxation and concentration techniques are "taught" in peaceful, often remote surrounds. Many people report that such a withdrawal from normal everyday life is a rich and rewarding experience.

Meditation and Buddhism

Meditation is also central to Buddhism. Indeed, in around 500 BC, the Indian prince Siddharta Gautama rejected the material world and attained enlightenment through meditation beneath a *bodhi* tree. Theravāda Buddhism advocates various meditative practices, but the two best known are Samadhi or "Concentrative Meditation" and Vipassana or "Mindfulness Meditation". Both are considered part of the eightfold path Buddhists must follow in order to achieve Nirvana.

At its most simple, concentrative meditation focuses attention on the breath, an image or a sound (mantra) in order to still the mind and allow a greater awareness and clarity to emerge. By focusing on the continuous rhythm of inhalation and exhalation, the mind becomes absorbed in the rhythm, breathing becomes slower and deeper, and the practitioner becomes more tranquil and aware. Mindfulness meditation, on the other hand, seeks to open up the mind's awareness. The practitioner sits quietly, simply witnessing whatever goes through the mind, thereby obtaining a more calm, clear and non-reactive state of mind.

Again, both types of meditation are open to non-Buddhists. Of particular note are the 10-day residential courses offered by the

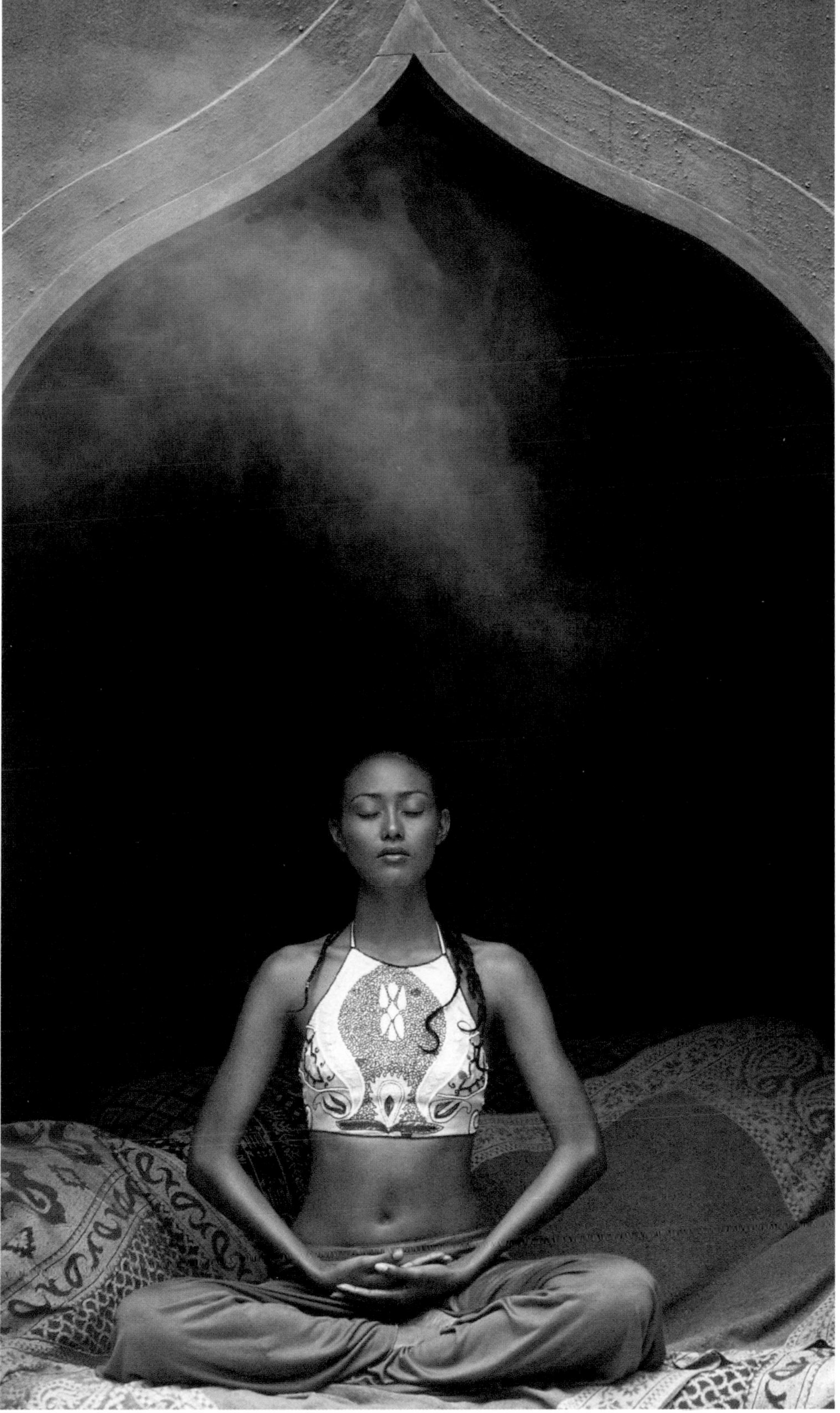

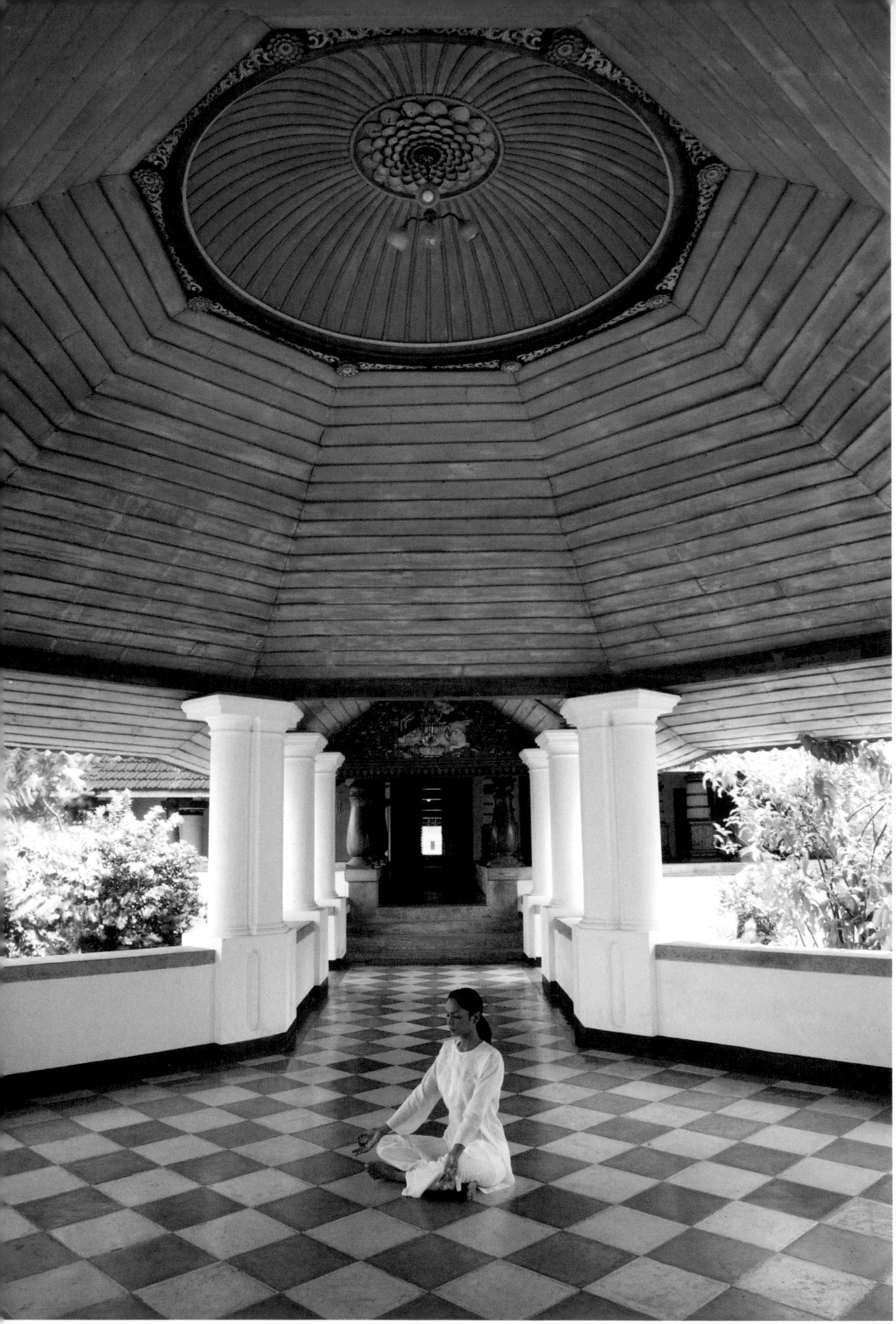

Many hotels, resorts and retreats offer meditation sessions in India. These may be group or solitary one-to-one "lessons" and are usually given early in the morning or at dusk. On **left**, we see a client in a meditative pose in a pavilion at the Ayurvedic retreat of Kalari Kovilakom; on **right**, a bamboo grove at Ananda, in the Himalayas, provides seclusion for a pair of devotees. A statue of the *nandi* or bull, the Lord Shiva's primary vehicle, forms a focus here.

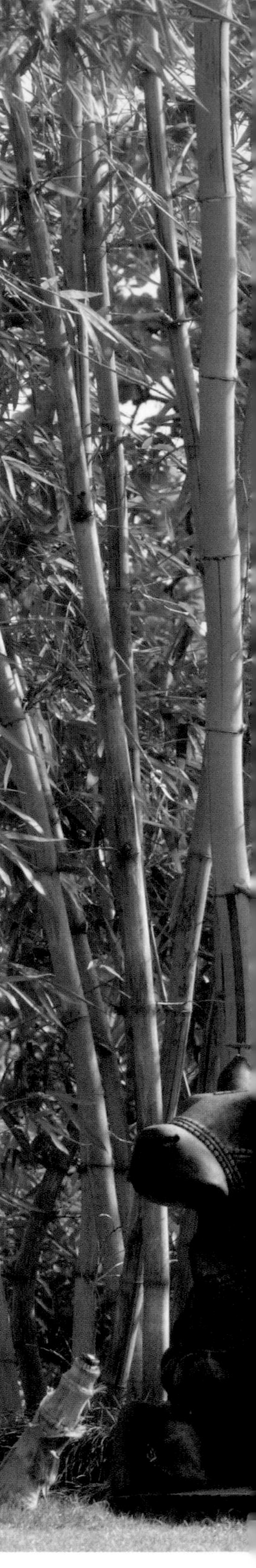

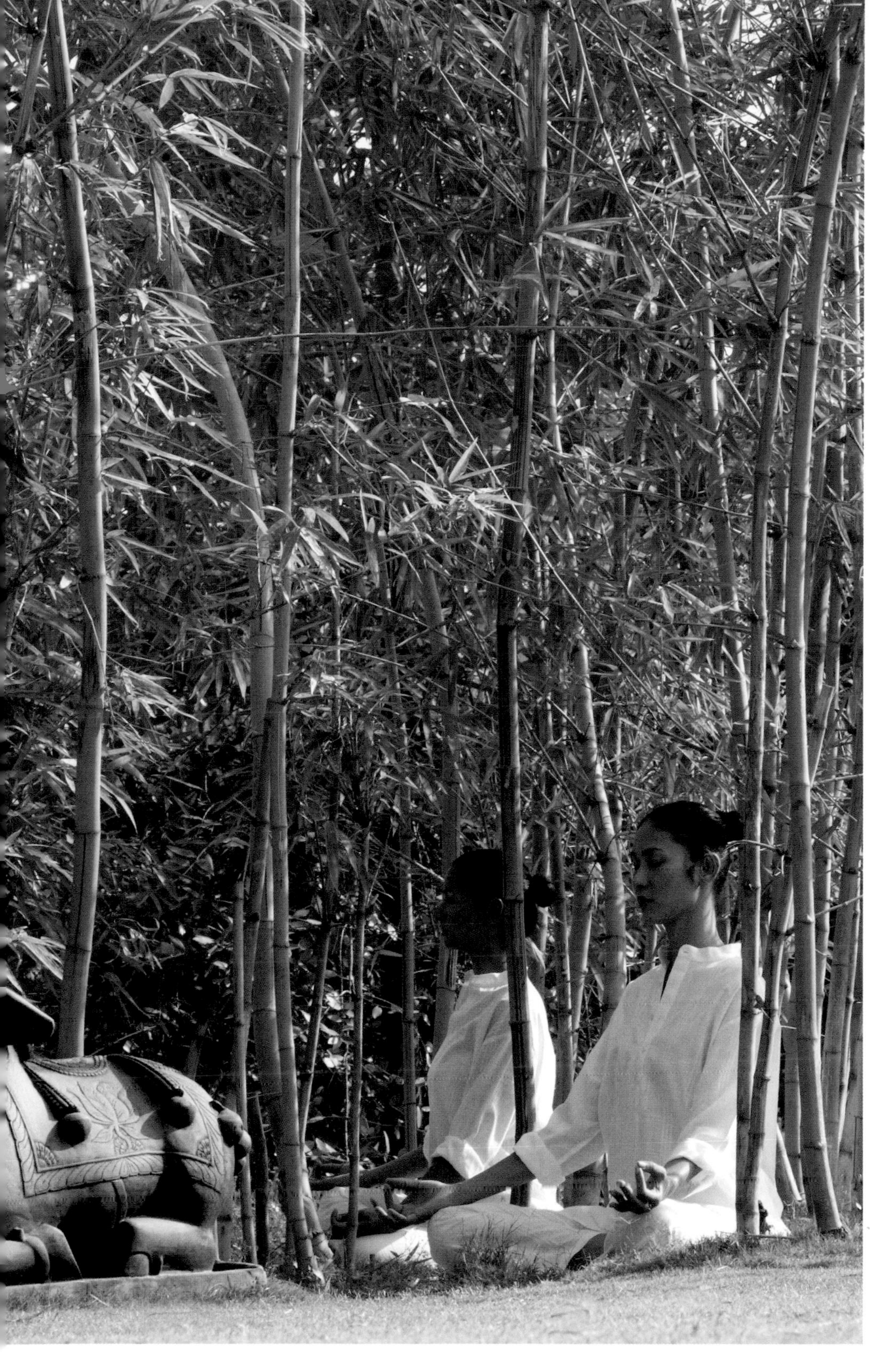

Vipassana Research Institute and patronized by clients from all over the world. Pioneered by S N Goenka, an Indian who learnt the technique in Burma, the courses are non-sectarian, as is Buddhism itself. Entirely free and funded by donations from previous attendees, they are silent meditative retreats aimed at enabling people to "see things as they really are".

Meditation in Spas, Resorts and Retreats

Of course, other religions including Islam, Christianity, Jainism and Sikhism advocate the use of meditation in one form or another as well. However, visitors to India are most likely to encounter Hindu and Buddhist meditation methods in a destination spa or retreat. Increasingly, such establishments include yoga, *pranayama* and meditation sessions to complement the other therapies on offer. Visiting "masters" often run specialized courses, while residential teachers are also on hand.

As Ayurvedic doctors have to study meditation as part of their medical degree, Ayurvedic retreats routinely include meditation sessions in their treatment schedules. For example, at Kalari Kovilakom guests are encouraged to start the day with a walking meditation known as *chandramanam*: As the unique property is criss-crossed with many secluded pathways, it is the perfect place to practice this technique. Walking purposefully, being aware of body and breath, all the while chanting a mantra, prayer or *sankalpa* (affirmation), guests are encouraged to open up to infinite possibilities. Similarly, afternoons are spent in yoga *nidra* sessions whereby a special meditative technique brings about deep relaxation.

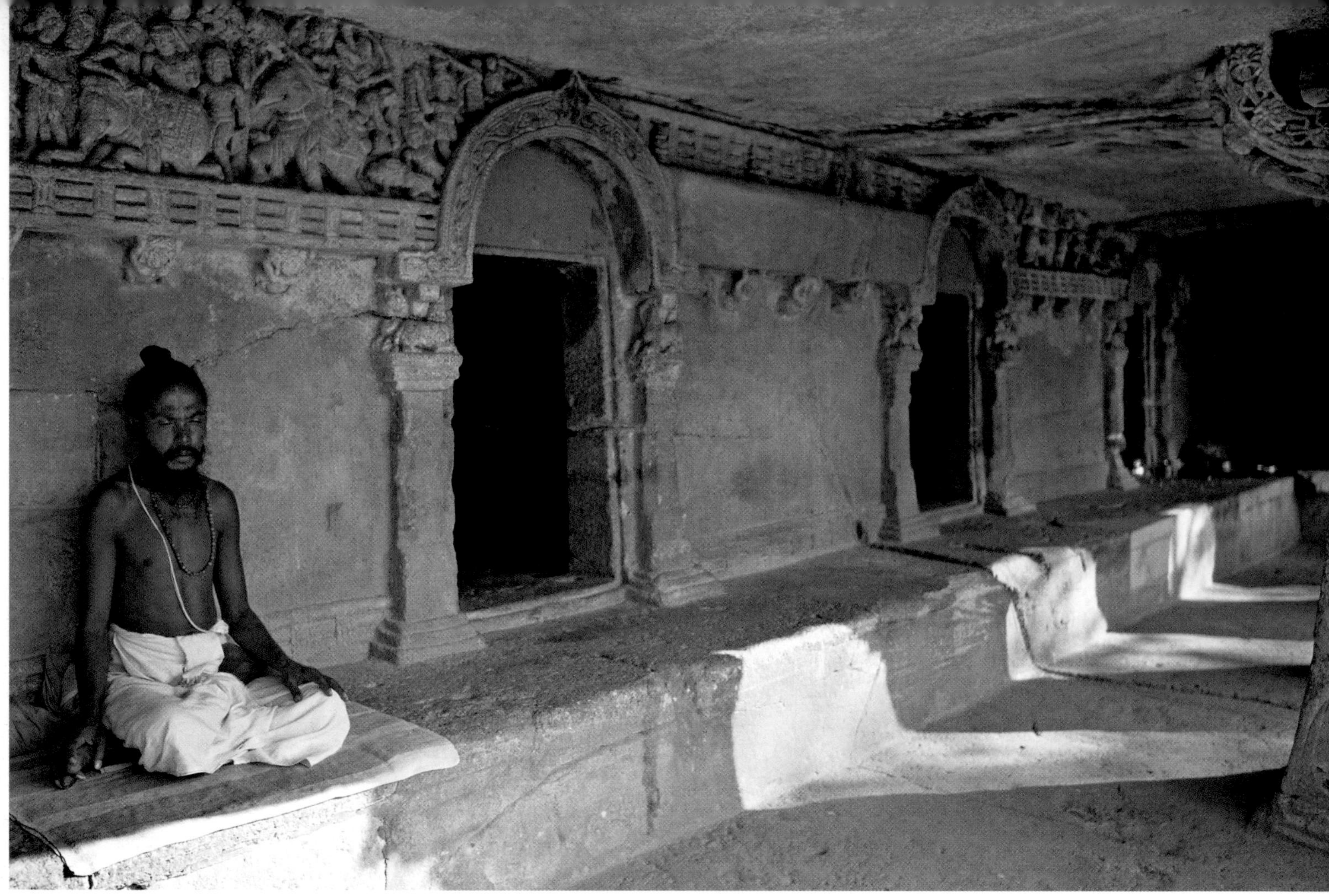

Another property that offers a unique meditation session is Amanbagh in the Rajasthani countryside near Jaipur. Designed to focus the mind through the continuous rhythm of *mantra* chanting and offering to fire, the Amanbagh's fire meditation is both a tribute to Indian culture and a celebration of the unique locale of the property. Fire is considered the purest of the five elements in Hinduism: it is used at auspicious occasions, such as weddings and homecomings, and is associated with the solar plexus area.

As the sun is setting behind the Aravali hills, a fire is lit beneath a marigold bedecked meditation pavilion situated on the property's roof. First comes the *vedi* or the decoration of the fire, then guests are blessed with a *tika* dot on the forehead. An *aarti* of incense begins the proceedings, then edible offerings are given up to the fire: rice, jaggery, sesame seeds and oatmeal.

Once the preliminaries are over, a meditation guide starts what is known as the *gayatri* mantra. Comprising 24 sounds that give homage to the mother of the tri-partite Hindu deity, the guide encourages guests to chant only five: *om*, *bhur*, *bhu*, *vah* and *swah*. Hindu philosophy advocates the use of sound, preferably in a low voice and a rhythmic manner, to facilitate concentration. In fact, many meditation techniques employ the repetitive chanting of simple sounds to clear the mind, open the heart and remove extraneous thoughts from the brain — and Amanbagh's mind-expanding ritual is no exception.

In addition to these traditional techniques, there is a plethora of what may be termed New Age meditation techniques. TM (Transcendental Meditation), Deeksha, Global Meditation through *sahaja* yoga, movement meditations such as 5 Rhythms, Active or Dynamic meditation, Tantric meditation and more . . . all are offered at a variety of venues in India. If you are serious about improving your health and wellbeing through this ancient practice, the sky — literally — is your limit in India.

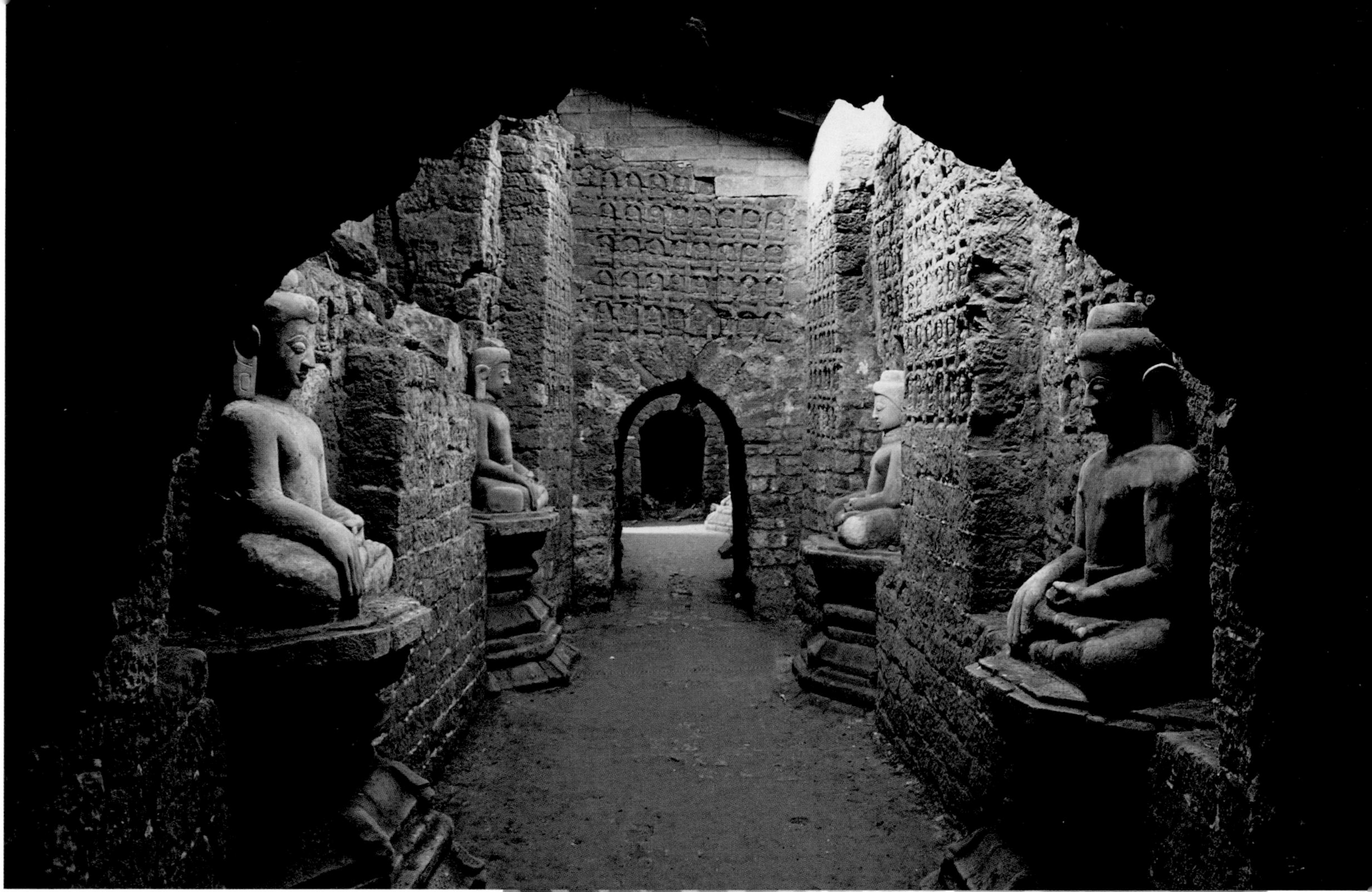

Opposite The ancient tradition of meditating in remote caves is illustrated by this Brahmin in Ranigumpha cave in Orissa. The cave dates from the 2nd century BC.
Above Statues of the Buddha in the ruins of Mrauk-U, Arakan, Myanmar.
Right Fire is used extensively in Hindu worship. In early Hindu mythology, Agni, the Hindu God of Fire is depicted as one of the most important of the Vedic gods. His role in sacrifices and rituals was unparalleled: as fire consumes everything, he was seen as a mediator between heaven and earth. Here a Jain priest conducts an *agni puja* (fire prayer).

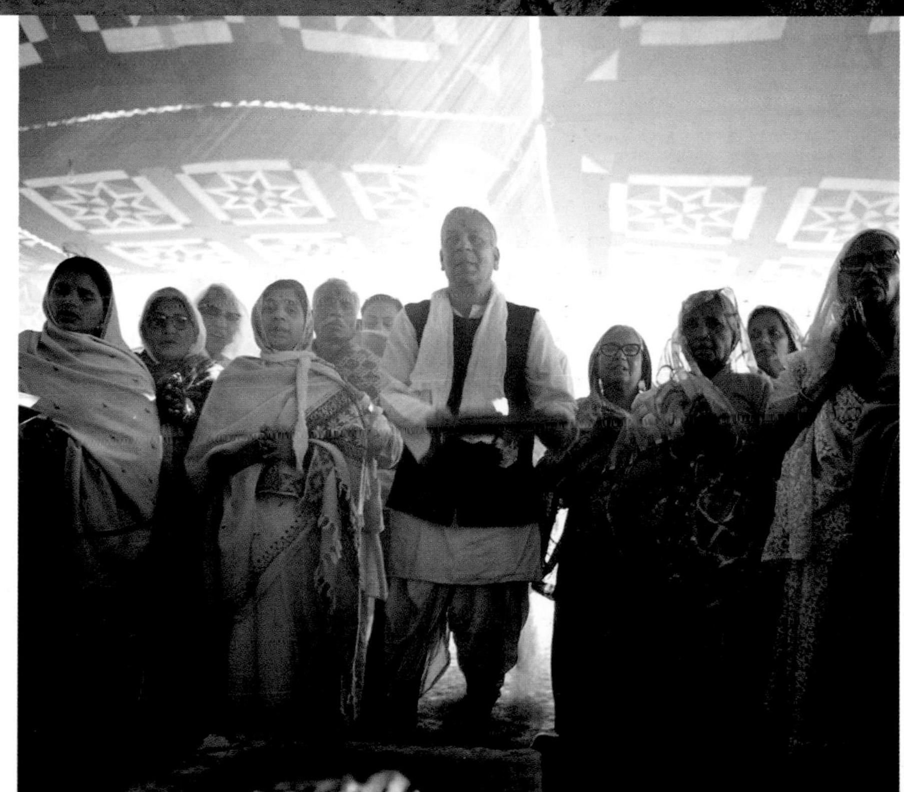

chakra therapy

YOGA IS INTERNALIZED WORSHIP WHICH LEADS TO UNION WITH GOD.

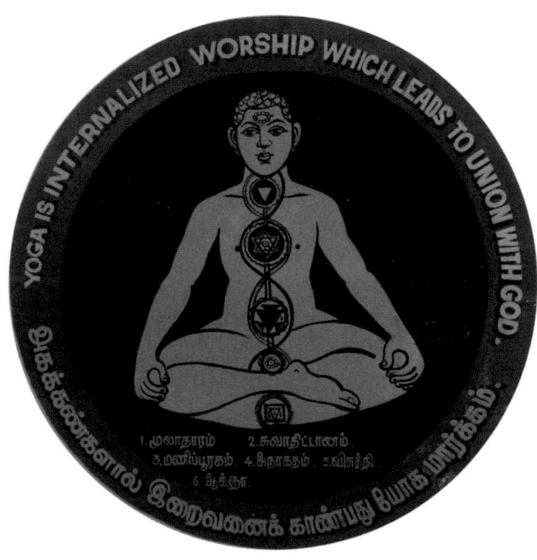

The term *chakra*, a Sanskrit word that literally means "wheel of light", refers to the seven basic energy centers in the body. In Indian philosophy, the *chakras* correlate to major nerve ganglia branching out from the spinal column, levels of consciousness, archetypal elements, developmental stages of life, colors, sounds, body functions and more. Some people reportedly see the *chakras*, describing them as spinning wheels of light and color located along the backbone, going from the base of the spine to the crown of the head.

Each of the seven *chakras* has a physical, an emotional, a creative and a spiritual component (see chart overleaf). Colin Hall, the spa manager at the Ananda, likens the spine to an elevator shaft of energy and the *chakras* as the various floors in the building of our body from which to view and experience life. When we rise from one floor to another within our consciousness, our perspective changes and expands.

"Based upon the area of consciousness that it influences, each *chakra* has its own purpose in the body," he explains. "In simple terms, we have a *chakra* for each issue that we commonly think about." He goes on to say that our thoughts have a direct relationship with our state of health. For example, love and faith based thoughts result in a smooth energy flow through the *chakras* and thus the physical body. Worry, obsession and fear based thoughts affect the *chakra* that relates to the issues we are thinking about, thus causing a blockage or restriction in the flow of energy to that part of the body.

Chakra therapists note that each *chakra* is found next to or near a hormonal gland in the body, so the *chakras* have the ability to push life energy or *prana* through the body to ensure vitality. These energy centers receive and radiate energy constantly, acting as storehouses and transmitters of universal energy as well. They say that it is necessary to balance the *chakras* from time to time to effectively regulate this flow.

According to yoga masters, disharmony on a physical, mental or spiritual level may be corrected by certain postures that concentrate the breath on the abdominal area. *Pranayama* is especially active on the *chakras*, while the Ayurvedic therapy of pouring medicated oils on to the *chakras* (*chakradhara*) also effectively regulates the proper flow *prana*. "It is particularly useful for people who have improper lifestyle habits," explains Ayurvedic physician, Dr Sreenarayanan, also of Ananda. "Their *chakras* are blocked as a result of stress, tension, bad diet, lack of exercise and so on. The therapy acts on the immune system, releasing energy flows, reducing anxiety and allowing the mind to become still and quiet."

Furthermore, *chakras* may be balanced by placing the hands gently over them, a few inches above the physical body. In this process, the recipient may be receptive to a flowing or warm sensation believed to be the transmission of universal energy. Known as Reiki in the West, practitioners say it helps harmonize the body's biological and emotional systems. As universal energy is received, the "doors" for self-healing are opened — and people use it for pain management and stress-relief as well as for more spiritual goals.

Left, top A figure in the lotus pose is illustrated with the seven *chakra* positions. Running from the base of the spine to the top of the head, they are seen as the body's energy centers. **Right** A *chakradhara* session at Ananda, in the Himalayas, concentrates on the fifth *chakra*, the one that is related to creativity and communication. *Chakradhara* is often recommended after a period of *panchakarma* (see pages 46–49), for patients with high cholesterol or diabetes and for those who suffer from anxiety and stress.

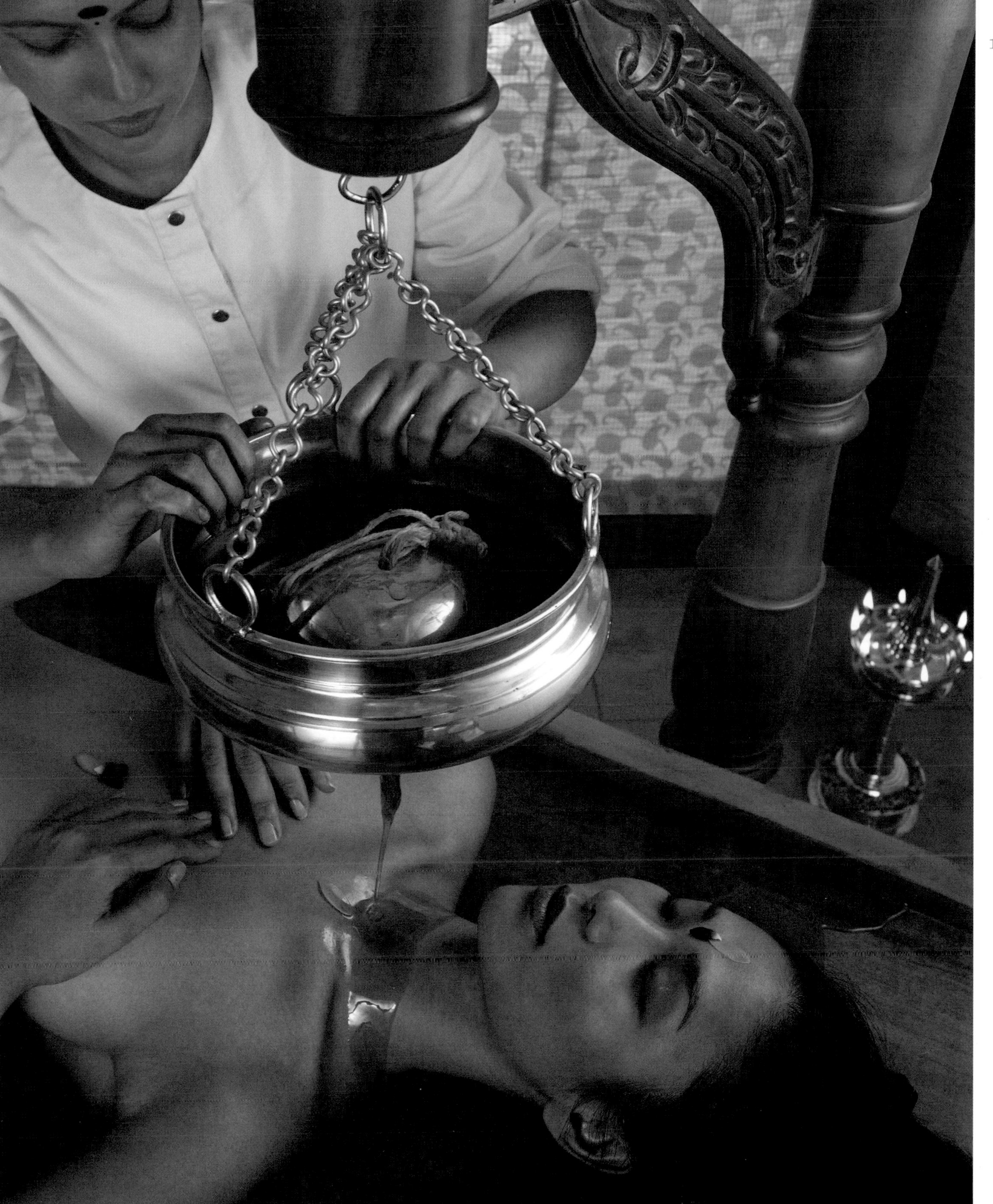

Below Some of the wold's principal oyster beds lie along the coasts of India, so references to mother-of-pearl and pearls are abundant in the Indian epics. They are potent when applied to the skin — as a powder or whole — especially on the *chakras*.

Right A Reiki master lays his hands above a client at Mandarin Oriental Dhara Devi. Both calming and spiritual, Reiki involves the laying of hands on, or above, the body's *chakras* to balance and heal.

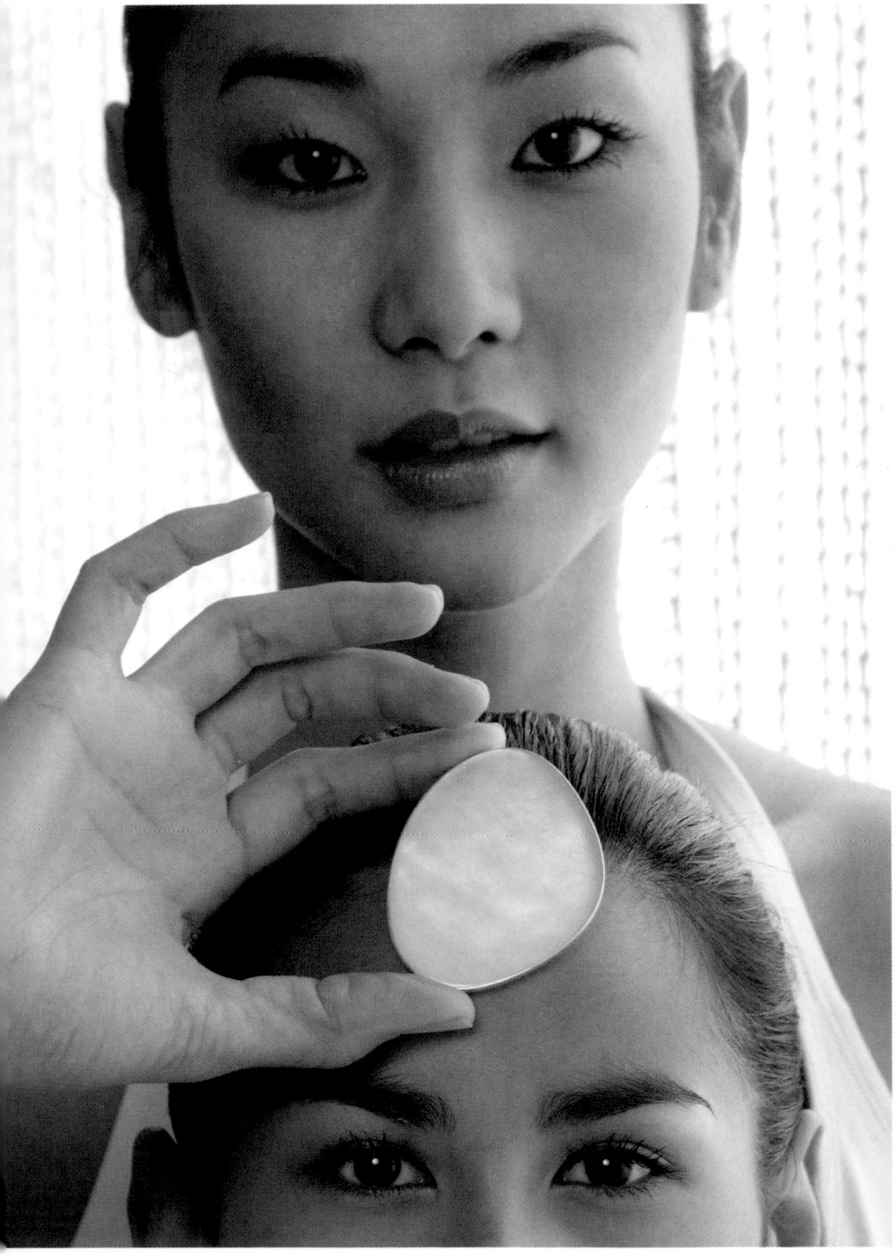

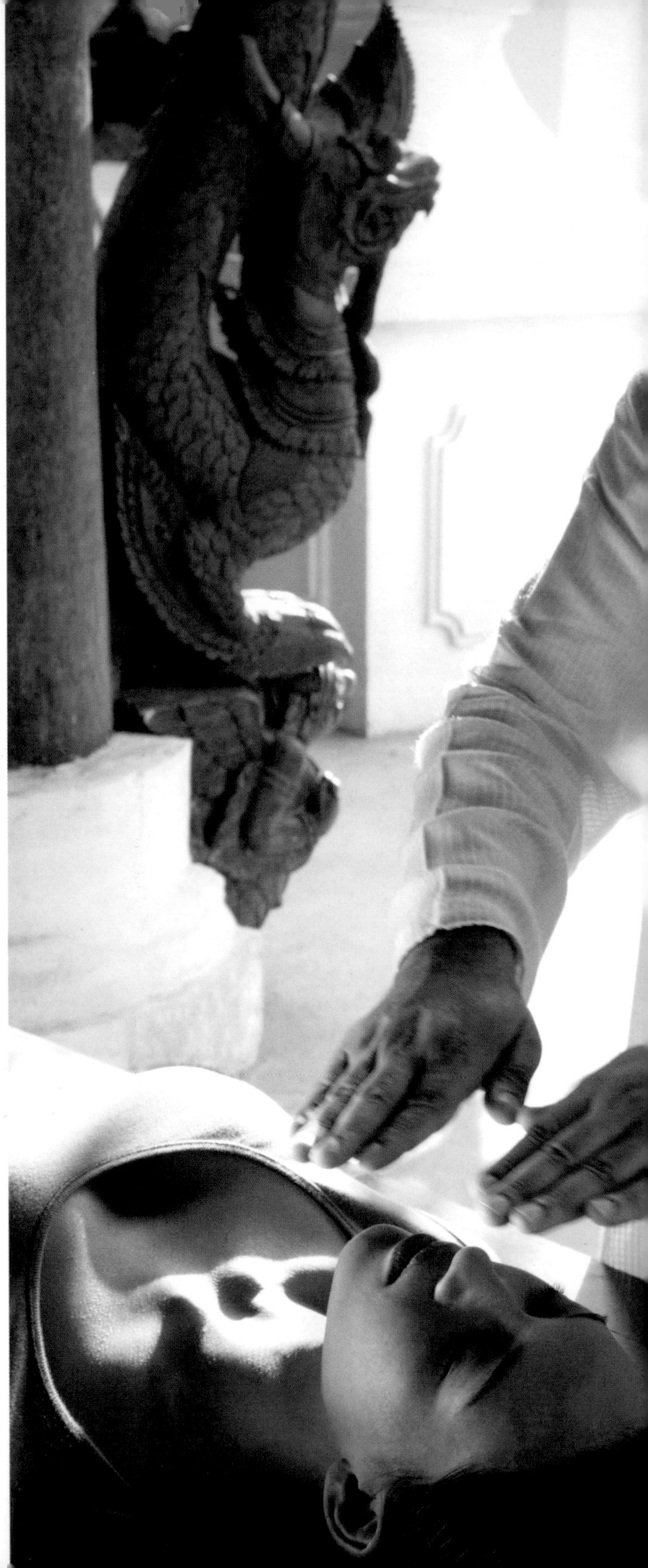

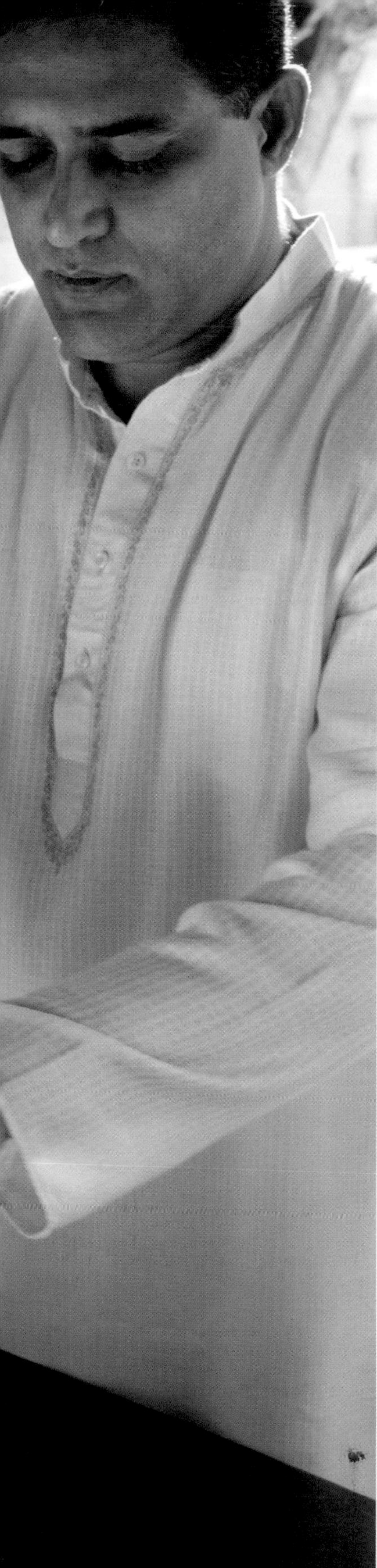

THE SEVEN CHAKRAS

Chakra Seven:
Thought, universal identity, oriented to self-knowledge
The crown *chakra* relates to consciousness as pure awareness. It is our connection to the greater world beyond, and, when developed, brings knowledge, wisdom, understanding, spiritual connection and bliss.

Chakra Six:
Light, archetypal identity, oriented to self-reflection
The brow *chakra* or third eye center is related to the act of seeing, both physically and intuitively. As such, it opens our psychic faculties and gives us greater understanding of "the big picture".

Chakra Five:
Sound, creative identity, oriented to self-expression
The throat *chakra* is related to communication and creativity. By experiencing the world symbolically through vibration (ie the vibration of sound representing language), a healthy fifth *chakra* results in expressiveness and erudition.

Chakra Four:
Air, social identity, oriented to self-acceptance
The heart *chakra* is the middle *chakra* in the system of seven. It is related to love and is the integrator of opposites in the psyche: mind and body, male and female, persona and shadow, ego and unity. A healthy fourth *chakra* allows us to love deeply, feel compassion and experience a profound sense of peace and centeredness.

Chakra Three:
Fire, ego identity, oriented to self-definition
Located in the solar plexus, this *chakra* is known as the power *chakra*. It rules our personal power, will and autonomy, as well as our metabolism. When healthy, it brings energy, effectiveness, spontaneity and non-dominating power.

Chakra Two:
Water, emotional identity, oriented to self-gratification
Located in the abdomen, lower back and sexual organs, the second *chakra* connects us to others through feeling, desire, sensation and movement. Ideally, this *chakra* brings us fluidity and grace, depth of feeling, sexual fulfillment and the ability to accept change.

Chakra One:
Earth, physical identity, oriented to self-preservation
Located at the base of the spine, this *chakra* forms our foundation. It is related to our survival instincts, our sense of grounding and to the physical plane. When healthy, this *chakra* brings health, prosperity, security and dynamic presence.

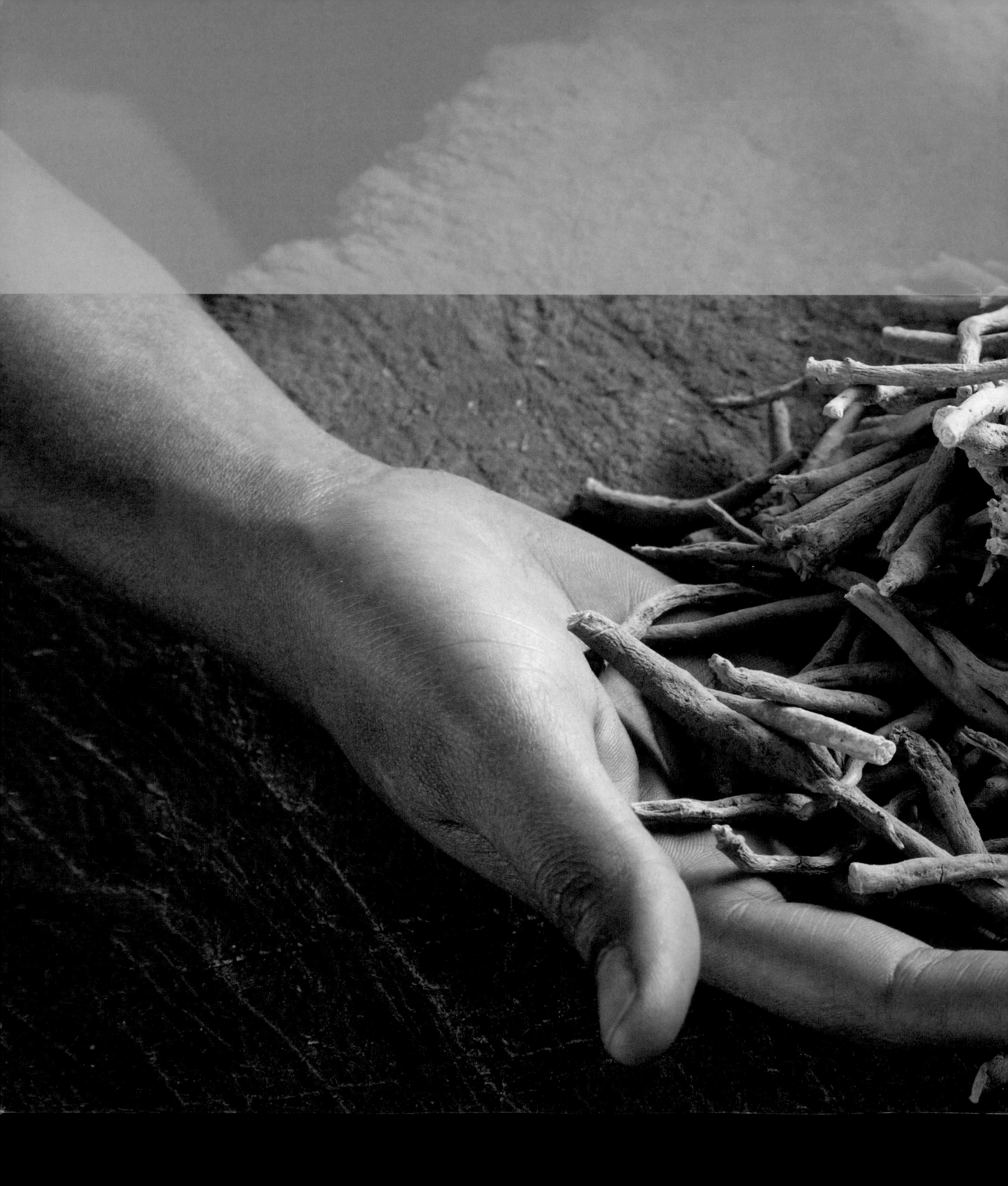

appendix

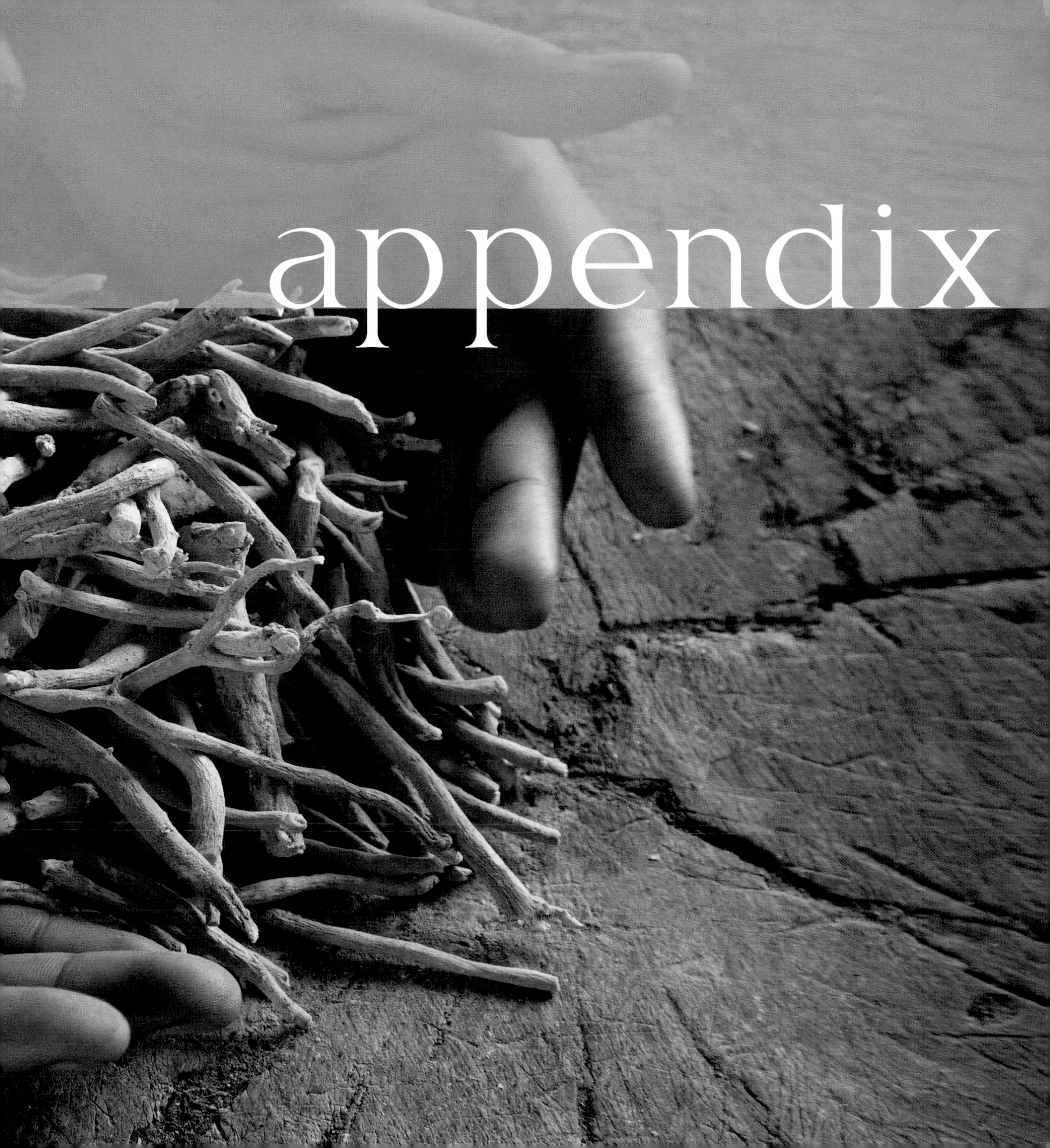

nattu vaidya

the barefoot doctor

Throughout India, people receive medical help from both qualified and non-qualified practitioners. As we have noted previously, there are four traditional systems practiced in India — Ayurveda, Siddha, Unani and Tibetan medicine — all of which are based on humoral pathology. Since Independence in the 1940s, each has built up a solid base of medical colleges imparting education in five-and-a-half year programs. They have been joined by a fifth: the study of Naturopathy. Currently, only graduates of such recognized medical schools are legally entitled to practice medicine, and it is believed that there are around 600,000 such licensed practitioners.

Be that as it may, there are, in addition, literally hundreds of thousands of non-qualified healers servicing the health and welfare needs of India's huge population. Often, they comprise families that have practiced their individual skills for centuries — and are well known in the community. Some such practitioners may have some rudimentary education as well, but economic and other factors may have resulted in their medical training being cut short. Others are completely unqualified on paper, indeed they may even be illiterate, but they are the recipients of countless generations of healing knowledge.

As such, they are hugely skilled — and a vital part of any community.

There are numerous examples of such traditional healers, all of whom fall into a category that can loosely be termed the "barefoot doctor" or *nattu vaidya*.

The village midwife:
Each village has at least one traditional birth attendant known as a *dai*. These women are skilled in delivering not only healthy babies, but have knowledge of breach births, stillborn fetuses and babies with umbilical

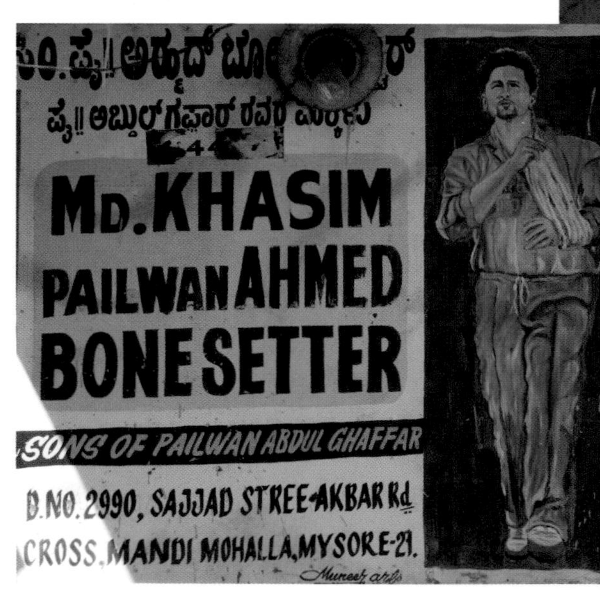

Left A sign by the door of Mysore-based Mohammed Khasim's practice. The son of Abdul Gafar, a renowned bone specialist who treated the Maharajah of Mysore's family, his skills have been handed down from father to son.

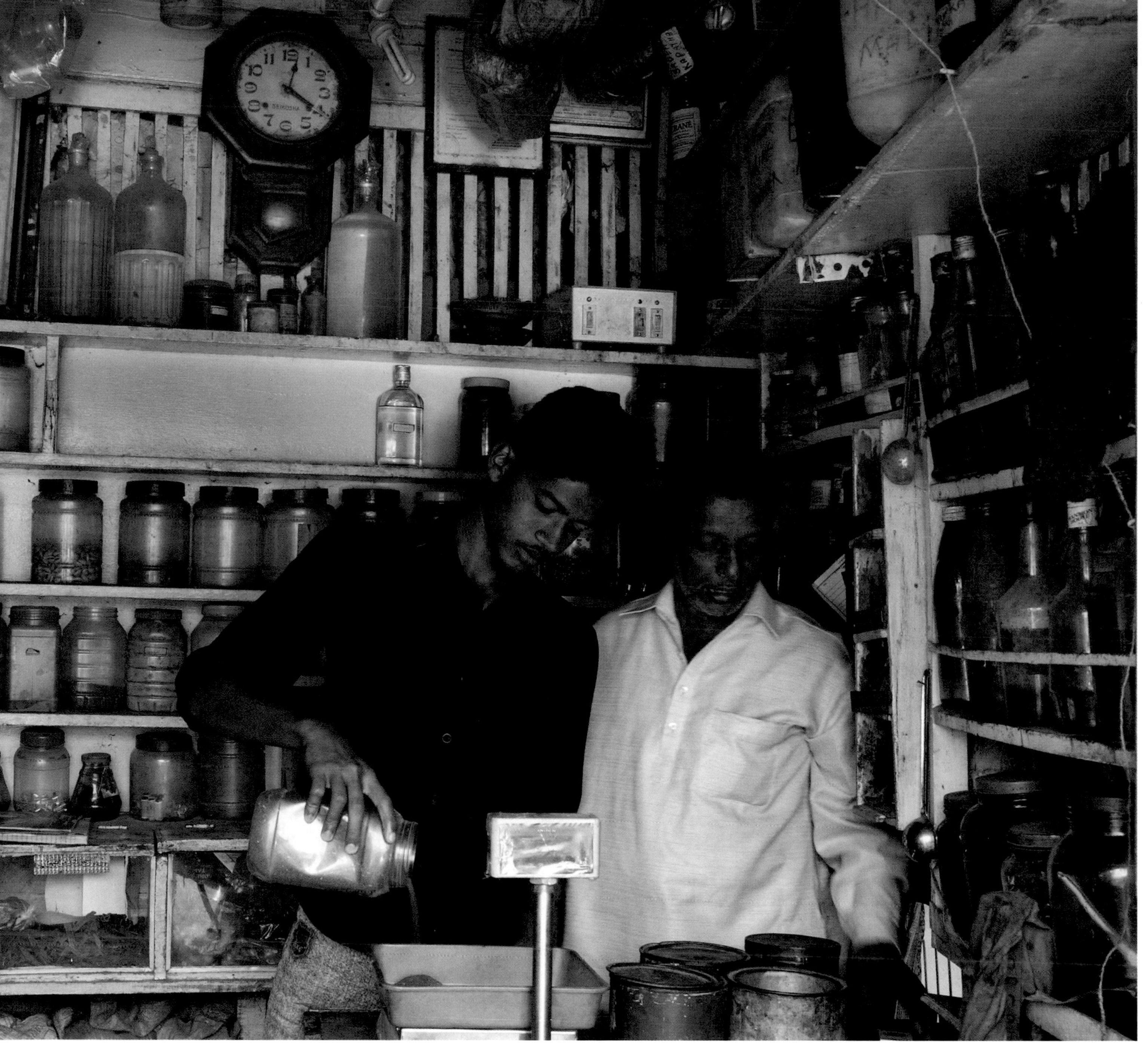

Above Even though there are thousands of Unani doctors, more than 100 medical colleges and a dozen major pharmaceutical companies in India, the roadside pharmacy overflowing with dusty medicine bottles, dried roots, powders and oils is a common sight. Here, a father and son (both unqualified) prepare prescriptions in their small shop. The boy's grandfather taught them all they know.

nattu vaidya

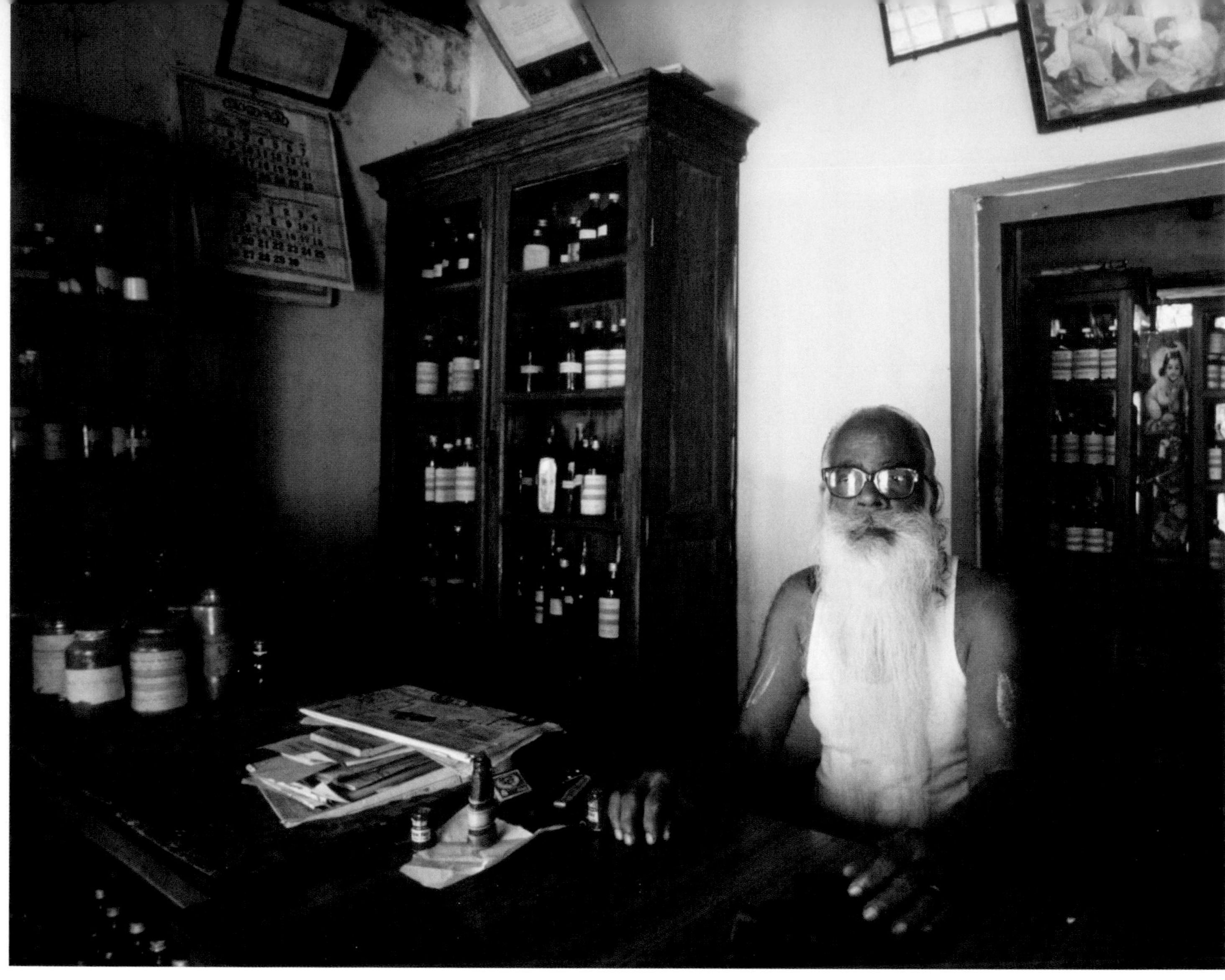

cords round their necks. Often coming from a family of midwives, they are skilled in ante-natal and post-natal care as well.

The bonesetter:

The traditional bonesetter or orthopedic healer is another example. In the countryside, such a person may look after the needs of the population of 20 villages or so, walking from one destination to the next to treat sprains, fractures, joint problems or muscle pain. A group involved in strengthening traditional systems of medicine called the Lok Swasthya Parampara Samvardhan Samithi (LSPSS) in Coimbatore estimates that there are over 60,000 bonesetters serving rural populations and, in cities, established practitioners may see up to 30 or 40 patients a day. It is estimated that over 50 percent of people with broken bones are treated by bonesetters in any given year.

The poison healer:

Snakebite is a common occurrence in rural India and traditional *visha vaidya* have specialist knowledge. They can differentiate between different snakebites, and they know which antidote works for which type of snake. Their remedies are almost always herbal and prescriptions include purgation, antidotes and topical application of specific plants. The *visha vaidya* is often called on in the case of rabid dog bites and scorpion bites too.

Many *nattu vaidya* learned their skills from their families. This physician is no exception. Although not formally qualified, he has practiced Ayurveda in Trivandrum for over 50 years and has many regular patients. He makes most of his prescriptions himself, to recipes that were handed down to him from his father.

Less clear cut, but nonetheless important, are people like oil producers, small-scale herbal medicine manufacturers, wandering monks with herbal knowledge, community elders who have specialist knowledge of herbal home remedies and nutrition, martial art masseuses, and *kannu vaidyas* or eye physicians who treat eye complaints even to the extent of giving cataract operations. There are also more general herbal medicine practitioners who specialize in such conditions as jaundice and paralysis, children's diseases and dentistry.

Such people may have very particular knowledge in *marmanam* (treatment of the vital points), *agni* and *kshara karma* (cauterization), *sodhana karma* (purification techniques) and *rasayana* (rejuvenation therapy) as well. According to the Foundation for the Revitalisation of Local Health Traditions (FRLHT) whose mission is to revitalize these health practices in four states in south India, there could be a million such practitioners catering to India's 4,600-odd ethnic communities.

Traditionally, many of these care-givers have a relationship with their "patients" and don't practice specifically for monetary gain. Rather, they place value on a code of ethics that includes service to others, the transference of skills, prayers for guidance and holistic health care for all. In some cases, practitioners accept a *kanikkae* (a kind of offering or a gratuity). Theirs is not a vocation; in fact, it is more than likely that they have another job, such as farmer or shopkeeper, as well.

Even though most of these people do not have legal status (or only semi-legal status) as medical practitioners, they are considered legitimate healers in their own right. Indeed, such organizations as the LSSPS are keen to tap into their specialist knowledge — some of which is invariably being lost with the passing of time. For a start, none of it is written down: Most barefoot doctors receive their healing knowledge orally via person-to-person transmission either in the form of the guru-*shishya* tradition (master/disciple), or commonly from father to son or mother to daughter. Secondly, with rapid industrialization and loss of rural land, vital herbs, plants and trees are being cut down in the name of "development". Thirdly, as India develops, a worrying trend has been recently noticed: such people are quite often over 40 years of age, and are often not handing down their skills to the next generation as they did in the past.

Below Dr S B Nithyanandam stands in the grounds of his local Shiva temple. A Siddha doctor, he learnt his trade from his father, but also trained at a Siddha medical college.
Bottom An example of the type of colorful billboards found all over India. This one is for a type of hair oil that contains *amla* or Indian gooseberry.

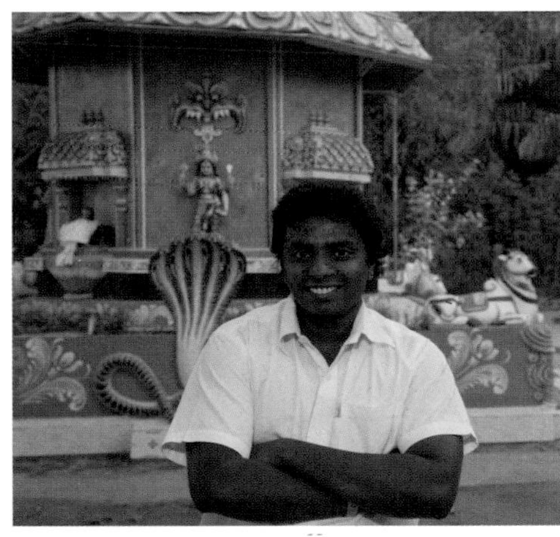

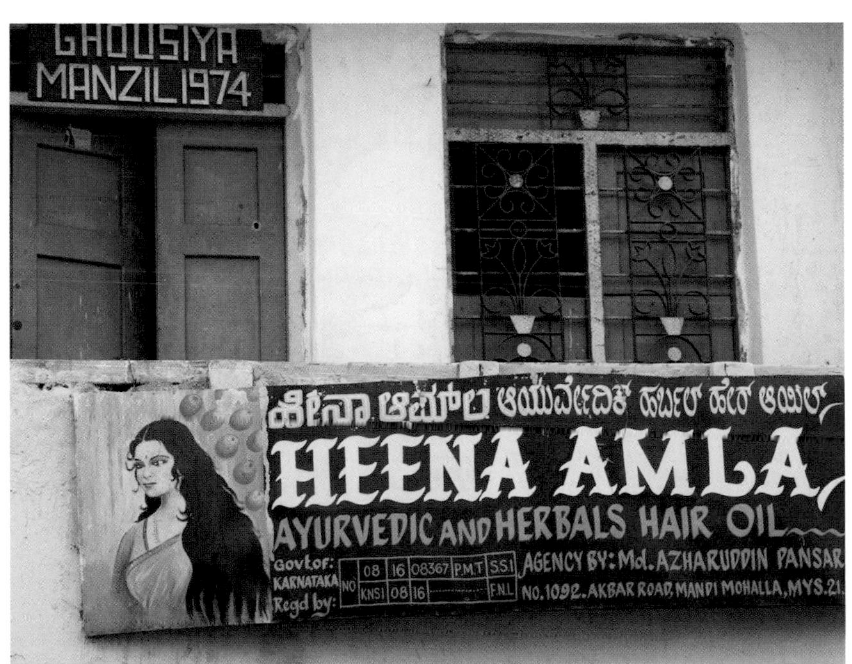

healing plants

India's creative healing systems are predominantly plant-based (although minerals have a role) and it is estimated that most households rely upon locally available plant material for their pharmacopeia. According to the World Health Organisation (WHO), between 35,000 and 70,000 plants have been used for medicinal purposes globally at one time or another — and in India today at least 20,000 species are found, 2,000 of which are efficacious in Ayurvedic formulations. Of these, about 600 are commonly used in oils (*tailam*), powders (*choornam*), internal medications, teas and tonics. We list some of the most important plants from the Ayurvedic pharmacopeia.

Lawsonia inermis **Henna**
Henna *(mehndi)* is commonly used as a dye and an anti-fungal. The leaves produce a red-orange dye molecule that has an affinity for bonding with protein, so has been used to dye skin, hair, fingernails, leather, silk and wool since the Bronze Ages. In India it is commonly used as a dye on hands, feet and hair, while henna essential oil is used as a scalp stimulator.

Centella asiatica **Asiatic pennywort**
Brahmi is a small herbaceous annual plant, the leaves of which are reported to be useful in abdominal disorders; a tea is made to help with dysentery in children. Scientific reports have documented its ability to aid wound healing, being particularly helpful with reduction of scarring, and it is also used in the treatment of leprosy, epilepsy, cardiac debility and more.

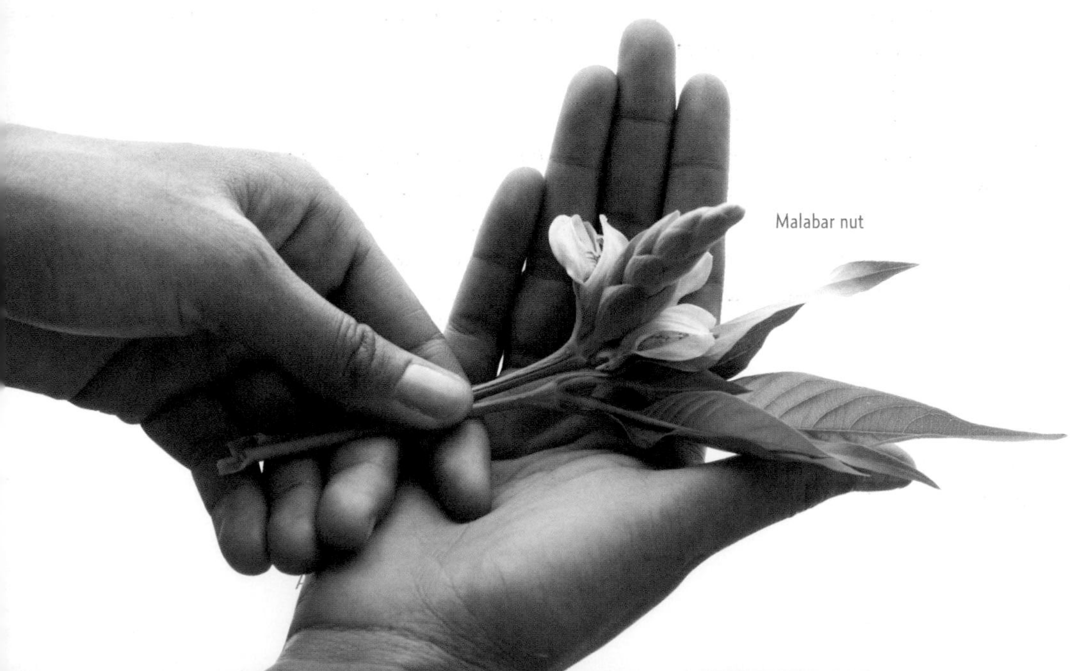

Malabar nut

Eclipta alba **False daisy**
Bhringaraja is an annual herb that is commonly used in the treatment of skin diseases and as an anti-inflammatory. It is also reported to be effective in blackening and strengthening the hair and is cooling on the head. It may also be taken as a tonic to help with liver and spleen enlargements.

Ocimum tenuiflorum **Holy basil**
Known as holy basil, *tulsi* is an important symbol in many Hindu religious traditions. It is mentioned in the *Rigveda* and the *Charaka Samhita*, and has been recognized by the *rishis* for thousands of years as a prime herb in Ayurvedic treatment. *Tulsi* extracts are used for common colds, headaches, stomach disorders, inflammation, heart disease, poisoning and malaria. *Tulsi* can be taken as an herbal tea, in dried powder form, fresh or mixed with ghee.

Adhatoda vasica **Malabar nut**
Also known as the Malabar nut tree, the *vasaka* shrub has leaves (see left) that are rich in vitamin C and carotene. Fresh or dried leaves are used to make a tea that is good for bronchial and asthmatic troubles. Powdered leaves are used on skin infections, and a preparation made from *vasaka* flowers is used to treat tuberculosis.

Chrysopogon zizanoides **Vetiver**
Native to India, vetiver is a Tamil name and old Tamil literature lists medicinal uses for the plant. Similar to other fragrant

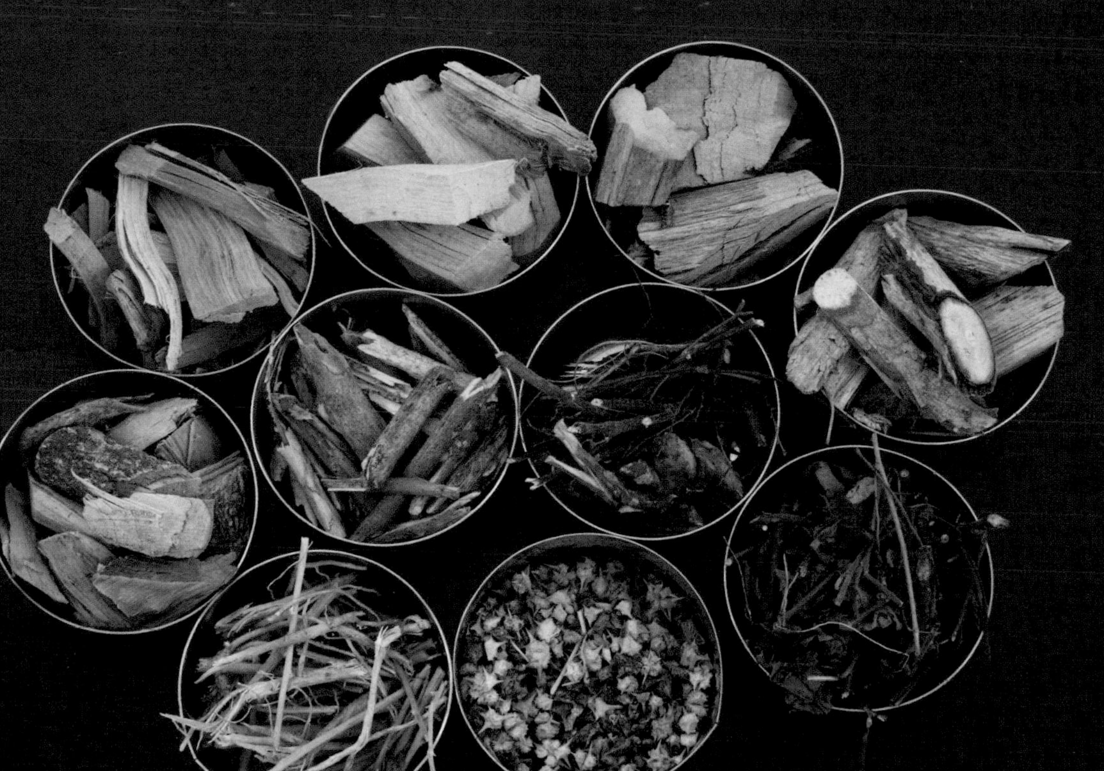

Dashmool "Ten Roots"

Solanum xanthocarpum
Poisonberry
This is one of the *dashmool* (ten roots) of Ayurveda and it is found in 50 percent of Ayurvedic preparations. It is a spiny diffuse herb that grows wild in India: The juice of the berries is used in sore throat. Roots and seeds are administered as an expectorant in cough, while the stem flowers and fruits are prescribed for relief in burning sensation in the feet. It is a nervous system regulator, good for the liver and asthmatic conditions.

Maranta arundinacea L.
Arrowroot
The creeping rhizome of the arrowroot is used to stop vomiting and it is good for the digestion. It helps relieve acidity, indigestion and colic and exerts a mildly laxative effect on the large bowel. When mixed with hot water, the root starch become gelatinous, so soothes irritated mucous membranes.

grasses such as lemongrass and citronella, *Chrysopogon zizanoides* is a perennial grass. The root has cooling and calming properties, so is effective in the treatment of burns, while oil of vetiver, known as the oil of tranquility, is a key ingredient in perfumes. Vetiver is antiseptic, sedative and stimulating also.

Datura stramonium L. **Thorn apple**
The thorn apple or *shivpriya* grows in India as a wasteland weed. Ancient Hindu physicians regarded it as intoxicant, emetic, digestive and heating. The dried leaves, flowering tops and seeds are used in indigenous medicine in the treatment of asthma and bronchitis, while the whole plant is used as a muscle relaxant. The fruits, when crushed, are used in a paste form to reduce swelling and pain.

Emblica officionalis **Indian gooseberry**
The Indian gooseberry or *amla* (overleaf) is a very important Ayurvedic fruit, used in the treatment of liver conditions, jaundice, anaemia and diabetes. It is an immune system booster and is high in vitamin C. *Triphala*, an Ayurvedic combination of *amla*, *haritaki* (*Terminalis chebula*) and *vibhitika* (*Terminalis belerica*) is used as a laxative and for headaches, biliousness, dyspepsia, constipation, piles and enlarged liver.

Coleus zeylanicus **No English name**
The *coleus zeylanicus* plant has anti-bacterial, deodorant and cooling properties, and is used in urinary infections and digestive problems. Known as *ambu* in Sanskrit and *hribera* in most other places in India, its flat silver leaves are used to reduce body temperature and fever.

Azadirachta indica **Neem**
The fast-growing neem tree (see page 140) has many medicinal properties, as it is a known purifier and antiseptic. Conditions ranging from digestive disorders to diabetes and from high cholesterol to cancer may be helped with neem, while purifying neem twigs are a traditional tooth cleaner in India. All parts of the tree are used; neem also makes fine soaps, shampoos, balms and creams.

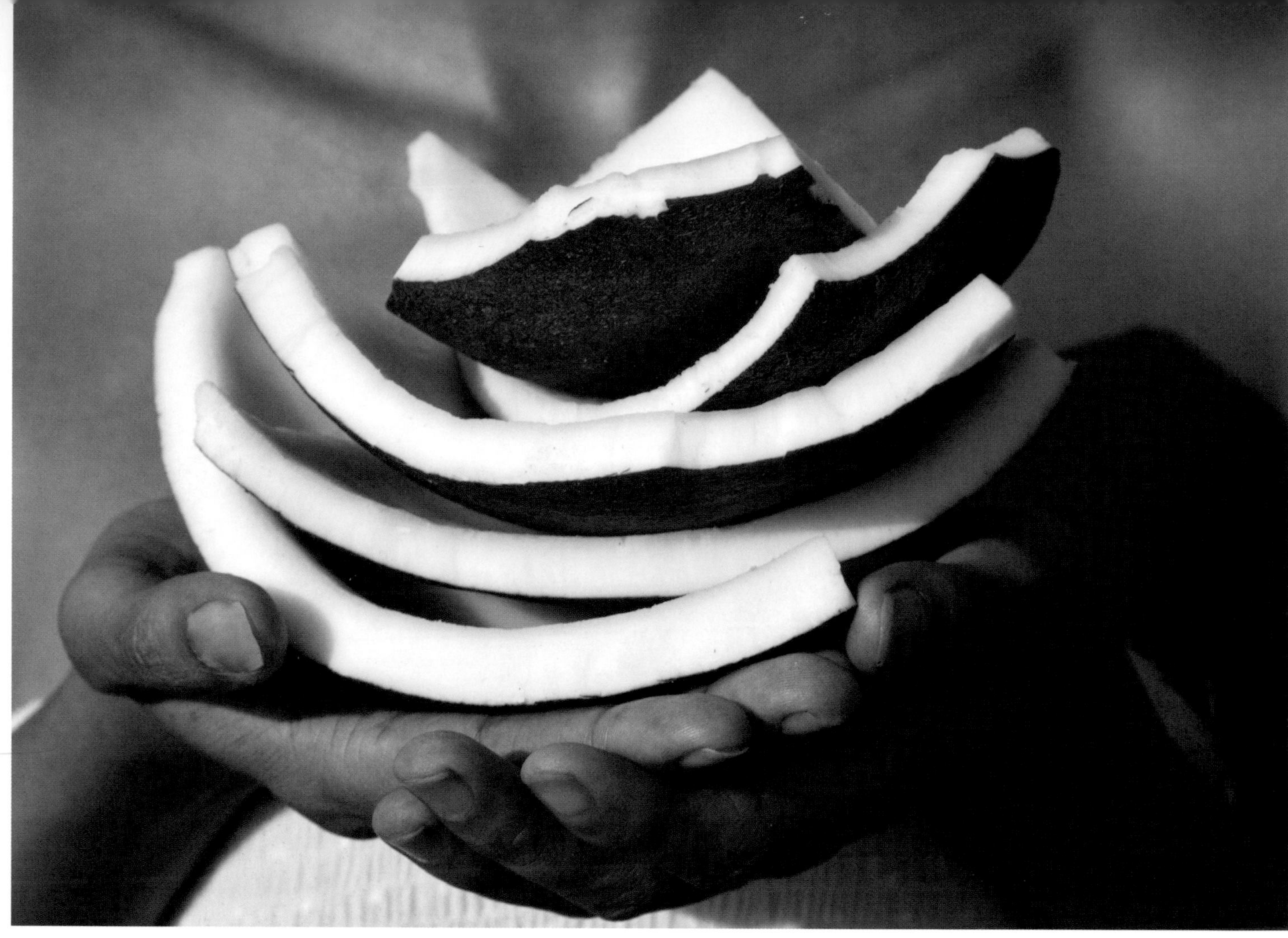

Coconut

Sida cordifolia **No English name**
The *bala* plant is associated with the Hindu Goddess of beauty and grace Parvati and it is part of the magical trio of herbs associated with women in Indian herbology (the other herbs that are recommended for beautifying women are *ashoka* and *shatavari*). *Bala* oil is recommended for all disorders produced by the derangement of *vata*, and recently an Ayurvedic *tailam* (containing *ashwagandha* and *bala* root and *Celastrus* oils) was clinically proven to be effective for neuralgia in controlled studies in Germany.

Cocos nucifera **Coconut**
The name for the coconut palm in Sanskrit is *kalpa vruksham* translating as "the tree which provides all the necessities of life". The term coconut refers to the nut (see above), which is widely used in Ayurveda both externally for its oil and internally as food. Charaka said that tender and half-mature coconuts increase the quantity and quality of all seven tissues and are *vata* pacifying, cooling and strengthening.

Oxalis corniculata **Yellow wood sorrel**
An annual herb, yellow wood sorrel or *puliyarila* has diuretic and refrigerant properties. It is used to treat disorders of the liver and digestive problems. The leaf pulp is applied over insect bites and burns. It has antibacterial properties and is high in Vitamin C.

Eupatorium triplinervie **No English name**
Known as *yapana*, the leaves of this ground-covering shrub are used for digestive disorders, piles (as it has haemostatic properties), nervine disorders and asthma. It is also used to bring down fevers as it is antipyretic.

Calycopteris floribunda **No English name**
Known as *pullani* or *ukshi,* this woody climber is used in Ayurvedic remedies for malaria, dysentery and snakebite. Its essential oil is supposed to be useful for depression as it has grounding properties.

Elaeocarpus sphaericus **No English name**
This small tree is famous for supplying the ridged fruits that are dried and used as medicinal "beads" in *rudraaksh* or garlands worn to stave off evil or illness. The fruits are used in Ayurveda for mental diseases, epilepsy, asthma, hypertension, arthritis and liver diseases.

Pandanus amaryllifolius **Pandan**
The long leaves of the pandan or screwpine plant known as *rumbha* in south Asia are used as a flavoring in food, but are also known medicinally for aiding digestion. The leaves are also believed to contain an anti-viral protein that may be useful in the case of influenza.

Bacopa monnieri **No English name**
Known as *bhrami* (as are some other herbs) this creeping herb has antioxidant properties and has been used for centuries in cases of epilepsy. It is believed to boost the memory, increase concentration and reduce anxiety. It forms part of an Ayurvedic cure for inflammatory bowel syndrome.

Melastoma malabathricum L. **Straits rhododendron**
A perennial shrub with bright purple flowers, this is used to treat diarrhea, dysentery and piles, and is also useful in uterine diseases.

Aloe barbadensis **Aloe vera**
Highly prized for the liquid contained in its thick, fleshy blades, aloe vera is revered for its cooling properties. It is used externally for skin rashes, sunburn, itchiness, scarring and psoriasis, as it is antibiotic and anti-septic in nature. It is also a purgative and anti-diabetic, so can be taken internally to aid the digestion.

Indian gooseberry

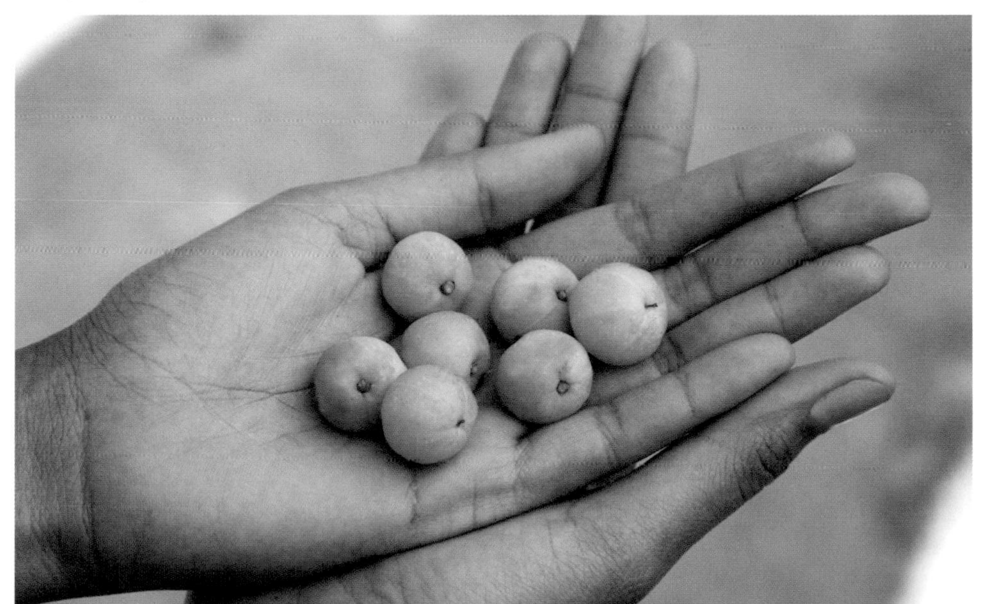

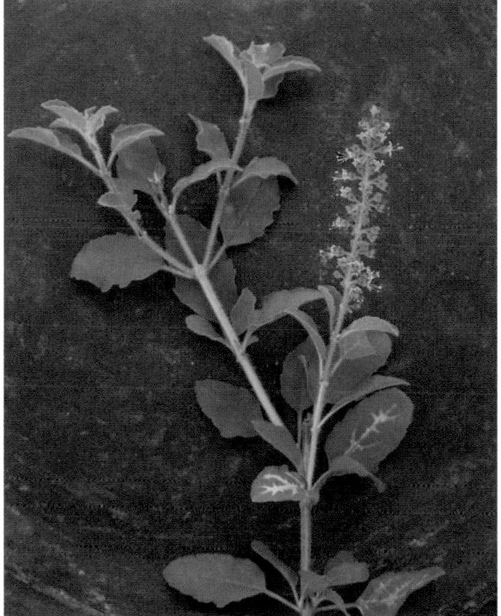

Holy Basil

Areca catechu **Areca nut**
Commonly known as betel, the areca nut comprises part of the Indian recreational digestive known as *paan*. The dried nut has stimulant and astringent properties and is used to sweeten the breath and strengthen the gums. It is used in Ayurveda to combat inflammatory bowel syndrome and the skin of the fruit is used as an anti-poisonous substance for insect bites.

Cinnamomum zeylanicum **Cinnamon**
A small bushy tree, the dried leaves and bark of the cinnamon tree are used as a spice, medicinally and for cosmetic purposes. The powdered bark is considered a brain tonic, while a decoction of the leaves aids the digestion. It is believed to alleviate anxiety and depression and helps clear the respiratory channels. In Ayurvedic beauty products, it improves the complexion and adds fairness to skin.

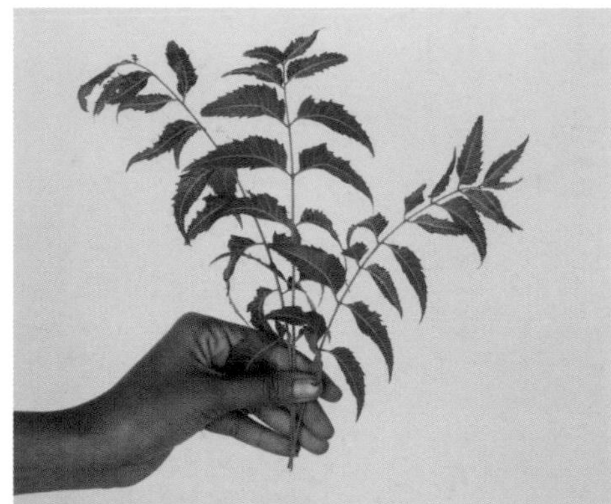

Neem

Caryophyllus aromaticus **Clove**
The dried unopened flower bud of a small tree, the clove has both culinary and medicinal uses. It is a stimulant and an antiseptic, so is used in a variety of Ayurvedic medicines: it helps gastric irritability, aids the digestion and enhances circulation and metabolism. The essential oil of clove is used to relieve pain from toothache and as an oral hygiene product.

Theobroma cacao **Cacao**
Used to make cocoa and chocolate, cacao beans also form the basis for cocoa butter, an all-natural vegetable fat. It is used in a variety of Ayurvedic beauty preparations as it is extremely rich. Often combined with jojoba oil, it is used for sunburn, as a skin softener and to reduce scar tissue and stretch marks from pregnancy.

Murraya koenigi **Curry leaf**
Found in many Indian backyards, the curry leaf plant is a staple in Indian cuisine. However, its leaves also aid the digestion as it is mildly laxative, and the powdered root and bark is used for relief from kidney pain. Traditional healers often used crushed leaves on topical applications of insect bites in the form of a poultice.

Zingiber officinale **Ginger**
Ginger is used widely in both Ayurvedic and Unani medicine. Charak, the ancient sage of Indian medicine, said: "Every good quality is found in ginger", and other texts suggest that everyone should eat fresh ginger before meals to enhance the digestion. It is also believed to clear the micro-circulatory channels of the body, help with joint pain and motion sickness and facilitate absorption of nutrients into the system.

Cymbopogon citrates **Lemongrass**
A medicinal plant, lemongrass is used in Ayurvedic herbal teas for *pitta* types, while the essential oil is a useful insect repellant. It is also widely used in perfumes and cosmetics, and Ayurvedic texts indicate that it is a useful stress-reliever and cleanser when placed with other herbs in a steam box.

Mentha arvensis **Mint**
Called *paparaminta* in Hindi, mint is indigenous to India and is widely distilled for its antiseptic and antispasmodic oil. Helpful for headaches, rheumatism and neuralgia, mint is also used in teas to

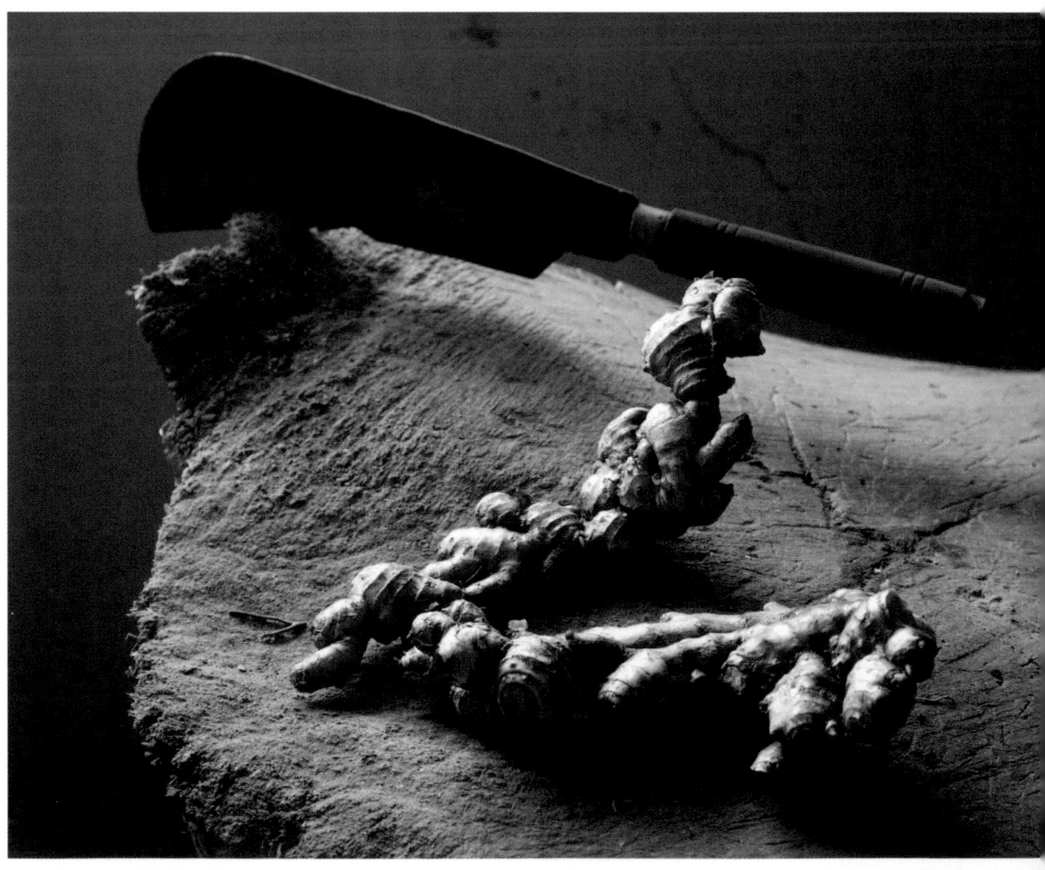

Ginger

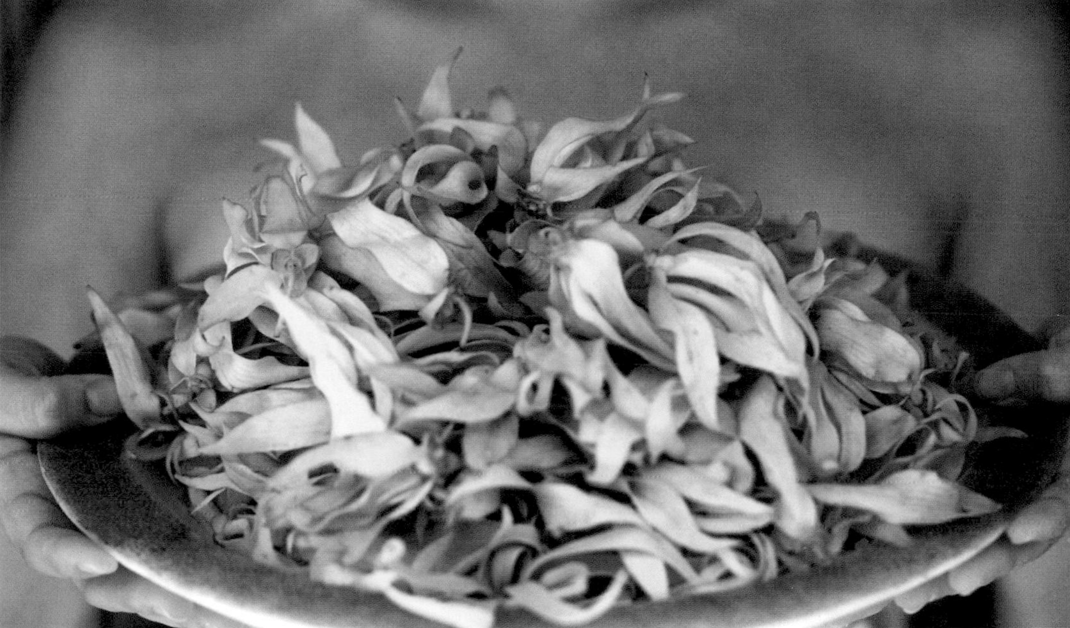

Ylang ylang

prevent vomiting and boost a weak digestive system. A popular ingredient in Ayurvedic herbal toothpastes and soaps, it is a cooling herb with a pungent aftertaste.

Curcuma domestica **Turmeric**
An all-round wonder rhizome, the majority of herbal healers use turmeric. Its benefits are too numerous to mention, but its most common uses are for detoxifying the liver, balancing cholesterol levels, fighting allergies, stimulating the digestion, boosting immunity and enhancing the complexion. Sushruta recommended it for epilepsy and bleeding disorders, while Charaka said it was useful in skin diseases, as a mind/body purifier and to help the lungs expel *kapha*.

Cananga odorata **Ylang ylang**
Oil from the greenish-yellow flowers of ylang ylang (see right, top) is relaxing and tension relieving. It is also recommended as an anti-depressant. It has an erotic, sweet, fruity smell so is widely used in perfumery. Ylang ylang is also believed to regulate and balance skin texture.

Withania somnifera **Indian winter cherry**
Also known as the Indian winter cherry, *ashwagandha* root (see page 130) is sometimes called Indian ginseng as it is used in Ayurveda extensively. It has antioxidant properties and is also an immune system booster; its anti-inflammatory and pain-reducing properties make it useful in the treatment of arthritis, and many Indians believe it promotes longevity.

Glycyrrhiza glabra **Licorice**
Famous for its distinctive flavor, licorice (see above) is used in traditional herbal medicine as a liver detoxifier and endocrine system booster. It is also useful for a variety of bronchial problems and in India licorice sticks were (and still are) commonly used as teeth-cleaners.

Licorice

Camellia sinensis **Tea**
Widely drunk throughout India, many people do not realize the medicinal benefits of this ubiquitous plant when they drink a cup of tea. Tea is an effective antioxidant; it stabilizes blood lipids, thus helping in reducing cholesterol; it helps with hypertension; and is an effective immune system booster.

Dashmool **"Ten Roots"**
The powder obtained from what is known in Ayurveda as *dashmool* or "ten roots" (see page 137) is used in over 50 percent of Ayurvedic preparations. The potent combination of these ten roots' properties has resulted in a powder that may be taken internally in the form of pills, rubbed on the body in the form of powders, or used externally and internally as an oil. *Dashmool* has exhaustive healing properties, balancing all three *doshas*, reducing *ama* disorders, reducing numbness and stiffness in the body, and helping with pain management.

ayurvedic preparations

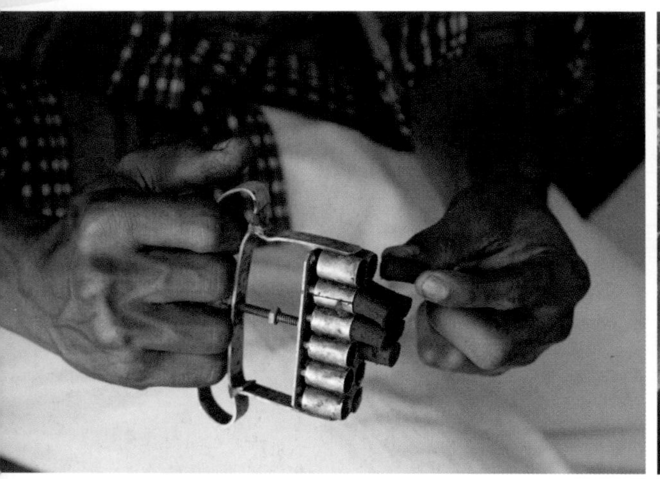

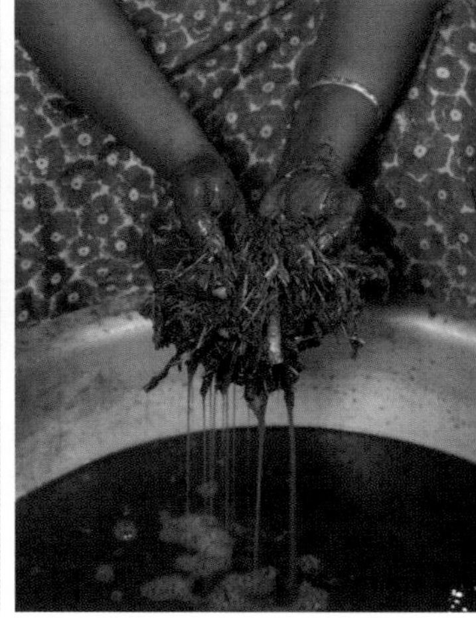

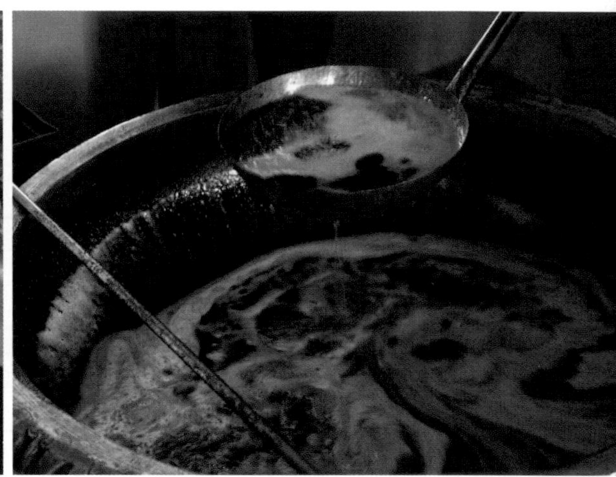

Ayurveda, Siddha, Unani and Tibetan traditional medicine all use materials from the earth in prescriptions. In most cases, the ingredients are not simply plucked and used, but undergo certain preparatory procedures before they are considered ready for use. Ayurvedic doctors stress the link between freshness and efficacy in the case of herbs and plants, whilst materials from the ground (metals, minerals and so forth) undertake complicated and time-consuming purification processes.

In Ayurveda, some preparations are used internally, others are reserved for external use and some can be used for both. For the most part, oils (*thailam*), powders (*choornam*), raw herbal pastes (*kalkam*) and processed herbal pastes (*leham*) are widely used as topical applications. Internal prescriptions include fermented preparations such as *asavam* and *arishtam* (both decoctions, the former made without heat, the latter with heat), medicated ghees or *gritham*, *bhasmas* (incinerated fine powders) and *gulikam* (pills). None are easy to make.

Depending on the size and scale of the Ayurvedic establishment, medicines and oils are either sourced from reputable manufacturing companies or pharmacies, or made on site. It is usually the smaller concerns that grow or locally source their own ingredients, and make their own medicines. Dr P Sathyanarayanan, a third-generation Ayurvedic doctor but also a qualified doctor from the Ayurvedic College in Coimbatore, runs an Ayurvedic homestay with his wife. "We have centuries of tradition behind us," he explains, "but also modern facilities and a home-away-from-home environment. All our medicines are made on site in our production facility, and we individually custom-make prescriptions for our patients."

Exploring the production facility is an eye-opener: each oil or powder or pill has to go through numerous processes before it is ready for use. The procedures are time-consuming, made-by-hand and labor-

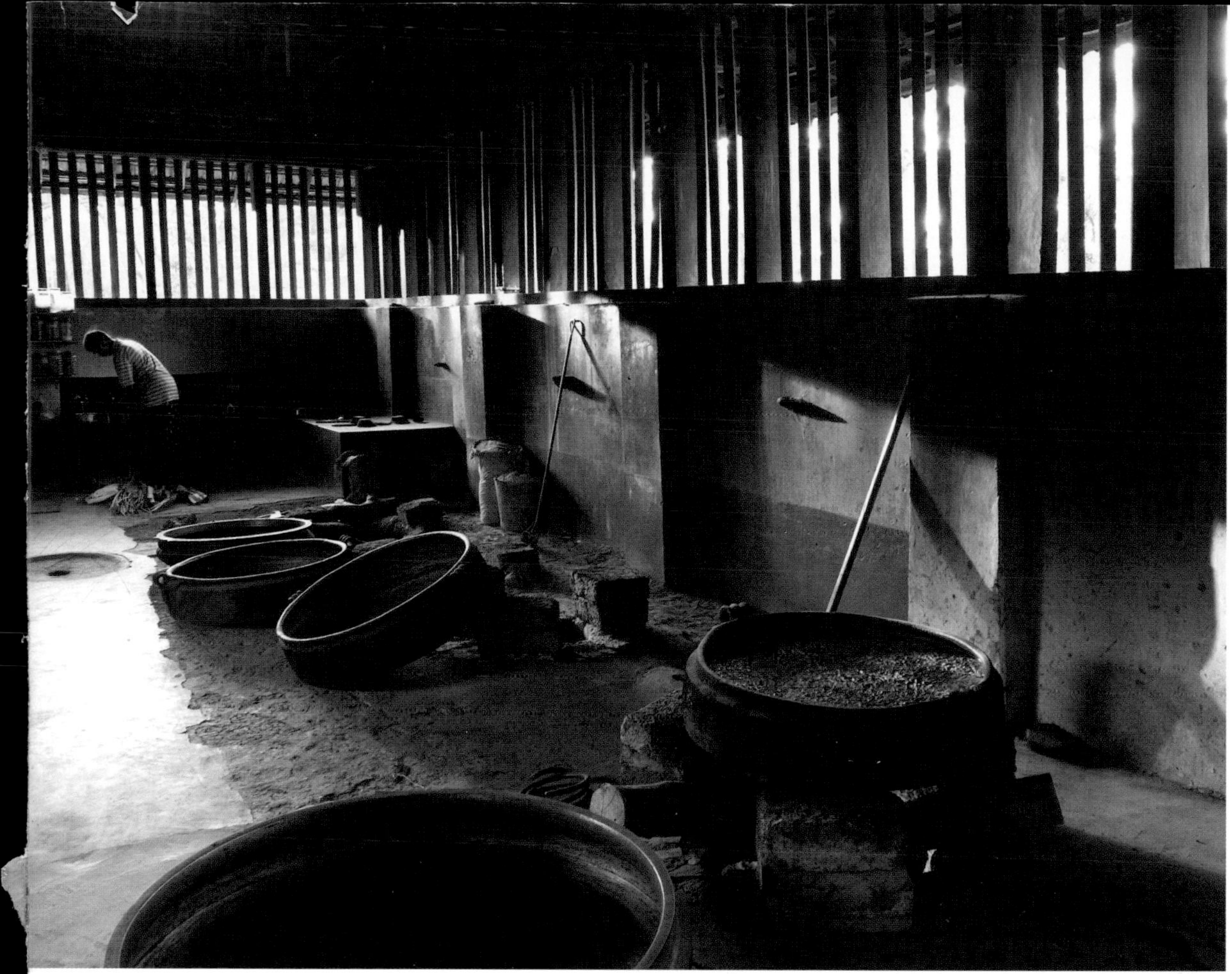

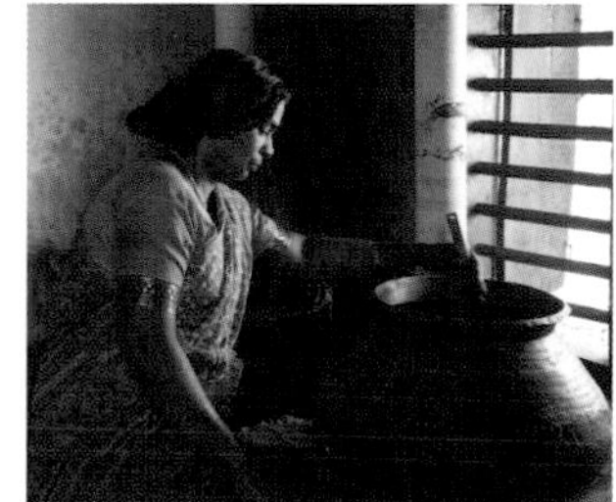

From left to right Ancient machinery grinds and reduces ingredients into a thick black paste-like consistency; this is then used to make pills or *gulikam*. *Sida cordifolia* roots are cut, washed, then crushed before being boiled and reduced (often many times); the result is a *bala* decoction. While boiling, oils have to be constantly stirred. Open fires at a production facility in Kerala. Brass, copper or large iron cauldrons are used for oil production.
Below The Aditya storage cupboard is constantly replenished. Ayurvedic preparations should always be stored in air-tight bottles.

intensive, but this "return to basics", in Dr Sathyanarayanan's opinion, is the true route for authentic Ayurveda.

Many agree with him. Punarnava, a Coimbatore-based Ayurvedic consultancy that helps link patients with suitable Ayurvedic doctors and homestays, embraces the concept of "living in the present but drawing on traditions from the past to look to the future." Their doctors believe that the "real" Ayurveda is a potent combination of ancient knowledge, logical, ethical and spiritual practice, a caring environment, correctly administered procedures and authentically prepared medicines. If all the above practiced, they believe that Ayurveda and Ayurvedic medicines have a bright future.

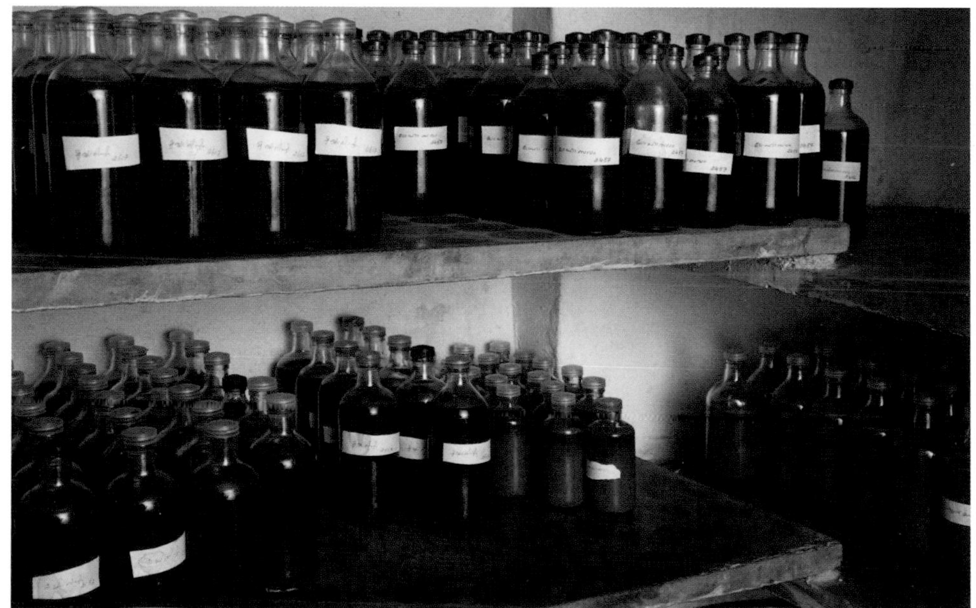

listings

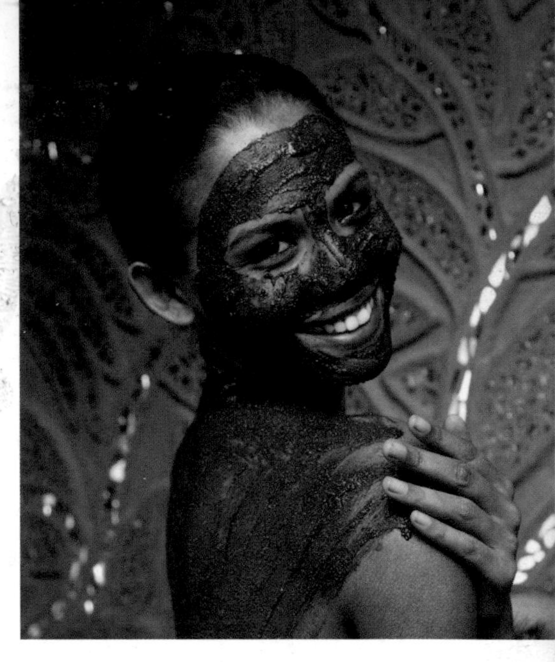

Ayurvedic Hospitals, Homestays and Treatment Centers:

Indus Valley Ayurvedic Center
http//:www.ayurindus.com

Kalari Kovilakom
http://www.kalarikovilakom.com

The Arya Vaidya Chikitsalayam
http//:www.avpayurveda.com

Keraleeya Ayurveda Samajam
http//:www.samajam.org

Kerala Ayurveda Ltd
http//:www.keralaayurveda.biz

Vasudeva Vilasam Ayurveda Pharmacy
http//:www.vasudeva.com

Aditya Ayurveda Hospital
email: sathyan12@sancharnet.in

Thulasi Ayurveda Chikitsalayam
email: ramananddr@ sancharnet.in

Swaasthya Ayurveda Village
http://www.swaasthya.com

Poomully Aramthampuran's Ayurveda Mana
http://www.ayurvedamana.com

Holistic Health Centers:

SOUKYA International Holistic Health Centre
http://www.soukya.com

Ayurvedic Consultants:

Punarnava Ayurveda Private Limited
http://www.punarnava-ayurveda.com

Hotels and Resorts with Spas:

Kumarakom Lake Resort
http://www.thepaul.in

Park Hotels
http://www.theparkhotels.com

Ananda – In The Himalayas
http://www.anandaspa.com

Taj Hotels, Resorts and Palaces
http://www.tajhotels.com

Neemrana "non hotel" Hotels & Resorts
http://www.neemranahotels.com

Shangri-La Hotels and Resorts
http://www.shangri-la.com

Mandarin Oriental Hotel Group
http://www.mandarinoriental.com

CGH Earth Hotels
http//:www.cghearth.com

JW Marriott Mumbai
http//:www.marriott.com

Aman Resorts
http://www.amanresorts.com

The Oberoi Group
http://www.oberoihotels.com

Yoga and Meditation Schools and Retreats:

Shreyas Reetreat
http://www.shreyasretreat.com

Mysore Mandala Yogashala
http://mandala.ashtanga.org

Ashtanga Yoga Research Institute
http://www.ayri.org

Vipassana Research Institute
http://www.dhamma.org

Swaswara Resort
www.swaswara.com

Salon, Spa and Product Companies:

Shahnaz Husain Group of Companies
http://www.shahnaz-husain.com

Sansha Spas
http://www.sanshaayurveda.com